FISH OILS
IN NUTRITION

FISH OILS IN NUTRITION

Edited by
Maurice E. Stansby
Scientific Consultant
Northwest Fisheries Center
National Marine Fisheries Service
Seattle, Washington

An *avi* Book
Published by VAN NOSTRAND REINHOLD
New York

An AVI Book
(AVI is an imprint of Van Nostrand Reinhold)

Copyright © 1990 by Van Nostrand Reinhold
Library of Congress Catalog Card Number 89-25101
ISBN 0-442-23748-0

Printed in the United States of America

Van Nostrand Reinhold
115 Fifth Avenue
New York, New York 10003

Van Nostrand Reinhold International Company Limited
11 New Fetter Lane
London EC4P 4EE, England

Van Nostrand Reinhold
480 La Trobe Street
Melbourne, Victoria 3000, Australia

Nelson Canada
1120 Birchmount Road
Scarborough, Ontario M1K 5G4, Canada

16 15 14 13 12 11 10 9 8 7 6 5 4 3 2 1

Library of Congress Cataloging-in-Publication Data

Fish oils in nutrition / edited by Maurice E. Stansby.
    p. cm.
    Includes bibliographical references.
    ISBN 0-442-23748-0
    1. Fish oils. 2. Fish oils in human nutrition. I. Stansby,
Maurice Earl, 1908–
TP676.F57 1990
641.1′4—dc20   89-25101
                                                    CIP

CONTRIBUTORS

Anthony P. Bimbo, Director of Applied Development, Zapata Haynie Corp., P.O. Box 175, Reedville, Virginia 22539. Chapters 6 and 7.

Diana H. Greene, Research Food Technologist, Utilization Research Division, Northwest Fisheries Center, National Marine Fisheries Service, P.O. Box 1638, Kodiak, Alaska 99615. Chapter 8.

Edward H. Gruger, Jr., formerly Research Chemist, National Marine Fisheries Service, 3727 NE 193rd Street, Seattle, Washington. Co-author Chapter 2.

Jeanne D. Joseph, Research Chemist, Biomedical Test Materials Program, Development Division, National Marine Fisheries Service, Charleston Laboratory, 217 Fort Johnson Road, Charleston, South Carolina 29412. Co-author Chapter 3.

Neva L. Karrick, formerly Assistant Laboratory Director, Food Science Pioneer Research Laboratory, National Marine Fisheries Service, 4926 52nd South, Seattle, Washington 98118. Chapter 9.

Judith Krzynowek, Research Chemist, Northeast Fisheries Center, Gloucester Laboratory, National Marine Fisheries Service, 30 Emerson Ave., Gloucester, Massachusetts 01930. Co-author Chapter 4.

William B. Nillson, Research Chemist, Utilization Research Division, Northwest Fisheries Center, National Marine Fisheries Service, 2725 Montlake Blvd. E., Seattle, Washington 98112. Co-author Chapter 4.

Hermann Schlenk, Professor of Biochemistry, The Hormel Institute, University of Minnesota, 801 16th Avenue NE, Austin, Minnesota 55912. Co-author Chapters 2 and 4.

Gloria T. Seaborn, Chemist, Lipid Analytical Services, Development Division, National Marine Fisheries Service, Charleston Laboratory, 217 Fort Johnson Road, Charleston, South Carolina 29412. Co-author of Chapter 3.

Maurice E. Stansby, Scientific Consultant, Northwest Fisheries Center, National Marine Fisheries Service, 2725 Montlake Blvd. East, Seattle, Washington 98112. Editor, Author Chapters 1, 5, 10, and 11, Co-author Chapter 2.

Virginia F. Stout, Research Chemist, Utilization Research Division, Northwest Fisheries Center, National Marine Fisheries Service, 2725 Montlake Blvd. E., Seattle, Washington 98112. Co-author Chapter 4.

PREFACE

Initially it had been planned for this book to be a second edition of the book *Fish Oils,* which I had edited and which was published in 1967. This book, long since out of print, covered all phases connected with fish oils. Upon further consideration it was realized that at present by far the principal interest in fish oils deals with aspects concerned with their nutritional properties.

The present book, therefore, entitled *Fish Oils in Nutrition,* lays special emphasis on nutritional aspects. Various other aspects closely related to nutritional properties, however, are included in the present book. Thus, four chapters are concerned with various aspects of fatty acids in fish oil since the nutritional properties are so closely concerned with such acids in the oil of fish. Two chapters deal with the commercial manufacture and processing of fish oil and one chapter is concerned with the role of fish oils in living fish. The last three chapters discuss in detail the nutritional properties of fish oils.

Today the general public very frequently sees items in newspapers and other popular publications about recent findings supporting the idea that consumption of fish or fish oils will lead to lower incidence of heart attacks or other disease conditions. These reports have led to the public misconception that those ideas are based only upon current research. How many such readers know that, as discussed in Chapter 10, more than 200 years ago results of a detailed 10-year study at a British hospital showed conclusively that arthritis symptoms could be eliminated by consumption of fish oil? Especially in the last three chapters of the book, the discussions on nutritional properties of fish oil have been written with a minimum of complicated scientific wording so as to be understandable to the general public.

The book, therefore, is of value not only to those in industry who may want either to promote the wider use of fish in the diet or to develop concentrates of fish oil fatty acids for medical application, but also for those in the general public who are interested in learning more about fish oils and nutrition.

Acknowledgment is made to Patricia Cook, librarian at the Northwest Fisheries Center, Seattle, for her tracking down many obscure scientific references not generally available in most libraries. Acknowledgment is also made to Susan Rose for her outstanding ability in keeping the preparation of the various chapters under way in a highly skillful manner.

Maurice E. Stansby

CONTENTS

FISH OILS
IN NUTRITION

Chapter 1
INTRODUCTION

Maurice E. Stansby

EARLIER BOOKS DEALING WITH FISH OILS

One of the first books containing information on fish oils was *Chemical Technology and Analysis of Oils, Fats and Waxes* (Lewkowitsch 1895). This book came out first in 1895, but there were several subsequent editions. In the fifth editions published in 1913, 68 pages dealt with fish oils. At that time very little was known about fatty acids in oils, so the different oils were characterized by various fat constants. It was apparently believed that an oil made from a given species of fish always had identical chemical components. The oil fat constants were, therefore, initially stated to values going to one or two digits beyond the decimal point. Thus, even in the 1913 edition, for example, iodine numbers were expressed as mackerel oil, 191.63; bonito oil, 208.92; and Japanese sardine oil, 176.78. Because of these erroneous ideas, books published around the turn of the century are of very limited value today.

Coming forward to a somewhat more recent period, probably the first book in English on fish oils was *Chemistry and Technology of Marine Animal Oils* (Brocklesby 1941).[1] This book, although dealing primarily with fish oils of Canada, was of a general enough nature that it soon became the best standard reference for all fish oils. It was revised by Bailey et al. (1952) and continued to be a major source of information on fish oils.

The next general book on fish oils was *Fish Oils* (Stansby 1967), subtitled *Their Chemistry, Technology, Stability, Nutritional Properties and Uses*. The present book was originally intended to be a revision of *Fish Oils*, but upon further consideration it was decided to write it to cover largely nutritional aspects and also to include certain other subjects that would be useful in connection with nutritional problems.

Various books dealing with fish oils have been published in recent years treating some limited aspect of the subject. For example, *Introduction to Fishery By-Products* (Windsor and Barlow 1981) covers a number of

---

[1]This bulletin was a greatly expanded version of a leaflet of Brocklesby and Denstedt (1933) (only 149 pages as contrasted to the 1941 bulletin's 442 pages).

1

products of which fish oil is an important one, but the discussion of any one product is brief (only 13 pages for fish oils). *Seafood Nutrition* (Nettleton 1985) covers not only that aspect of fish relating to the nutrition of the oil but also a wide variety of other components such as protein and mineral content. *Fish and Human Health* (Lands 1986) gives an excellent presentation with respect to the mechanism whereby the fish oil reacts to bring about favorable health effects. This book, however, does not attempt to cover various related effects such as chemical methods for concentrating and analyzing fatty acids in fish oil, nor does it provide information on such other aspects such as fish oil stability. A paperbound booklet, *Fatty Fish and Human Nutrition Resource Notebook* (Miller, 1984), which is based on a special study carried out by Ted Miller of Marine Chemurgics and several associates at Clemson University, contains 171 pages of important information dealing especially with the value of relatively high-fat species of fish upon health.

COVERAGE OF CHAPTERS 2 THROUGH 11

In 6 of the 11 chapters in this book the senior authors are individuals who authored chapters in the 1967 book on fish oils. This does not, by any means, indicate that the present book is a second edition of the 1967 book. Whereas the earlier book covered almost all aspects of fish oils, this one relates to those aspects important in providing properties that contribute to important nutritional benefits.

Chapter 2, "Fatty Acid Composition of Fish," corresponds to Chapter 1 in the 1967 book. The first part of this older chapter, written by Edward Gruger and dealing with general aspects of fatty acids, has been used with only a few changes. A new section of furan fatty acids, written by Dr. Hermann Schlenk of Hormel Institute, has been added. Very little was known about furan fatty acids and their occurrence in fish oils in 1967; in fact they were not even mentioned. Much of the recent research on this subject has been carried out since 1967 by Hermann Schlenk and co-workers. The final section of Chapter 2 deals with the fatty acid content of oils from different species of fish, and this section replaces all that was contained in the 1967 book on this aspect. In 1967 it was not fully realized that there is a tremendous difference in the fatty acid content of different oils of the same species when the oil is made from fish caught at different times and places. The values that investigators had been reporting had been based on very inadequate samples where only a few fish of the given species (often all caught at the same time and place) had been used; yet the authors often implied that their results were typical for any or all other oil samples made from the same species. It was therefore necessary to completely rewrite this section, which was done by Maurice Stansby.

Chapter 3, on analyses of marine fatty acids, covers procedures (some of which were mentioned in Chapters 4 and 5 of the 1967 book) but includes much new information. The authors of this new chapter have been working for quite a few years at their agency's Charleston, South Carolina, laboratory where much of the government analyses of fatty acid content of fish oils has been done in recent years. They are therefore highly knowledgeable in this field.

Chapter 4, on fractionation, was authored by Stout, Nilsson, Krzynowek, and Schlenk, and it covers the same subject as that in Chapter 6 by Schlenk and Sands in the 1967 book. Although, in general, the outline of the 1967 chapter was followed, so much new material was involved that the chapter was completely rewritten.

Chapter 5, "Deterioration," includes much of the information discussed in Chapters 9 through 12 of the 1967 book. This chapter was completely rewritten.

Chapter 6, 7, and 8, on fish oil production and processing, and on lipid metabolism in fish, have been completely updated and rewritten by authors who did not participate in the writing of corresponding Chapters 13, 15, and 21 in the old book. Chapter 9 in this book, "Nutritional Value as Animal Feed," has been updated by the original author (Neva Karrick) with some additional information added on the value of fish oil for hatchery-grown fish. The final two chapters, on nutritional value for humans, are new chapters not covered as such by chapters in the 1967 book.

CLASSES OF LIPIDS IN FISH

In the 1967 book a separate chapter covers the classes of lipids in fish. In this new book some of this information is included in various chapters. A little general information on this subject is, however, included here.

Figure 1-1 lists the principal different classes of compounds occurring in fish oils. Triglycerides occur in all fish oils, and in nearly all cases triglycerides are the principal class that occurs. Also, in nearly all fish oils, various phospholipids always occur, usually in amounts considerably less than those of the triglycerides. Among the various phospholipids that may occur in fish, lecithins (phosphatidyl cholines) occur to the greatest extent, with phosphatidyl ethanolamines (cephalins) being the second most common class.

The other three main classes of lipids are wax esters, diacyl glyceryl ethers, and hydrocarbons. The latter two of these classes occur both in the flesh and in liver, primarily in certain sharks, and sometimes to a very

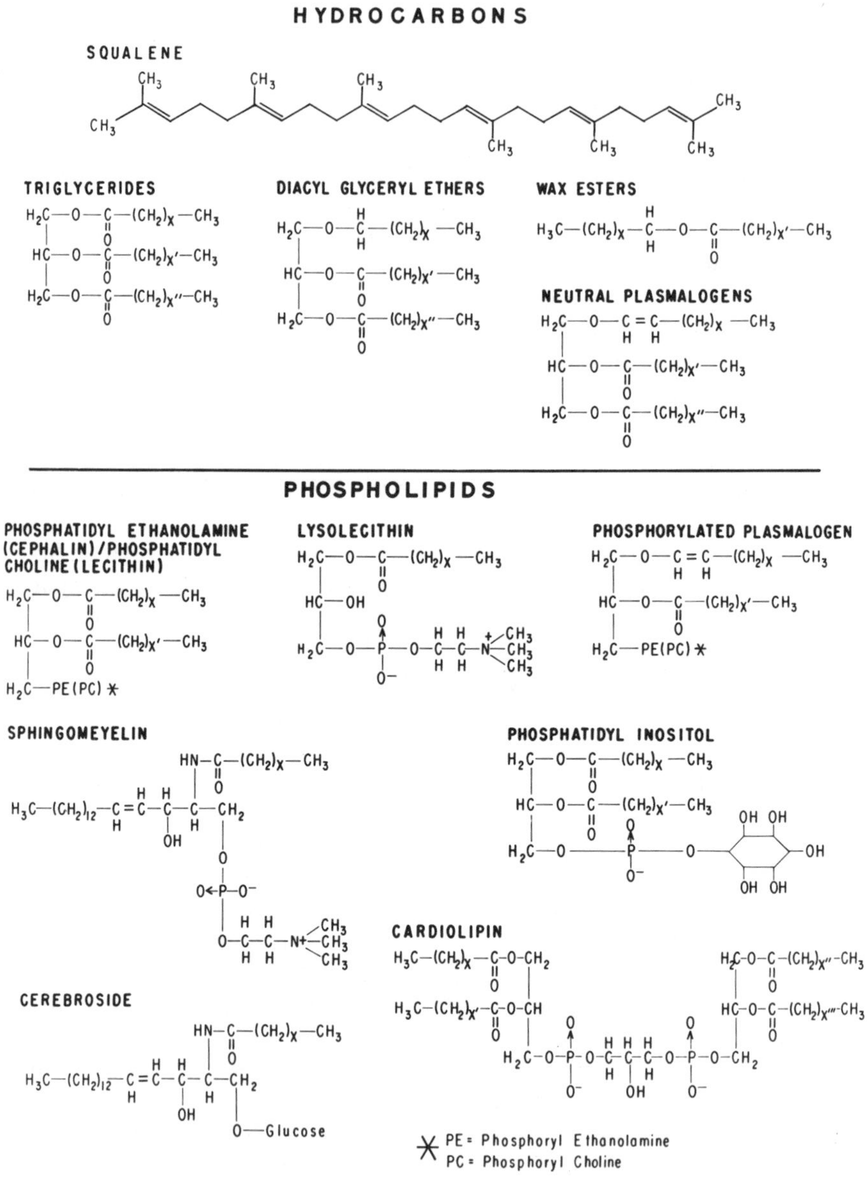

HYDROCARBONS

SQUALENE

TRIGLYCERIDES

DIACYL GLYCERYL ETHERS

WAX ESTERS

NEUTRAL PLASMALOGENS

PHOSPHOLIPIDS

PHOSPHATIDYL ETHANOLAMINE (CEPHALIN)/PHOSPHATIDYL CHOLINE (LECITHIN)

LYSOLECITHIN

PHOSPHORYLATED PLASMALOGEN

SPHINGOMYELIN

PHOSPHATIDYL INOSITOL

CEREBROSIDE

CARDIOLIPIN

PE = Phosphoryl Ethanolamine
PC = Phosphoryl Choline

Fig. 1-1. Classes of lipids in fish.

high extent, for example, up to 90% squalene (Heller et al. 1957) in the liver. The wax esters occur in a wide range of species, mostly species not used as a food. In one species, the castor oil fish (*Ruvethus pretiosus*), the lipid of the muscle was found to contain over 90% wax esters (Nevenzel, Rodegker, and Mead (1965).

REFERENCES

Bailey, B. E., Carter, N. M., and Swain, L. A. 1952. *Marine Oils with Particular Reference to Those of Canada*. Ottawa: Bulletin 89. Fisheries Research Board of Canada.

Brocklesby, H. N. 1941. *The Chemistry and Technology of Marine Animal Oils with Particular Reference to Those of Canada*. Ottawa: Bulletin 59. Fisheries Research Board of Canada.

Brocklesby, H. N., and Denstedt, O. F. 1933. *The Industrial Chemistry of Fish Oils with Particular Reference to Those of British Columbia*. Ottawa: Bulletin 37. Biological Board of Canada.

Heller, J. H., Heller, M. S., Springer, S., and Clark, E. 1957. Squalene content of various shark livers. *Nature* 179:919–920.

Lands, W. E. M. 1986. *Fish and Human Health*. Orlando, Fla.: Academic Press.

Lewkowitsch, J. 1895. *Chemical Technology and Analysis of Oils, Fats and Waxes*. London: McMillan and Co.

Miller, T. M. 1984. *Fatty Fish and Human Nutrition Resource Notebook*. Newport, N.C.: Marine Chemurgics.

Nettleton, J. A. 1985. *Seafood Nutrition*. Huntington, N.Y.: Osprey Books.

Nevenzel, J. C., Rodegker, W., and Mead, J. F. 1965. The lipids of *Ruvettus pretiosus* muscle and liver. *Biochemistry* 4:324–330.

Stansby, M. E. 1967. *Fish Oils*. Westport, Conn.: Avi Publishing Co.

Windsor, M., and Barlow, S. 1981. *Introduction to Fishery By-Products*. Farnham, Surrey, England: Fishing News Books, Ltd.

Chapter 2
FATTY ACID COMPOSITION OF FISH

Maurice E. Stansby, Hermann Schlenk,
and Edward H. Gruger, Jr.

INTRODUCTION

The history and early developments of research on the fatty acid composition of fish oils are well documented by Hilditch and Williams (1964) and by Bailey et al. (1952). Also, Lovern (1942, 1964) has reported extensive investigations during the early era. Recent investigations continue to add to current understanding of fish oils, and one now finds renewed interest in the many types and classes of compounds associated with fatty acids of marine life.

Nature of Fatty Acids and Chemical Distribution[1]

Fish oils and marine-animal oils are generally characterized by a rather large group of saturated and unsaturated fatty acids, which are commonly associated with mixed triglycerides. In addition to triglycerides, body oils from fish and marine animals usually include minor amounts of fatty acids as substituents of phospholipids and other lipids. In comparison to body oils, on the other hand, liver oils and oils from particular parts of fish and marine animals can often contain large amounts of fatty acids associated with phospholipids, glyceryl ethers (alkoxydiglycerides), and wax esters, depending on the source of oils and lipids (Lovern 1962).

Nature of Fatty Acids. The fatty acids derived from fish oils are of three principal types: saturated, monounsaturated, and polyunsaturated. The

---

[1] The material under this heading and under the subsequent two headings, "Origin of Fatty Acids in Fish" and "Environmental Influence on Fatty Acid Composition," was written by Dr. Edward H. Gruger, Jr., and appeared in Chapter 1 of the earlier book (Stansby 1967). The text in these sections appears here with almost no changes over that in the 1967 book.

6

formula,

$$CH_3(CH_2)_x(CH{=}CHCH_2)_n(CH_2)_yCOOH$$

where $n = 0$ to 6, illustrates the type of fatty acid structures common to fish oils.

The saturated fatty acids have carbon chain lengths that generally range from C_{12} (lauric acid) to C_{24} (lignoceric acid). Also, traces of C_8 and C_{10} acids may be found in some fish oils. A C_5 acid (isovaleric), however, occurs in jawbone oil of dolphin and porpoise.

The monounsaturated type is comprised of monoethenoic acids, and the polyunsaturated type is comprised of polyethenoic acids that contain from two to six ethylenic bonds per acid. The carbon chain lengths of the unsaturated acids range generally from C_{14} (9-tetradecenoic acid) to C_{22} (4,7,10,13,16,19-docosahexaenoic acid). Small amounts of C_{10} and C_{12} monoenoic acids have been found in some fish oils. There are no naturally occurring acetylenic acids and hydroxy carboxylic acids presently known in fish oils.

Even-numbered carbon fatty acids make up about 97% of the total fatty acids, with a few notable exceptions. It was relatively recently that odd-numbered carbon fatty acids were generally acknowledged to be part of all fish oils. Branched-chain odd-carbon acids were isolated by Morice and Shorland (1956) from shark liver oil. They isolated 13-methyltetradecanoic acid, (+)-12-methyltetradecanoic acid, and (+)-14-methylhexadecanoic acid, and found that together these acids comprised 0.1–0.2% of the liver oil fatty acids. Earlier work by Morice and Shorland (1952) demonstrated the presence of other branched-chain acids in shark liver oil that resembled 2,3-dimethyloctadecanoic acid and 2,3,4-trimethylhexadecanoic acid. The application of gas-liquid chromatography by Farquhar et al. (1959) to the analysis of menhaden oil fatty acids has also demonstrated the existence of straight-chain and branched-chain odd-carbon acids of fish oils. Saturated and unsaturated odd-carbon fatty acids were isolated from menhaden oil by Gellerman and Schlenk (1959) and from mullet oil by Sen and Schlenk (1964), respectively. Normal and branched-chain odd-numbered fatty acids in fish depot fats, seal blubber, and whale blubber were examined by Ackman and Sipos (1965). These workers noted the ratios of *iso* and *anteiso* fatty acid to be comparable in the fish and seal samples, but differed in a whale sample. (See also the discussion under the heading "Fish Diets").

The nature of the ethylenic bonds in the unsaturated acids from fish oils has been known for many years to be of the *cis* geometric configuration. In addition, however, evidence has been sufficient only recently to prove as far as is known that the carbon-carbon atom separations of the ethylenic bonds of polyunsaturated acids are of a methylene-interrupted type (Klenk 1958; Farquhar et al. 1959; Kayama et al. 1963B). This type of separation is also referred to as a divinylmethane structure. Numerous investigators have shown that the divinylmethane structure is common as far as we know for individually isolated polyunsaturated acids of fish oil. Among these investigators, Silk and Hahn (1954) positively identified a 6,9,12,15-hexadecatetraenoic acid (C_{16} acid) in South African pilchard oil. The work of Klenk and Brockerhoff (1957) and Matic (1958) revealed the presence of a 6,9,12,15-octadecatetraenoic acid (C_{18}) in herring oil and South African pilchard oil, respectively. The structures of 5,8,11,14,17-eicosapentaenoic acid (C_{20}), 7,10,13,16,19-docosapentaenoic acid (C_{22}), and 4,7,10,13,16,19-docosahexaenoic acid (C_{22}) were determined by such workers as Whitcutt and Sutton (1956), Whitcutt (1957), Klenk and Brockerhoff (1958), Toyama et al. (1959), Farquhar et al. (1959), Ackman and Jangaard (1963), and Ackman (1964). Ahrens et al. (1959) were the first to point out that menhaden (*Brevoortia tyrannus*) oil is composed of at least 44 different fatty acids.

Other workers have approached the problem of proving the general divinylmethane structure by analyzing mixtures of fish oil fatty acids. Privett (1956) investigated the effects of lipoxidase-catalyzed oxidations on concentrates of fatty acids, and demonstrated the 1,4-diene nature of the double-bond structures. More conclusively, however, Hashimoto et al. (1963) proved the gross divinylmethane structure in fish oil polyunsaturated acids by analysis of nuclear magnetic resonance spectra.

Chemical Distribution of Fatty Acids.   There are differences in the natural distribution of fatty acids associated with lipids such as triglycerides and phospholipids. For example, it is generally believed that phospholipids, such as lecithins and cephalins, contain more polyunsaturated fatty acids than do the triglycerides when isolated from the same oil or tissues. Also, it is believed generally that depot fats consist largely of triglycerides, while the total lipids of various body organs and muscle tissues can by comparison contain large proportions of phospholipids. The reasons for such distributions are the subject of much research, which will not be discussed here. It is only important to point out some examples of these differences in order to understand better the composition of fish oil fatty acids.

To aid the following discussion, examples of the molecular structures of triglycerides and phospholipids may be represented by the formulas for β-oleodipalmitin and α'-oleyl-β-eicosapentaenyl-α-lecithin, respectively, as follows:

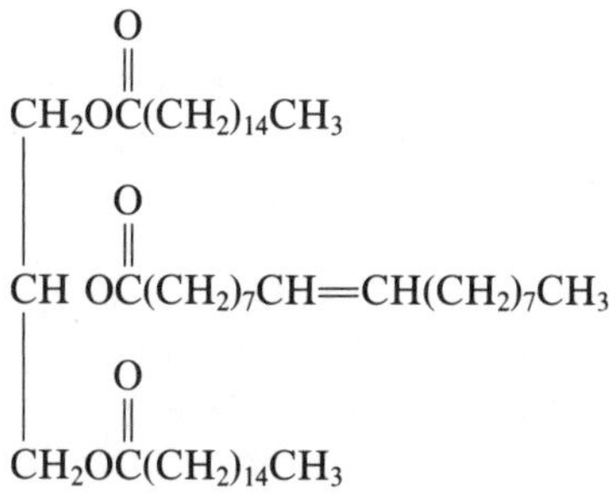

$$O$$
$$\parallel$$
$$CH_2OC(CH_2)_{14}CH_3$$
$$\mid \quad O$$
$$\quad \parallel$$
$$CH\ OC(CH_2)_7CH=CH(CH_2)_7CH_3$$
$$\mid \quad O$$
$$\quad \parallel$$
$$CH_2OC(CH_2)_{14}CH_3$$

β-oleodipalmitin

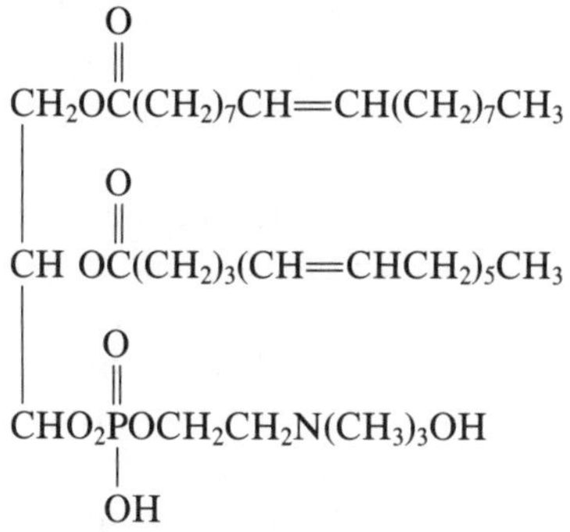

$$O$$
$$\parallel$$
$$CH_2OC(CH_2)_7CH=CH(CH_2)_7CH_3$$
$$\mid \quad O$$
$$\quad \parallel$$
$$CH\ OC(CH_2)_3(CH=CHCH_2)_5CH_3$$
$$\mid \quad O$$
$$\quad \parallel$$
$$CHO_2POCH_2CH_2N(CH_3)_3OH$$
$$\mid$$
$$OH$$

α′-oleyl-β-eicosapentaenyl-α-lecithin

Additional information about the kinds of lipids associated with fatty acids may be found in such texts as those by Deuel (1951), Gunstone (1958), and Hanahan (1960).

Fatty acids of the triglycerides, lecithins, and phosphatidyl ethanol-amines (cephalins) from livers of cod and lobster and from muscles of cod and scallop were analyzed by Brockerhoff et al. (1963). They demon-strated that the polyunsaturated fatty acids were preferentially located in the β position of both the triglycerides and the lecithins. The phosphatidyl ethanolamines were also found to be highly unsaturated.

Brockerhoff and Hoyle (1963) analyzed the fatty acid distribution in the α and β positions of triglycerides from fish body and liver oils, and found that the polyenoic acids were preferentially distributed in the β position. They also analyzed seal blubber and whale oils, and found that the polyenoic acids occurred in the α position rather than in the β position of the blubber triglycerides.

Lecithin fractions from tuna, salmon, and menhaden muscle were shown by Menzel and Olcott (1964) to have fatty acids distributed similarly to the lecithins isolated from muscle tissues by Brockerhoff et al. (1963). For the three species, 91–99% of the fatty acids in the β position were unsaturated and 36–86% of the fatty acids in the α position were saturated. Tuna lecithin, for example, had 8.4% 20 : 5[2] acid and 39% 22 : 6 acid in the α position and 15% 20 : 5 acid and 48% 22 : 6 acid in the β position. In another investigation, Schuster et al. (1964) showed that white muscle of five species of tuna contained cephalins and lecithins having 47% and 50% of the 22 : 6 acid, respectively. Other instances of fatty acid distributions in fish phospholipids are cited by Schuster et al. (1964).

An interesting investigation of the triglycerides of sablefish (*Anaplopoma fimbria*) was begun by Dolev and Olcott (1965A), in which they found much less polyunsaturated fatty acids in the total triglyceride fraction than is customarily found in most marine oils. The most recent results of this work demonstrated that some of the α- and β-substituent fatty acids of sablefish triglycerides do not follow the usual distributional patterns (Dolev and Olcott 1965B). In this species, they observed, for example, that 18 : 3, 20 : 3, and 20 : 4 occur mainly in the α, α' positions compared to 14 : 0, 16 : 0, and 16 : 1, which occur mainly in the β position. The 18 : 0 and 18 : 1 acids appeared to be distributed evenly. Notably important was the finding that 22 : 6, which was present in the glycerides, was not detected as free fatty acid from hydrolysis by lipase.

Origin of Fatty Acids in Fish

It has been known for many years that the nature of fat in fish diets can influence the proportionate distribution of fatty acids in fish oils (Lovern 1942). Natural oils in marine plant life, planktonic crustacea, and other plankton are consumed by fish in varying degrees depending on feeding habits. Feeding habits of fish can vary according to such factors as avail-

---

[2]It has become common practice to use abbreviations when referring to particular fatty acids (Farquhar et al. 1959). Generally, the abbreviation is written as two numbers separated by a colon. The first number designates the number of carbon atoms in the fatty acid molecule and the second number (after the colon) designates the number of methylene-interrupted *cis* ethylenic bonds. In addition, polyunsaturated fatty acids may be regarded according to families of which the terminal structures are the same. For this reason, the position of the ethylenic bonds along the carbon atom chains may be designated by the Greek letter omega, or ω, and a number that refers to the number of carbon atoms separating the terminal methyl group from the ethylenic bond nearest the terminal methyl (Mohrhauer and Holman 1963). For example 18 : 3 ω3 stands for 9,12,15-octadecatrienoic acid (linolenic acid), and fish oil fatty acids designated with an ω3 are said to belong to the linolenic acid family. Similarly, endings of ω6 and ω9 refer to the linoleic and oleic acid families, respectively. Another way of designating the location of the first double bond substitutes "*n*-" for omega. Thus, 18 : 3ω3 would be written as 18 : 3 *n*-3.

ability of food, which may be a geographic factor, periods of fasting, and spawning cycles. The food fat metabolism in fish is being investigated continuously in order to understand better the origin of the unique fatty acids in fish oils. To illustrate how the fatty acids of fish can change according to dietary fats, some findings are discussed.

Fish Diets. Experiments by Kelly et al. (1958A) with mullet (*Mugil cephalus*) gave indications that fish, like land animals, probably convert fatty dienoic acid into tetraenoic, pentaenoic, and hexaenoic acids. Unlike land animals, however, the mullet seemed capable of converting $18:2\omega6$ acid to a fatty trienoic acid. Other experiments have shown that young freshwater fish on low fat or cottonseed oil diets had no significant change in fatty acids, but when these fish were fed a diet containing other fish oil the fatty acids of the freshwater species changed to resemble the dietary fish oil (Kelly et al. 1958B). Similar results have been observed by Brenner et al. (1960, 1963), Mead et al. (1960), and Brockerhoff et al. (1964).

In another instance, rainbow trout were fed for 103 days on a diet containing soybean oil. Results showed that no $20:4$, $20:5$, and $22:6$ acids could be detected in the trout oil after such treatment (Toyomizu et al. 1963).

Work on goldfish (*Carrassius auratus*) by Reiser et al. (1963) demonstrated that controlled diets depleted of polyunsaturated fatty acids, but containing principally $18:0$, $18:1$, $18:2$, and $18:3$, produced changes after 76 to 120 days in fatty acids of both triglycerides and phospholipids. It appears from their data that the triglycerides in these fish showed significantly less $20:5$ and $22:6$ acids when compared to the phospholipids.

Marine plankton, as a major food source for fish, have commanded the attention of scientists in recent years. Crabs and shrimps, which when immature are included in the crustacean class of plankton, are known to exhibit fatty acid changes in body fats analogous to fish, depending on their diets (Kelly et al. 1959). Klenk and Eberhagen (1962A, B) isolated from marine plankton a group of polyunsaturated fatty acids, which are like those found in fish and marine animal oils. Others have also shown the similarities between the fatty acids of fish oils and plankton oil fatty acids (Farkas and Herodek 1962, 1964; Lewis 1962; Kayama et al. 1963A).

Ackman and Sipos (1965) examined a number of samples of fish oil fatty acids and made a detailed study of the saturated fractions. They noted that the normal odd-numbered fatty acids found in marine lipids originate in phytoplankton, but that there is little evidence to indicate that branched-chain fatty acids are prominent in these plankton. It is suggested that branched-chain fatty acids are formed to some degree in zooplankton.

Environmental Influence on Fatty Acid Composition

It has been observed in the past that environmental factors such as geographic locations of catch and seasons of the year, which may be related to water temperatures, are related to the proportions of fatty acids of fish oils (Lovern 1942; Swain 1953). Reevaluations of these factors have been important in light of modern instrumentation like gas-liquid chromatography (GLC) (Farquhar et al. 1959). Seasonal variations in fatty acids of commercial cod liver oils were investigated by DeWitt (1963). He observed a range in iodine values, 146 to 168, for GLC-analyzed fatty acids of the liver oils sampled from May to November.

The influence of season, as well as water temperatures and pressure effects, was observed by Lewis (1962) on fatty acids of Arctic plankton. When comparing plankton fatty acids from Arctic plankton and California coastal plankton, Lewis (1962) found two changes in the fatty acids, namely, an increase in the degree of unsaturation and a reduction in chain length with a reduction in environmental temperature.

It is unfortunate that Lewis (1962) reported for some two dozen species only those fatty acids with GLC retention times up to that of 20:1. Rodegker and Nevenzel (1964) point out that this indicates only about 45–90% of the total component fatty acids to be anticipated. Lewis (1962) proposed the ratio of 16:0 to 16:1 acids as a valuable index of the temperature of the habitat of marine ectotherms. However, in the work by Rodegker and Nevenzel (1964) on fatty acids of mussel, barnacle, and starfish, only one of their samples agreed with the 16:0 to 16:1 ratio reported by Lewis. They suggested that problems may be due to attempts to compare fatty acids of different tissue types and, hence, different lipids which may have different biological functions. Rodegker and Nevenzel (1964) suggest that a clear picture of temperature effects, etc., would be anticipated from analyses of the same type of lipid fatty acid source, say, for example, the muscle phospholipids.

The effects of temperature on growing mullet (*Mugil cephalus*) and goldfish (*Carrassius auratus*) were investigated by Reiser et al. (1963). They concluded from analyses of fish raised in water at 13°C and at 23°C that these temperatures had little or no influence on the deposition or interconversion of polyunsaturated acids in the mullet. These findings were surprising. Based on controlled diets, they reasoned that possibly saturated fatty acids (12 : 0 and 14 : 0) are not absorbed at the lower temperature, thereby causing a lack of significant influence on the unsaturated fatty acids. Contrary to these findings, however, Kayama et al. (1963A) have demonstrated that guppies (*Lebistes reticulatus*) raised in water at 17°C possessed more 22 : 6 acid in the oil than did guppies raised in water at 24°C.

In other work, Farkas and Herodek (1964) showed that the amount of C_{20}–C_{22} polyunsaturated acids in freshwater planktonic crustacea increased with decreasing temperatures, and in some species these acids exceeded the values common to marine animals. The fatty acids of freshwater fish that fed on these crustacea resembled fatty acids of marine fish. One might say, then, that temperature had an indirect influence on the fatty acids via the food chain.

FURANOID FATTY ACIDS[3]

A group of acids that have a furan ring as part of their chain should not be omitted in an inventory of fatty acids of fish oils. These furanoid fatty acids (often referred to as F acids) were discovered in liver and testis lipids of freshwater fish as constituents of the cholesteryl esters and triglycerides (Glass et al. 1974). Soon they were recognized also in cod liver and other marine oil sources (Gunstone et al. 1976). Further studies revealed their presence in terrestrial animals, plants, and algae, indicating that their occurrence is much wider than anticipated. The furanoid fatty acids are mentioned briefly in some reviews (Jacini 1986; Henderson and Tocher 1987) and they are the topic of a review focused mainly on their reactions (Spiteller 1987).

The novelty, unusual structure, and properties warrant a discussion of the F acids that goes beyond listing their occurrence in fish. In addition, some details on their structure, on analytical methods, and on biological aspects will be presented here, instead of grafting such topics into chapters that deal with the common, more familiar fatty acids.

Structure

The furanoid acids most commonly encountered in fish are listed in Table 2-1. Mass spectra and other spectral characteristics are in full agreement with these structures, which originally were established by

---

[3]This section was prepared entirely by Dr. Hermann Schlenk. Since furanoid fatty acids were first noted in fish in 1974, they were, of course, not mentioned at all in the earlier book (Stansby 1967).

Table 2-1. F Acids in Fish Lipids

$$
\begin{array}{c}
R_1 \qquad\qquad R_2 \\
\diagdown \qquad\quad \diagup \\
C\text{---}C \\
\| \qquad \| \\
HOOC(CH_2)_m\text{---}C \qquad C\text{---}(CH_2)_n CH_3 \\
\diagdown \quad \diagup \\
O
\end{array}
$$

ACID	CARBON CHAIN LENGTH	m	n	R_1	R_2	TERMINAL CHAIN	ABBREVIATED TERM
F_1	16	8	2	CH_3	CH_3	propyl	diMeF(9,3)
F_2	18	8	4	CH_3	H	pentyl	MeF(9,5)
F_3	18	8	4	CH_3	CH_3	pentyl	diMeF(9,5)
F_4	18	10	2	CH_3	CH_3	propyl	diMeF(11,3)
F_5	20	10	4	CH_3	H	pentyl	MeF(11,5)
F_6	20	10	4	CH_3	CH_3	pentyl	diMeF(11,5)
F_7	22	12	4	CH_3	H	pentyl	MeF(13,5)
F_8	22	12	4	CH_3	CH_3	pentyl	diMeF(13,5)
Reference[a]	18	7	5	H	H	hexyl	F(8,6)

[a] Example for synthetic model compounds lacking methyl substituents. Reported from *Exocarpus* seed oil (see text).

chemical degradation (Glass et al. 1975) and some of which have also been confirmed by synthesis (Rahn et al. 1979).

The numbering of the furanoid acids, F_1, F_2, . . . , originated from the sequence of elution in GLC, and it persists in the literature. Indeed, F_6 acid is a more expedient term than 11-(3,4-dimethyl-5-pentyl-2-furyl)undecanoic or 12,15-epoxy-13,14-dimethyleicosa-12,14-dienoic acid. For cases where the topic requires structural identification, an abbreviated nomenclature has been suggested (Rahn et al. 1981) which, with the examples given in Table 2-1, is self-explanatory. It implies that the proximal (alkylcarboxyl) and the terminal (alkyl) chains are always in the α positions, and that one methyl substituent, as in F_5, is always in the β position of the furan ring. Two methyl substituents are in β and β' positions.

In Table 2-1 is also indicated a classification, as propyl- and pentyl-furanoid acids. Biological conversions between these structures would be rather unexpected.

Furanoid acids without methyl substituent have not been encountered in fish lipids. However, this may not be final, since the possibility for biomethylation of the furan ring has been demonstrated in vitro. Accordingly, such acids may occur as precursors of the commonly found F acids with methyl groups at the ring.

An unsubstituted furanoid fatty acid, F(8,6), has been reported from *Exocarpus* seed oil as the first fatty acid of furanoid type (Morris et al. 1966) (see also Table 2-1). However, in contrast to those to be discussed here, it is a hexyl-furanoid acid and likely is an artifact from an associated oxygenated acetylenic fatty acid (Gunstone et al. 1978). F(8,6) is, however, easily accessible by chemical synthesis and has served as a model in several investigations on biological F acids.

Identification and Analysis

Mass spectrometry (MS), mostly in conjunction with GLC, is the method of choice for identification of F methyl esters. They are obtained from biological materials together with esters of the other fatty acids by the usual preparations of analytical samples.

The mass spectrum of F_6 methyl ester in Fig. 2-1 serves as a typical example for the fragmentation of F esters. The oxygen ring exerts a stabilizing effect, so that the molecular ion, in this case m/z 364, is pronounced. It is accompanied by m/z 333 ($M^+ -31$), but other ions characteristic for fatty esters are suppressed.

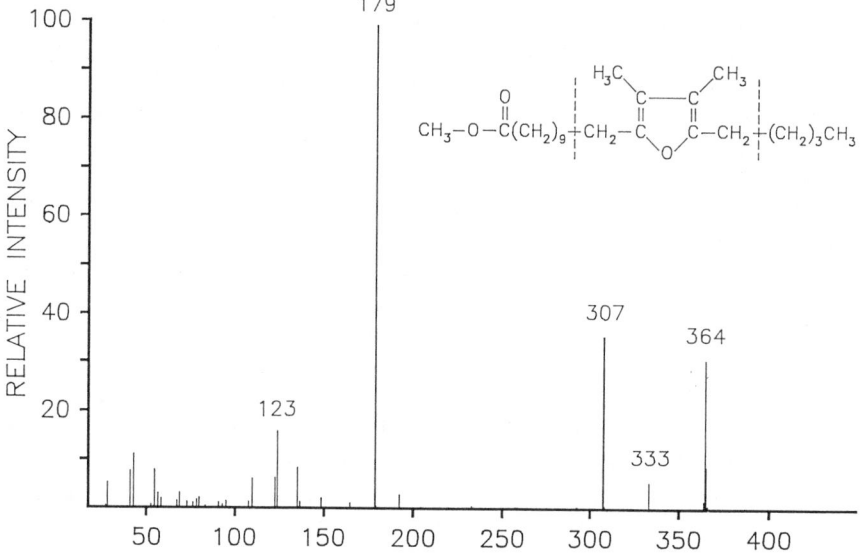

Fig. 2-1. Mass spectrum of F_6 methyl ester (EI, 70 eV).

The base peak from F_6 ester, m/z 179 (M^+ -185, $C_{11}H_{21}O_2$) is due to cleavage in the proximal chain, in allylic position. Corresponding cleavage occurs in the terminal chain, leading to m/z 307 (M^+ -57, C_4H_9). Both cleavages lead, with H rearrangement, to m/z 123 (M^+ $-(185 + 57) + 1$), a fragment representing the ring with methyl substituents and the first methylene of the chains in α and α' positions. When there is only one methyl substituent, MS leaves undecided the β or β' position of this group, but the β position has been ascertained by chemical degradation (Glass et al. 1975) and is, by implication, accepted for all monomethyl furanoids.

F esters mostly are only a small percentage of esters in biological samples. In GC they are eluted in the range of noncyclic fatty esters and can easily be obscured. For their analysis, simplification of the mixture and prefractionation for enrichment of F esters are desirable, if not necessary. Several methods are available to such ends.

The ring of F esters is not as readily hydrogenated as are the olefinic bonds of other fatty esters (Glass et al. 1974; Gunstone et al. 1978; Sand et al. 1983; Ishii et al. 1988A, B), so selective hydrogenation of the latter is possible, greatly simplifying the pattern of peaks in GC and the monitoring by MS. Any olefinic bond in F esters, however, may be prone also to be hydrogenated in such a procedure.

By virtue of the bulky substituted ring structure in the chain, F esters are not bound by urea (Glass et al. 1974, 1975; Scrimgeour 1977; Gunstone et al. 1978; Ishii et al. 1988A), so in crystallization of a mixture with urea, the F esters are enriched in the mother liquor while saturated esters are depleted there by precipitation. However, the unsubstituted ring of F(8,6) can be adapted in the urea inclusion structure (Schlenk and Sand, unpublished) and such F esters may be incorporated in the solid phase.

In argentation chromatography, F esters migrate between saturated and monounsaturated esters (Glass et al. 1975, 1977; Scrimgeour 1977; Gunstone et al. 1978). This offers another method to eliminate polyunsaturated components.

The use of high-pressure liquid chromatography (HPLC) for enrichment of F esters so far has been reported only once (Puchta et al. 1988).

In another approach to analytical differentiation, the F esters are hydrogenated (Gorst-Allmann et al. 1988; Puchta and Spiteller 1988; Puchta et al. 1988). With Rh/Al_2O_3 as catalyst, one of the predicted isomeric tetrahydrofuran derivatives is consistently predominant. Tetrahydro F esters are more polar than the common fatty esters and can be well separated from them by thin-layer chromatography (TLC) for subsequent GC-MS.

Preparation of F Esters

Some of the above methods have been used for preparation of F esters as a group, essentially free of other esters (Sand et al. 1983). Preparative separation of F esters from each other has received little attention. F_6 can be separated from others by preparative GC, but this involves considerable loss. Preparative HPLC might be a preferable method to single out some of the F components.

Chemical syntheses were and will be required for research on F acids, including the use of proper internal standards for quantitation of small amounts. The reader is referred to a thorough review of chemical syntheses of F acids (Lie Ken Jie 1981). Linoleic or ricinoleic acids may be starting materials, and chemical methods for introducing the methyl substituents are available. Synthetic methods that are more flexible in regard to chain length and position of the ring begin with easily accessible furan compounds which allow introduction of the desired terminal (alkyl) and proximal (alkylcarboxyl) substituents. In addition to the literature already reviewed (Lie Ken Jie 1981), an improved method leading to F_3 (Schoedel and Spiteller 1985) and the use of $^{14}CH_2N_2$ for labeling F acids (Rahn et al. 1981) may be quoted.

Occurrence of F Acids

In comparison to common fatty acids, information on F acids in fish is still sketchy. They were discovered in fish, and their enrichment in liver—at times also in testis or roe lipids—led to analyses of mainly these organs. Data on other organs, muscle, and depot fat are even more scant. With Table 2-2 an attempt is made to give account of present knowledge about F acids in marine fish lipids.

The number of species and often the number of specimens analyzed are low. There is, however, no reason to conclude that the F acids do not occur, if only at low level, in many other marine species. One may expect that with refined and more standardized analytical procedures, these gaps will narrow.

Higher percentages of F acids have been found in freshwater fish. They represented up to 43% of acyls in liver and/or testis lipids from 20 species (Glass et al. 1977). Outstanding, with levels about 10% F, were big mouth buffalo (*Ictiobus cyprinellus*), bluegill (*Lepomis macrochirus*), northern black bull head (*Ictalurus melas*), northern rock bass (*Ambloplites rupestris*), brook trout (*Salvelinus fontinalis*), northern pike (*Esox lucius*), carp (*Cyprinus carpio*), and bowfin (*Amia calva*) (all from the Minneapolis,

Table 2-2.   Occurrence of F Acids in Marine Fish Lipids

NAME	ORGAN	% OF TOTAL FATTY ACIDS	REFERENCE
Dog fish (*Squalus acanthias*)	liver	0.6	1
Cod (*Gadus morhua*)	liver	1	1
Ice fish (*Chaenocephalus aceratus*)	liver	4	1
Salmon (*Salmo salar*)[a]	liver	2	1
Sardine[b]	liver	0.6	2
Sea bream	liver	0.1	2
	roe	<0.1	
Mackerel	muscle	0.8	2
	liver	—	
Bonito	liver	0.7	2
Halfbeak	roe	0.9	2
Yellowtail	liver	0.2	2
Flounder	liver	0.5	2

References: 1, Gunstone et al. 1978; 2, Yoshioka 1981.
[a] Sampled from marine waters.
[b] Zoological names are not given in reference 2.

Minnesota area). Some of these occurrences have been confirmed in the literature, but such high levels have not been reported. They are verified, however, by preparative isolation in close to 100% yield from carp and northern pike lipids (Mississippi River, La Crosse area), where according to analyses about half of all acyls were F acids (Sand et al. 1983). Reasons for such unusual accumulation are not known.

In regard to other aquatic species, F acids have been reported, at low levels, from tissues of crayfish (*Procambarus clarkii*) (Okajima et al. 1984; Ishii et al. 1988A), octopus (*Eledone cirrhosa*) (Gunstone et al. 1978), sea squirt and scallop (Yoshioka 1981), and soft corals (*Sacrophytum glaucum* and *gemmatum*) (Groweiss and Kashman 1978). The enumeration can be expanded to amphibia with bullfrog, and reptiles with turtle as examples (Ishii et al. 1988A). However, of greater significance is their occurrence in plants.

A single furanoid acid, MeF(9,5) (F_2), had been identified from latex of the rubber tree (*Hevea brasiliensis*), where it represents >90% of acyls in the triglycerides (Hasma and Subramaniam 1978; Lie Ken Jie and Sinha 1981). Not until more recently were several F acids recognized as constituents of lipids from numerous other plants, and from algae and yeast (Hannemann et al. 1989). The levels were relatively high in photosynthetic tissue. In algae (*Chlorophyta* sp.) about 0.15 mg F acids/g of dry material were found.

The landmarks set for the occurrence of F acids in nature suggest their presence also in mammalian lipids, if not by de novo synthesis at least by transmittance with the diet. Indeed, F acids have been identified from bovine liver (Schoedel and Spiteller 1987) and human blood (Puchta et al. 1988; Puchta and Spiteller 1988).

After the preceding survey of occurrence, some more specific features of F acids in fish should be discussed, with the restraint that meager data impose on generalizations. A study over several years on F acids in freshwater fish (Glass et al. 1974; 1977) led to the following observations:

1. F acids occur foremost in males of a species but are occasionally found also in females, e.g., in northern pike.
2. Their amounts fluctuate during the year, in some species synchronic with the reproductive cycle.
3. They occur preferentially in liver and/or testis, but are found also in muscle, heart, and blood lipids.
4. Among lipid classes, they are at their highest levels in cholesteryl esters, next in triglycerides, but they are found also in phospholipids when high in the former two classes.
5. F_6 is prominent among the F acids, regardless of species, tissue, or lipid class.

It should be noted that these observations are from freshwater fish, which often have a much higher content of F acids than so far encountered in marine fish. By far not as many data are available for the latter, but some cautious comments may be made regarding the extent to which the above points may also be valid for them. (1) Preference for males seems not to apply, and such a generalization has been questioned also for freshwater fish. (2) Data for evaluating seasonal fluctuations in marine fish have not been reported. (3) Accumulation in liver and occurrence in other tissues and (4) the high relative level of F_6 in cholesteryl esters and their occurrence in other lipid classes have been confirmed. (5) The predominance of F_6 among F acids appears to be very common. Some examples for this point are compiled in Table 2-3. Rather consistently, diMeF(11,5) (F_6) acid is at the highest level, followed by diMeF(11,3) (F_4) acid, and this has been encountered also in sources other than fish.

Environment, diet, and physiological state of the fish doubtlessly affect the furanoid lipids, but only one such factor has been addressed in a controlled experiment. F acids in liver oil from fed and starved cod were compared (Gunstone et al. 1976, 1978), and the results are given in Table 2-4 in slightly condensed form.

Table 2-3. Composition of F Acids from Fish Lipids

SOURCE	F_1	F_2	F_3	F_4	F_5	F_6	F_7	REF.
Dog fish liver[a]	2	10	3	10	5	29	1	1
Cod liver[a]	1	10	3	12	9	43	1	1
Ice fish liver[b]	3	4	5	33	1	18	—	1
Salmon egg[c]	0.3	0.8	0.7	15.3	6.2	75.7	—	2
Kokanee testis[d]	0.2	0.5	0.3	1.8	0.7	7.1	<0.1	3
Northern pike testis[e]	1.5	3.1	—	5.5	4.9	14.7	—	4
Northern pike liver[e]	1.2	2.2	—	6.5	1.7	14.8	—	4
Crayfish hepato pancreas[f]	2.0	1.6	6.8	3.5	0.9	11.9	—	5

References: 1, Gunstone et al. 1978; 2, Ishii et al. 1988B; 3, Ota and Tagaki 1983; 4, Glass et al. 1974; 5, Ishii et al. 1988A.
[a] % F acids in an enriched fraction, which represented 1% of total acyls.
[b] % F acids in an enriched fraction representing 6% of total acyls.
[c] % F total acyls of the phospholipid fraction, which represented 30% of total lipids. Six additional F acids were detected, 1.4%.
[d] % F in acyls of triglycerides.
[e] % F in total acyls.
[f] % F in acyls of cholesteryl esters, which represented 19% of total lipids. Altogether, 24 additional F acids were detected, 2.8%.

With the decrease in total lipid and class amounts, starvation changed greatly the relative amounts and distribution of F acids. The lipid content of liver was reduced to 10% of the reference value, but the percentage of F acids in total acyls increased by a factor of 50–100. Similar to essential fatty acids, they seem to be spared in the catabolism of lipids during starvation, but the possibility of their being catabolized and newly formed is not ruled out. The enrichment is foremost in cholesteryl esters, probably by a shift from triglycerides. F_6 remained the major F acid, but the relative amounts of others seemed to be affected by the hunger period (values not quoted here).

Table 2-4. F Acids in Liver Lipids from Fed and Starved Cod[a]

	FED[b]	STARVED[c]
% lipid in liver (LL)	56	5
% F in LL acyls	0.5	48
% CE in LL	1	57
% F in CE acyls	<3	84
% TG in LL	80	6
% F in TG acyls	<4	—
% PL in LL	15	37
% F in PL acyls	<1.4	1

[a] LL, liver lipids; CE, cholesteryl esters; TG, triglycerides; PL, phospholipids.
[b] One fish, fed with herring and other small fish.
[c] Two fish, starved for five months.

In this experiment, the level of F acids in the fish fed in captivity was in agreement with that found in commercial cod liver oil, and other experiments confirmed that refining the oil is not destructive to them (Scrimgeour 1977).

Interconversions of F Acids

Comparison of the structures of F acids suggests interrelationships by chain elongation and shortening of the alkycarboxyl chain, and by methylation (Glass et al. 1977). Bis-homologous relationships in chain length were verified by administering F acids specifically labeled with ^{14}C to carp and blue gill (Sand et al. 1984). The tracer indicated conversion of MeF(11,5) to MeF(13,5) and to MeF(9,5), and of diMeF(9,5) to diMeF(11,5). In experiments with gourami (*Trichogaster cosbi*), the biological reduction of labeled F(9,5) acid to the corresponding F alcohol was demonstrated. Accordingly, reactions common for the carboxyl group of straight-chain fatty acids are not prevented by the furan ring. However, methylation of the ring or desaturation of the chain were not detected in these in vivo experiments.

Biosynthesis of F Acids

It is most reasonable to assume polyunsaturated acids, in particular of $\omega 6$ and $\omega 3$ type, as precursors of F acids. Accordingly, F acids, like the surmised precursors, would not be de novo synthesized in fish, and this was confirmed by giving ^{14}C-acetate to northern pike and brook trout (Sand et al. 1984). Radioactivity was incorporated into the F acids, but detailed chemical degradation showed ^{14}C to be exclusively located in the proximal chain, apparently introduced into an existing precursor by chain elongation. The conclusion is that, like essential fatty acids, the F acids were not de novo synthesized. However, it still leaves open the possibility that the furan moiety was synthesized in the fish from the dietary polyunsaturated acids.

Nevertheless, the result gives credence to the assumed precursor-product relationship, although this has not been directly demonstrated. Chemical formation of the furan ring from a peroxide of linoleic acid has been cited as model for the possibility of biological cyclization (Gunstone and Wijesundera 1979). Peroxides of linoleic and linolenic acids may lead to pentyl- and propyl-furanoid acids, respectively, which then are substrates for methylation(s) to yield parent acids for the chain-homologous F acids (Gorst-Allmann et al. 1988).

The assumed methylation as a late step in the biosynthesis found experimental support (Dietel and Spiteller 1988) by incubation of synthetic F(9,4) with a subcellular preparation obtained from beef liver homogenate by centrifugation. In the presence of S-adenosylmethionine, F(9,4) yielded diMeF(11,4) together with its vinylogous F acids. The essential point made by this experiment is that methylation of the ring has taken place.

The scheme proposes furanoid acids without ring-methyl as intermediates, but such acids have not been encountered in analyses aimed at the biological F acids. The structure of certain urinary metabolites provides an argument for their existence (Bauer and Spiteller 1985A).

Catabolism of F Acids

Independent of investigations on F acids, furanoid dicarboxylic acids had been identified from human blood and urine (urofuran acids) (Spiteller et al. 1980; Pfordt et al. 1981; Bauer and Spiteller 1985A), and a somewhat different type of such acids was discovered in bovine urine (Bauer and Spiteller 1985B). Their structures resemble those of the furan moieties in F acids, and feeding experiments revealed two pathways for the catabolism of F acids, summarized in Fig. 2-2.

A mixture of F acids fed to rats led to urinary acids of mainly type B (Sand et al. 1983), while in humans the prominent products are of type A (Schoedel et al. 1986). The two pathways have in common the β-oxidation of the proximal chain. It is brought to a halt in the vicinity of the furan ring, similar to the classical results from ω-phenylalkylcarboxylic acids (Knoop 1904). The catabolism is supplemented by methyl oxidation, predominant in humans, or by ω-oxidation, predominant in rats and cattle. A

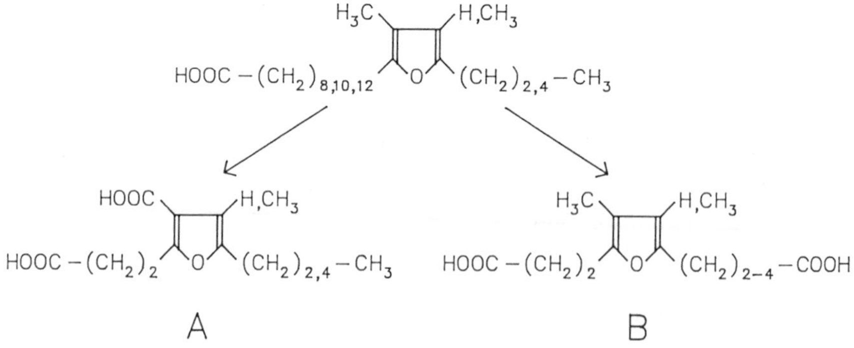

Fig. 2-2. Catabolism of furanoid fatty acids to dicarboxylic furanoid acids.

species preference for type A or B is obvious. Without implying a generalization for fish, mainly type B was found in urine of northern pike (Spiteller, Schlenk, and co-workers, unpublished).

These catabolic reactions are rather conventional, but as characteristic metabolites the products were important indicators for the unexpected presence of F acids in dietary material (Gorst-Allmann et al. 1988; Hannemann et al. 1989).

Conversions Involving the Furan Ring.   The furan ring is retained in the above dicarboxylic acids, and they are not necessarily ultimate products of F acid catabolism. However, of greater interest are conversions of the furan ring where the fatty acid chain is retained. The key to such reactions is the oxidative opening of the ring by lipoxygenases (Boyer et al. 1979). This was found with F(9,5) methyl ester as a model compound. It was oxidized by soybean lipoxygenase I, preferably with linoleate as co-oxidant, to 10,13-dioxo-*trans*-11-octadecenoate, presumably via the *cis* isomer. Leaving aside discussion of a possible mechanism, the oxidation of the ring can be presented as:

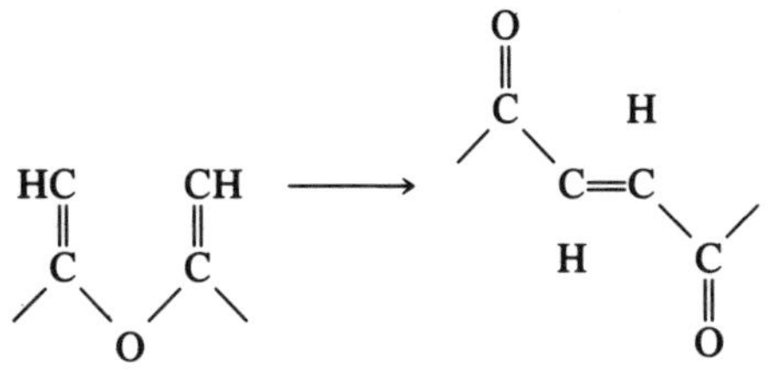

Reactions of dioxoenoic acids derived by enzymatic oxidation from model and biological F acids involve intramolecular cyclizations and the formation of S-conjugates and of sequential compounds.

Figure 2-3 describes cyclizations that were found from aqueous beef liver homogenate, taking F_3 as an example for a precursor. Alkaline workup yielded isomeric cyclopentene structures, due to intramolecular aldol condensation (Schoedel and Spiteller 1985; Spiteller 1987). Acidic workup gave isomeric olefin-furanoid acids (Schoedel and Spiteller 1987), by recyclization to the furan ring, with introduction of a conjugated double bond. This reaction is known also from other compounds featuring an oxo-ene-oxo structure (Ernest and Stanek 1959).

Extractive homogenization of liver with chloroform-methanol, followed by equal treatments for analysis, did not lead to such products and revealed only the presence of F acids. Apparently, the organic solvents are destructive to enzymes prerequisite for liberating F acid from lipid

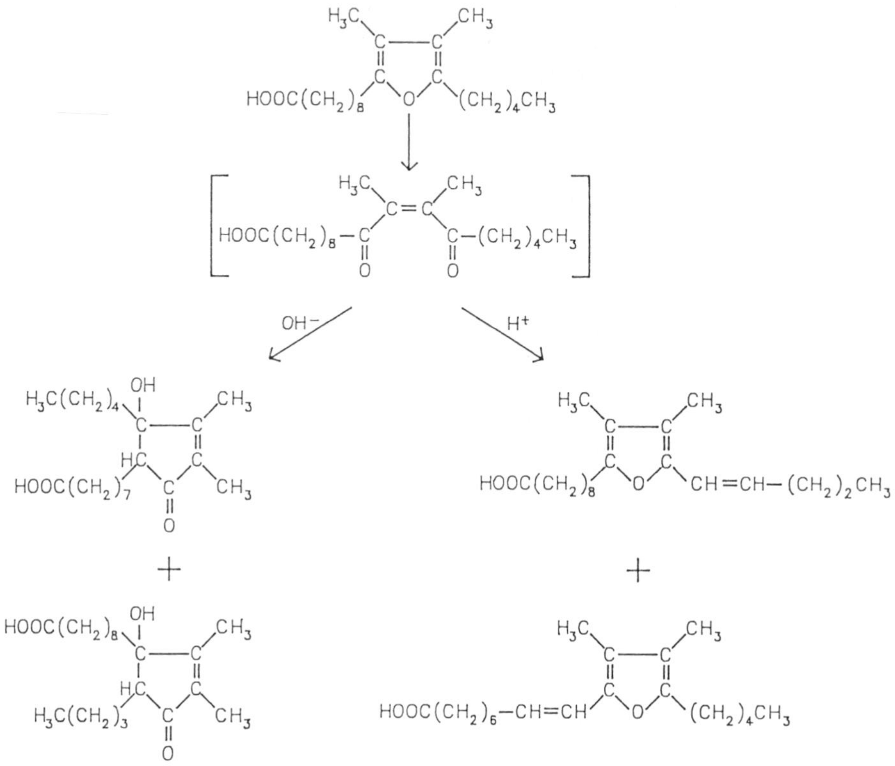

Fig. 2-3. (Hydroxy-oxo-cyclopentenyl) alkanoic acids (left) and olefin-furanoid acids (right) from F_3 acid after enzymic oxidation of the furan ring.

and for oxidizing it. The expected intermediate, a dimethyldioxo-ene, in contrast to the dioxo-ene from model F acid, is not sufficiently stabile for isolation and analysis but the products prove such a structure as a precursor. The cyclizations (Fig. 2-3) discussed for these experiments are by chemical treatment, but other experiments indicate that they can occur also under biological conditions (Dietel and Spiteller 1988).

The conjugated oxo-ene-oxo structure is chemically highly reactive and is active also in biological systems. Compounds containing it have been studied in great variety for their inhibitory effect on the growth of some bacteria, on sulfhydryl enzymes, and on the aggregation of blood platelets (Geiger 1948; Skoda et al. 1961; Graff et al. 1984). Inhibitors of platelet aggregation included the product from the above model, F(9,5), and similar dioxoenoic acids. A reaction of sulfhydryl groups with the inhibitors has been quoted as the most likely explanation for the inhibitory mechanism in these biological tests.

The compounds readily react with sulfhydryl groups, yielding thioethers (S-conjugates) in place of the double bond. In vitro reaction of 10,13-dioxo-*trans*-11-octadecenoic acid with mercaptoethanol or, more pertinent, with glutathione, gave the expected isomeric conjugates (Graff et al. 1984; Jandke et al. 1988).

$$\underset{\substack{\\ }}{HOOC(CH_2)_8} - \overset{\overset{O}{\|}}{C} - CH_2 - \overset{\overset{SR}{|}}{CH} - \overset{\overset{O}{\|}}{C} - (CH_2)_4CH_3$$

$$+ \; HOOC(CH_2)_8 - \overset{\overset{O}{\|}}{C} - \overset{\overset{SR}{|}}{CH} - CH_2 - \overset{\overset{O}{\|}}{C} - (CH_2)_4CH_3$$

(—SR = mercaptoethanol or glutathione conjugate component)

In an approach to a possible in vivo situation, F_3 acid was subjected to enzymic oxidation in the presence of these sulfhydryl compounds, to react in situ with the elusive dimethyldioxo-ene from that acid (Jandke et al. 1988). S-Conjugates were obtained, but their structures did not conform with the indicated scheme. Apparently, the methyl substituents steered, likely via en enol form, the addition of —SR to the chain carbon adjacent to the dioxo-ene system. Recyclization of the 1,4-dioxo compound followed and gave isomeric S-conjugates of the original F acid.

Accordingly, sulfhydryl groups of glutathione, cysteine, and likely also proteins, can be masked by metabolites of F acids. This may be of crucial importance for biological reactions where a certain sulfhydryl status is essential.

Several other lines of products from F acids can be mentioned. For example, incubation of the model acid F(9,5) with certain subcellular fractions from bovine liver led to acids that have a pyrrole instead of a furan ring as part of the chain (Dietel and Spiteller 1988). It is assumed that the N of the new heterocycle is introduced after oxidation, by transamination before cyclization. Pyrrole fatty acids with double bonds, methyl, hydroxyl, or oxo groups have been identified from these experiments.

Concluding Remarks

Furanoid acids seem to be rather common, normally minor constituents in many lipids, similar to odd-numbered fatty acids. In contrast to the latter, the F acids exhibit properties and reactions that are analytically and biologically more challenging for research. In these aspects, they resemble rather the polyunsaturated fatty acids. The array of products that can derive from F acids is already quite large. The field is open for speculation and experimentation in regard to any physiological importance they might have. One should expect that the wide occurrence of F acids is not merely a metabolic oddity.[4]

FATTY ACID CONTENT VARIATION IN OIL FROM A SINGLE FISH SPECIES[5]

At the time Edward Gruger, Jr., wrote Chapter 1, entitled "Fatty Acid Composition," in the book *Fish Oils* (Stansby 1967), virtually nothing was known about the extent of variation of the fatty acid content in the oil from different samples of fish of the same species. At that time, although it was recognized that there probably was some variation in fatty acid composition in oils within samples of the same species, the general belief was that such variation was relatively small. As a result nearly all the investigations up to that time that involved analyses of fatty acid content of the oil of a given species of fish were carried out using only a few individual fish generally all taken at the same time and location.

Today we know that there can be a huge variation in fatty acid content of the oil of different individual fish of the same species. Most of the early publications, where only a very few individual fish of the same species

---

[4]Research on F acids in the Hormel Institute was supported by Grant #HL08214 and by the Hormel Foundation.
[5]This section was written entirely by Maurice E. Stansby.

were used, do not at all represent the fatty acid content of the oil of that species of fish. In Chapter 1 of the book *Fish Oils* therefore, the values reported in Tables 1 through 3 for fatty acid composition of the oils from the flesh or liver of many species of fish or shellfish are for the most part quite misleading.

In the late nineteenth century, oils were ordinarily described by certain oil or fat constants such as the iodine value. In that early era it was assumed that all samples of a given fish oil of the same species would always have the same oil constant value. Iodine numbers were established by chemists in leading oil laboratories and were reported often to two digits beyond the decimal point. If anyone else later found a different iodine number for such an oil, it was believed that the difference was dependent not upon the oil varying from one lot to another but rather to inept analysis by the one carrying out the test. These ideas persisted into the early 1900s. One of the best treatises on oils and fats was that by Lewkowitsch in three volumes, which first came out about 1883. By the time its fifth edition was printed in 1913, the iodine values for most oils of fish still were given as if there was no variation from lot to lot, for example, salmon oil 161.42, and sturgeon oil 125.3. Two industrial oils, however, menhaden and herring, were reported as having ranges of iodine numbers, menhaden 139–173 and sardine 161–193. Nevertheless, extending well into the twentieth century, most workers with fish oils had the general idea that there was no particular difference in the chemical makeup of one lot of oil from a given species of fish to another lot of oil from the same species.

After the introduction of gas-liquid chromatography in the 1950s, the use of fat constants such as iodine numbers was largely superceded by use of the fatty acid analyses of the various fish oils. Many papers have been appearing since then purporting to give the fatty acid composition of fish oils from many different species of fish. Unfortunately, these older ideas suggesting that the chemical composition of fish oils varies by only a small amount among different lots of oil of the same species have still persisted. As a result, many papers are still being published in which the fatty acid content was determined from just a few fish of the same species, usually all individual fish having been taken at the same time and place.

One such study, however, which has been going on for a long time, has been made by Zapata-Haynie Corporation in which entirely adequate sampling has been used. Samples of commercial menhaden oil are being taken from several areas in the Gulf of Mexico and along the American Atlantic Coast. Samples have been taken at different times of the year for 12 years (1977–1988). Each sample analyzed for fatty acid content repre-

Table 2-5. Range of Fatty Acid Content in Large Batches of Commercial
Menhaden Oil Taken Annually from 1977 Through 1988

FATTY ACID	RANGE % OF TOTAL FATTY ACIDS	RATIO HIGHEST TO LOWEST
C14:0	7.2–12.1	1.7
C15:0	0.4–2.3	5.8
C16:0	15.3–25.6	1.7
C16:1	9.3–15.8	1.7
C16:2	0.3–2.8	9.4
C16:3	0.9–3.5	3.9
C16:4	0.5–2.8	5.6
C17:0	0.2–3.0	15.0
C18:0	2.5–4.1	1.6
C18:1	8.3–13.8	1.7
C18:2	0.7–2.8	4.0
C18:3	0.8–2.3	2.9
C18:4	1.7–4.0	2.4
C20:0	0.1–0.6	6.0
C20:4	1.5–2.7	1.8
C20:5	11.1–16.3	1.5
C22:1	0.1–1.4	10.0
C22:5	1.3–3.8	2.9
C22:6	4.6–13.8	3.0

Source: Zapata-Haynie Co., Anthony Bimbo, laboratory director.

sented millions of individual menhaden fish. The results of this long-term survey are shown in Table 2-5.

In spite of the fact that each sample analyzed was taken from oil representing millions of individual fish, there was a huge variation from lot to lot in the amount of each of the separate fatty acids that were determined. Undoubtedly had the sample size been small, such as only a few individual fish for each sample (such as ordinarily in the past had been used in papers reporting on the fatty acid content of oil from one species of fish), the variation would have been a great deal larger. Of the 20 fatty acids considered, only three had as little as a 50% difference between the maximum and minimum. At the other extreme, two fatty acids had a 10- to 15-fold difference. Eleven of the fatty acids had a variation greater than $2\frac{1}{2}$ times, and in this category was the important $\omega 3$ fatty acid, DHA ($C_{22}:6$).

Unfortunately, the results mentioned above have never been published other than in brief mention of a part of the entire program. However, in addition to this work, a shorter (two-year) study on commercial menhaden oil fatty acid composition was carried out in considerable detail (Joseph 1985.) This study is much more complete than that of the fatty acid makeup of the oil of any other species of fish, and fortunately it has been published. In it, very large amounts of menhaden oil produced in 1982 and 1983 were analyzed for fatty acid content employing up-to-date analytical techniques. There were 65 commercially produced oils made in 1982 and 63 such samples produced in 1983. Samples were collected monthly and also from menhaden oil manufactured from plants located at three different areas on the Atlantic Coast and nine different areas on the Gulf Coast. As was the case in the much longer (12-year) unpublished study cited above, there was considerable variation in the amount of several of the fatty acids determined. For example, the C22 : 6 fatty acid for samples produced on the Atlantic Coast varied from 7.3 to 13.1%, and for those manufactured on the Gulf Coast the variation for C22 : 6 was from 4.2 to 8.2%.

No other fish oil besides commercial menhaden oil has had anywhere near such a thorough examination of its fatty acid variation. The questions arise as to whether such large variation is one peculiar to menhaden oil or to commercial fish oils in general and also whether oils from food fish show similar large variation in fatty acid makeup.

There are two other fish oils for which examination has been made of fatty acid variability at a much lesser extent than menhaden oil, yet which is thorough enough to give us some idea as to what the situation is. One of these is a commercial oil, herring; the other is the oil of a food fish, mullet. Studies have been made to a limited extent on the variability of fatty acids from commercial herring oil prepared from fish caught in the Pacific and Atlantic oceans off the coasts of North America. These studies have shown a high variability in fatty acid content of commercial herring oil (e.g., C22:6 varying from 2.0 to 7.8% and C20:5 from 3.9 to 15.2% (Stansby 1981) (see Table 2-6).

A fairly extensive survey has been made of fatty acid variation in mullet (Table 2-7). This study (Deng et al. 1976) was made not in connection with nutritional properties (such as ω3 fatty acids) but rather because the oil from mullet, unlike that of oil from other fish, often has considerable quantities of odd-chain-length fatty acids (e.g., sometimes more than 10 times as much C17 fatty acids occur than in other species). This study showed that not only did the odd-carbon-chain fatty acids vary widely (e.g., C17:1 from 1.7 to 8.2%), but also most other fatty acids varied considerably (e.g., C20:5 from 3.9 to 15.2 and C22:6 from 0.7 to 3.9%).

Another consideration relating to variation in fatty acid composition of a species is whether the oil is produced as a by-product in the manufacture of both fish meal and oil or whether the oil is extracted by solvents and the resulting oil analyzed for fatty acid content. A comparison of menhaden oils fatty acid composition made by each way reveals the fact

Table 2-6. Range of Fatty Acid Composition of Commercial North
American Herring Oils

FATTY ACID	RANGE % OF TOTAL FATTY ACIDS
C14:0	4.6–8.4
C16:0	10.1–18.6
C16:1	6.2–12.0
C18:0	0.7–2.1
C18:1	9.3–25.2
C18:2	0.1–0.6
C18:3	0.0–1.1
C18:4	1.1–2.8
C20:1	7.3–19.9
C20:5	3.9–15.2
C22:1	6.9–30.6
C22:5	0.3–1.3
C22:6	2.0–7.8
C24:1	0.2–1.3
C24:5	0.0–0.5

that quite different values are obtained in the two cases. For example, C22:6 in commercial menhaden oil varies from 4.7 to 12.2%. Yet the oil of menhaden when solvent extracted has about twice as much C22:6, in one determination ranging from 11.0 to 18.75. It is not known why this should occur. One possibility is that during the industrial manufacture of fish oil a considerable proportion of the C22:6 fatty acid (probably occurring largely as phospholipids) is not removed with the oil but rather remains behind in the portion of the oil that is contained in the fish meal. At any rate, this situation shows that fatty acid composition of industrial fish oils can not be used as a measure of the fatty acid content of the oil in the fish of the same species and where the oil is removed by solvent extraction.

In 1981 a paper was published (Stansby 1981) pointing out in considerable detail the many errors that were being made by the publication of fatty acid compositions based on erroneous fatty acid makeup of oils for which only a few individual fish were used. Nevertheless, this paper got little or no attention, and most subsequent papers on the fatty acid content of fish continued to assume that there is little variation in fatty acid content of different lots of fish oil from the same species even though woefully inadequate numbers of individual fish were used to represent the species. More recently, in a chapter in a book, this problem was pointed

Table 2-7. Range of Fatty Acid Composition of Mullet Oil

FATTY ACID	RANGE % OF TOTAL FATTY ACIDS[a]
C14:0	4.6–11.5
C15:0	3.2–12.4
C15:1	0–1.2
C16:0	20.2–33.7
C16:1	13.4–29.3
C17:0	0–2.5
C17:1	1.7–8.2
C17:2	0.0–4.4
C18:0	1.8–5.4
C18:1	7.1–13.6
C18:2	0.7–2.7
C18:3	0.3–1.3
C18:4ω3	0.7–2.2
C18:4ω6	0.1–2.3
C19:1	0–2.5
C20:0	0.0–3.9
C20:3ω3	0.1–0.8
C20:3ω6	0.0–1.7
C20:4ω3	0.3–0.6
C20:4ω6	1.6–3.8
C20:5ω3	4.6–8.1
C22:3ω3	0.0–0.2
C22:4ω3	0.2–0.6
C22:5ω3	1.3–3.6
C22:5ω6	0.4–1.0
C22:6ω3	0.7–3.9

[a]Data from Deng et al. (1976).

out with a suggestion as to how, as an interim measure pending vast amounts of analytical analyses with proper sampling, an approximation could be reached as to the ranges of ω3 fatty acids in oils from different fish species (Stansby 1986).

This suggestion was based on the far greater role of the oil content in a given species in controlling the amount of a given fatty acid in the fish than was the effect of the amount of fatty acid in the particular oil. The oil content of nearly all species of fish varies over a very wide range from a few tenths of one percent to 25% (sometimes even much higher amounts). Recently the problem has arisen of which species of fish are the best source of ω3 long-chain fatty acids (which are believed to have beneficial health effects). The sum of the three most important ω3 fatty acids— C20:5ω3, C22:6ω3, and C22:5ω3—varies for most all species between

17.5% and 35% a factor of only 2. The fat content of a large proportion of the various species of fish varies from 1 to 13%, a factor of 13. Thus it is apparent that the major factor is the oil content (not the fatty acid content of the oil of fish), which should be given greater consideration in the selection of desirable species of fish as a source of ω3 fatty acids. Of course the oil content of a given species may vary considerably from samples taken at different seasons of the year. Nevertheless a great deal more is known about such variation than is the case with the fatty acid content of the oils of different species of fish. The species that vary in oil content to the greatest extent are mostly ones in which the fish undergo long spawning migrations. The fat content of the flesh of such fish is built up prior to the start of such migration. During the spawning migration, the fish eat very little food; rather they depend on metabolism of their body fat as a major energy source during migration. Examples of species that undergo spawning migration with resulting high variation in their body fatty content are mackerel, herring, and the various species of salmon. As an example, the common mackerel (*Scomber scombrus*) living in waters along the American Atlantic Coast may have a fat content in their flesh in early spring of only about 4%. As the season progresses, this fat content rapidly increases, reaching maximum values as high as 20% or more by midsummer (Stansby and Lemon 1941).

Because there is a lack of reliable knowledge on fatty acid contents of oil for nearly all species of fish, it is not possible at this time to compile any meaningful table of fatty acid ranges by species. There are, however, a few facts known about some species. For example, the C22 : 6 fatty acid is often considerably higher in the oils of various species of tuna (fresh tuna, not canned tuna) than in that of most species. The long-chain monoene (C20 : 1) is usually very high in the oil of herring.

A good example of the lack of reliable information on fatty acid content in the flesh of different species of fish is that occurring for salmon. No reliable information is available on the fatty acid makeup in the oils of any of the five species of salmon caught on the Pacific Coast or for the Atlantic Coast species. Nevertheless, in recently published tables there often appears fatty acid makeup of something sometimes listed as "salmon." Often there is neither an indication of the species of salmon nor a suggestion of whether the oil is made from whole fish or from waste from salmon canneries or whether it is the oil in the flesh of salmon; furthermore, it is frequently assumed that there may be no difference in fatty acid content from the oil among the various species of salmon.

We do know that there can be a big difference in the makeup of the oil in different species of salmon. A very good study was carried out between 1936 and 1939 on the oil from many tins of canned salmon. This study

(Stansby 1952) involved examination of the oil from over 2000 cans of salmon divided among the five Pacific species.

Each year for many years the National Food Processors Association held in Seattle a salmon can cutting at which many cans of fish that had been canned the previous season were examined. At that time it was not common to run fatty acid analyses; instead, refractive indices were run. From the refractive index the iodine number can be calculated. Iodine numbers give a measure of the degree of unsaturation of an oil which is brought about by the presence of different amounts of highly polyunsaturated fatty acids.

From these studies it was apparent that the oil from the five different Pacific Coast species each differed in iodine numbers (and hence must have varied in fatty acid composition). The species, listed in order of increasing iodine value, are (1) chinook (or king), (2) sockeye or red, (3) chum or keta, (4) silver or coho, and (5) pink or humpback. These results are also confirmed by the degree of oxidation taking place when the fish is frozen, packaged, and held in cold storage. King salmon held in this way will keep in good condition for up to a year or more without developing any extensive rancidity. Pink salmon becomes rancid after just a few weeks in cold storage and is quite inedible after two to three months.

It is unfortunate that we must rely on old data based on fat constants such as iodine numbers to differentiate the properties of salmon oils of different species. A few analyses of the fatty acids in some species of salmon have been run, but the number of fish used has been quite inadequate. One such study is that of Gruger et al. (1964), which measured the fatty acid makeup of a number of species of fish including four Pacific Coast salmon species. In this study, for each species of salmon, only five fish—all taken at the same time and caught at the same place—were used. This investigation was made not in any way to establish the fatty acid ranges for salmon of different species or other fish. Rather it was undertaken in the 1950s, when gas-liquid chromatography was first being introduced, to look into whether gas chromatography might be readily applicable for using in future studies. In their paper, Gruger et al. (1964) very clearly stated that the results in no way represented the reported species composition: "No attempt was made to prepare composite samples representative of the particular species variations from one time of year to another or from one catching area to another. In this respect, the sampling was definitely inadequate to be representative of the species under any conditions except those that prevailed at the time of sampling." In spite of this clear warning, the results for the five species of salmon as well as those of most of the other species listed in this paper have appeared in many tables of fatty acid composition of fish species as being *the* composition for that species, with no suggestion that the species as a whole undoubtedly had a range of fatty acid composition values whose average was certainly not that reported.

For the many species of fish besides salmon (with the exception of commercial menhaden and herring oils and of the oil in mullet) there are no adequate data for which one can get any idea of the range of fatty acid content representative for a given species.

It is for this reason that fatty acid content values are not included in this book for species other than commercial menhaden and herring and for the food fish, mullet. In all probability, sometime in the future reliable data based on adequate sampling will become available. However, until this occurs, it is not desirable to set up meaningless tables of fatty acid composition of fish species where quite erroneous values would to a large extent appear.

REFERENCES

Ackman, R. G. 1964. Structural homogeneity in unsaturated fatty acids of marine lipids. A review. *J. Fisheries Res. Board Can.* 21:247–254.

Ackman, R. G., and Jangaard, P. M. 1963. On the occurrence of 4,7,10,13-16-docosapen-taenoic acid in saury (*Coloabis saira*) oil. *J. Fisheries Res. Board Can.* 20:1551–1552.

Ackman, R. G., and Sipos. 1965. Isolation of the saturated fatty acids of some marine lipids with particular reference to normal odd-numbered fatty acids and branched-chain fatty acids. *Comp. Biochem. Physiol.* 15:445–456.

Ahrens, E. H., Jr., Insull, W., Jr. Hirsch, J., Stoffel, W., Peterson, M. L., Farquhar, J. W., Miller, T., and Thomasson, H. J. 1959. The effect on human serum-lipids of a dietary fat, highly unsaturated, but poor in essential fatty acids. *Lancet* 1959:115–119 (Jan. 17).

Bailey, B. E., Carter, N. M., and Swain, L. A. 1952. *Marine Oils, with Particular Reference to Those of Canada.* Ottawa: Bulletin 89. Fisheries Research Board of Canada.

Bauer, S., and Spiteller, G. 1985A. Identification and synthesis of previously unknown furancarboxylic acids from human urine (in German). *Liebigs Ann. Chem.* 1985:813–821.

Bauer, S., and Spiteller, G. 1985B. Furancarboxylic acids in cattle urine (in German). *Helv. Chim. Acta* 68:1635–1638.

Boyer, R. F., Litts, D., Kostishak, J., Wijesundera, R. C., and Gunstone, F. D. 1979. The action of lipoxygenase-1 on furan derivatives. *Chem. Phys. Lipids* 25:237–246.

Brenner, R. R., Mercui, O., de Tomas, M. E., and Peluffo, T. O. 1960. Effect of the natural diet on the depot fats of the Rio de la Plata freshwater fish *Pimelodus* maculatus. Proc. Intern. Conf. Biochem. Lipids, 6th Marseilles. 101–108 (Pub. 1961).

Brenner, R. R., Vazza, D. V., and de Tomas, M. E. 1963. Effect of fat-free diet and of different dietary fatty acids (palmitate, oleate and linoleate) on the fatty acid composition of freshwater fish lipids. *J. Lipid Res.* 4:341–345.

Brockerhoff, H., Ackman, R. G., and Hoyle, R. J. 1963. Specific distribution of fatty acids in marine lipids. *Arch. Biochem. Biophys.* 100:9–12.

Brockerhoff, H., and Hoyle, R. J. 1963. On the structure of the depot fats of marine fish and mammals. *Arch. Biochem. Biophys.* 102:452–455.

Brockerhoff, H., Hoyle, R. J., and Ronald, K. 1964. Retention of the fatty acid distribution pattern of a dietary triglyceride in animals. *J. Biol. Chem.* 239:735–739.

Brockerhoff, H., Yurkowski, M., Hoyle, R. J., and Ackman, R. G. 1964. Fatty acid distribution of lipids of marine plankton. *J. Fisheries Res. Board Can.* 21:1379–1384.

Deng, J. C., Ortholfer, F. T., Dennison, R. A., and Watson, M. 1976. Lipids and fatty acids in mullet (*Mugil cephalus*): Seasonal and locational variations. *J. Food Sci.* 41:1479–1483.

Deuel, H. J., Jr. 1951. *The Lipids, Their Chemistry and Biochemistry*, vol. 1. New York: Interscience.

DeWitt, K. W. 1963. Seasonal variations in cod liver oil. *J. Sci. Food Agric.* 14:92–98.

Dietel, P., and Spiteller, G. 1988. Incubation of 2,5-disubstituted F acids with bovine liver homogenate (in German). *Liebigs Ann. Chem.* 1988:397–403.

Dolev, A., and Olcott, H. S. 1965A. Triglycerides of sable fish (*Anaplopoma fimbria*). I. Quantitative frationation by column chromatography on silica gel impregnated with silver nitrate. *J. Am. Oil Chemists' Soc.* 42:624–627.

Dolev, A., and Olcott, H. S. 1965B. The triglycerides of sable fish (*Anaplopoma fimbria*). II. Fatty acid distribution in triglyceride fractions as determined with pancreatic lipase. *J. Am. Oil Chemists' Soc.* 42:1046–1051.

Ernest, I., and Stanek, J. 1959. Decomposition of diazoketones with cupric oxide. V. A new reaction of unsaturated aliphatic γ-diketones (in German). *Coll. Czech. Chem. Commun.* 24:530–535.

Farkas, T., and Herodek, S. 1962. Origin of the characteristic fatty acid composition of aquatic organisms. *Magy. Tud. Akad, Tihanyl Biol. Kutatoint, Evkonyve* 29:79–83.

Farkas, T., and Herodek, S. 1964. The effect of environmental temperature on the fatty acid composition of crustacean plankton. *J. Lipid Res.* 5:369–373.

Farquhar, J. W., Insull, W., Jr., Rosen, P., Stoffel, W., and Ahrens, E. H., Jr. 1959. The analysis of fatty acid mixtures by gas-liquid chromatography: Construction and operation of an ionization chamber instrument. *Nutrition Rev.* 17, Pt. II:1–30.

Geiger, W. B. 1948. Antibacterial unsaturated ketones and their mode of action. *Arch. Biochem. Biophys.* 16:423–435.

Gellerman, J. L., and Schlenk, H. 1959. Column chromatography of lipids—odd-numbered straight chain fatty acids of menhaden oil. *Experientia* 15:387–388.

Glass, R. L., Krick, T. P., and Eckhardt, A. E. 1974. New series of fatty acids in northern pike (*Esox lucius*). *Lipids* 9(12):1004–1008.

Glass, R. L., Krick, T. P., Olson, D. L., and Thorson, R. L. 1977. The occurrence and distribution of furan fatty acids in spawning male freshwater fish. *Lipids* 12(10):828–836.

Glass, R. L., Krick, T. P., Sand, D. M., Rahn, C. H., and Schlenk, H. 1975. Furanoid fatty acids from fish lipids. *Lipids* 10(11):695–702.

Gorst-Allmann, C. P., Puchta, V., and Spiteller, G. 1988. Investigations of the origin of the furan fatty acids (F-acids). *Lipids* 23(11):1032–1036.

Graff, G., Gellerman, J. L., Sand, D. M., and Schlenk, H. 1984. Inhibition of blood platelet aggregation by dioxo-ene compounds. *Biochim. Biophys. Acta* 799:143–150.

Groweiss, A., and Kashman, Y. 1978. A new furanoid fatty acid from the soft corals *Sarcophyton glaucum* and *gemmatum*. *Experientia* 34:299.

Gruger, E. H., Jr., Nelson, R. W., and Stansby, M. E. 1964. Fatty acid composition of oils from 21 species of marine fish, freshwater fish and shellfish. *J. Am. Oil Chemists' Soc.* 41:662–667.

Gunstone, F. D. 1958. *The Chemistry of Fats and Fatty Acids*. New York: Wiley.

Gunstone, F. D., and Wijesundera, R. C. 1979. Fatty acids, part 54. Some reactions of long-chain oxygenated acids with special reference to those furnishing furanoid acids. *Chem. Phys. Lipids* 24:193–208.

Gunstone, F. D., Wijesundera, R. C., Love, R. M., and Ross, D. 1976. Relative enrichment of furan-containing fatty acids in the liver of starving cod. *J. Chem. Soc. Chem. Commun.* 1976:630–631.

Gunstone, F. D., Chaska, R., Wijesundera, R. C., and Scrimgeour, C. M. 1978. The compo-nent acids of lipids from marine and freshwater species with special reference to furan-containing acids. *J. Sci. Food Agric.* 29:539–550.

Hanahan, D. J. 1960. *Lipid Chemistry.* New York: Wiley.

Hannemann, K., Puchta, V., Simon, E., Ziegler, H., Ziegler, G., and Spiteller, G. 1989. The common occurrence of furan fatty acids in plants. *Lipids* 24(4):296–298.

Hashimoto, T., Nukada, K., Shina, H., and Tsuchiya, T. 1963. On the structure of highly unsaturated fatty acids of fish oils by high resolution nuclear magnetic resonance spectral analysis. *J. Am. Oil Chemists' Soc.* 40:124–128.

Hasma, H., and Subramaniam, A. 1978. The occurrence of a furanoid fatty acid in *Hevea brasiliensis* latex. *Lipids* 13(12):905–907.

Henderson, R. J., and Tocher, D. R. 1987. The lipid composition and biochemistry of freshwater fish. In *Progress in Lipid Research,* ed. R. T. Holman, W. W. Christie, and H. Sprecher, pp. 281–347, esp. p. 294. New York: Pergamon Press.

Hilditch, T. P., and Williams, P. N. 1964. *The Chemical Constitution of Natural Fats,* 4th ed. New York: Wiley.

Ishii, K., Okajima, H., Koyamatsu, T., Okada, Y., and Watanabe, H. 1988A. The composi-tion of furan fatty acids in the crayfish. *Lipids* 23(7):694–700.

Ishii, K., Okajima, H., Okada, Y., and Watanabe, H. 1988B. Studies on furan fatty acids of salmon roe phospholipids. *J. Biochem.* 103:836–839.

Jacini, G. 1986. Furanoid fatty acids and lipids. *Fette, Seifen, Anstrichm.* 88(8):290–292.

Jandke, J., Schmidt, J., and Spiteller, G. 1988. The behavior of F acids in the oxidation with lipoxidase in the presence of SH-containing compounds (in German). *Liebigs Ann. Chem.* 1988:29–34.

Joseph, J. D. 1985. Fatty acid composition of commercial menhaden (*Brevoortia* spp.) oils: 1982 and 1983. *Marine Fisheries Rev.* 47(3):30–37.

Kayama, M., Tsuchiya, Y., and Mead, J. F. 1963A. A model experiment of aquatic food chain with special significance in fatty acid conversion. *Bull. Japan. Soc. Sci. Fish.* 29:452–458.

Kayama, M., Tsuchiya, Y., Nevenzel, J. C., Fulco, A., and Mead, J. F. 1963B. Incorpora-tion of linolenic-1-C^{14} acid into eicosapentaeonoic and docosahexaenoic acids in fish. *J. Am. Oil Chemists' Soc.* 40:499–502.

Kelly, P. B., Reiser, R., and Hood, D. 1958A. The origin and metabolism of marine fatty acids: The effect of diet on the depot fats of *Mugil cephalus* (the common mullet). *J. Am. Oil Chemists' Soc.* 35:189–192.

Kelly, P. B., Reiser, R., and Hood, D. W. 1985B. The effect of diet on the fatty acid composition of several species of fresh water fish. *J. Am. Oil Chemists' Soc.* 35:503–505.

Kelly, P. B., Reiser, R., and Hood, D. W. 1959. The origin of the marine polyunsaturated fatty acids. Composition of some marine plankton. *J. Am. Oil Chemists' Soc.* 36:104–106.

Klenk, E. 1958. The polyenoic acids of fish oils. In *Essential Fatty Acids,* ed. H. M. Sinclair. New York: Academic Press.

Klenk, E., and Brockerhoff, H. 1957. The occurrence of 6,9,12,15-octadecatetraenoic acid in herring oil and its isolation. *Z. Physiol. Chem.* 307:272–277.

Klenk, E., and Brockerhoff, H. 1958. The C_{18}- and C_{22}-polyenoic acids in herring oil. *Z. Physiol. Chem.* 310:153–170.

Klenk, E., and Eberhagen, D. 1962A. About the composition of the fatty acid mixture of various fish oils. *Z. Physiol. Chem.* 328:180–188.

Klenk, E., and Eberhagen, D. 1962B. Unsaturated C_{16} fatty acids of marine plankton and the occurrence of Δ 6,9,12,15-hexacatetraenoic acid. *Z. Physiol. Chem.* 328:189–197.

Knoop, F. 1904. Degradation of aromatic fatty acids in animals (in German). *Beitr. Chem. Phys. Path.* 6:150–162.

Lewis, R. W. 1962. Temperature and pressure effects on the fatty acids of some marine ectotherms. *Comp. Biochem. Physiol.* 6:75–89.

Lewkowitsch, J. 1914. *Chemical Technology and Analysis of Oils, Fats, Wares,* 5th ed., vol. 2, pp. 405–472. London: Macmillan and Co.

Lie Ken Jie, M. S. F. 1981. Chemical synthesis of furanoid fatty acids. In *Methods in Enzymology,* vol. 72, ed. J. M. Lowenstein, pp. 443–471. New York: Academic Press.

Lie Ken Jie, M. S. F., and Sinha, S. 1981. Fatty acid composition and the characterization of a novel dioxo C_{18}-fatty acid in the latex of *Hevea brasiliensis. Phytochemistry* 20(8):1863–1866.

Lovern, J. A. 1942. The composition of the depot fats of aquatic animals. Food Investigation Special Report 51, Dept. Scientific and Industrial Research, H. M. London: Stationary Office, York House, Kingsway.

Lovern, J. A. 1962. The lipids of fish and changes occurring in them during processing and storage. In *Fish in Nutrition,* ed. E. Heen and R. Kreuzer. London: Fishing News Ltd.

Lovern, J. A. 1964. The lipids of marine organisms. *Oceanogr. Mar. Biol. Ann. Rev.* 2:169–191.

Matic, M. 1958. South African pilchard oil. 7. The isolation and structure of an octadecate-traenoic acid from South African pilchard oil. *Biochem. J.* 68:692–695.

Mead, J. F., Kayama, M., and Reiser, R. 1960. Biogenesis of polyunsaturated acids in fish. *J. Am. Oil Chemists' Soc.* 37:438–440.

Menzel, D. B., and Olcott, H. S. 1964. Positional distribution of fatty acids in fish and other animal lecithins. *Biochim. Biophys. Acta* 84:133–139.

Mohrhauer, H., and Holman, R. T. 1963. Effects of linolenic acid upon the metabolism of linoleic acid. *J. Nutrition* 81:67–74.

Morice, I. M., and Shorland, F. B. 1952. The isolation from shark (*Galeorhinus australis*) liver oil of a multi-branched C_{18} saturated fatty acid fraction. *Chem. Ind. (London)* 52:1267–1268.

Morice, I. M., and Shorland, F. B. 1956. The isolation of iso- and (+)-anteiso-fatty acids of the C_{15} and C_{17} series from shark (*Galeorhinus australis*) liver oil. *Biochem. J.* 64:461–464.

Morris, L. J., Marshall, M. O., and Kelly, W. 1966. A unique furanoid fatty acid from *Exocarpus* seed oil. *Tetrahedron Lett.* 36:4249–4253.

Okajima, H., Ishii, K., and Watanabe, H. 1984. Studies on lipids of crayfish, *Procambarus clarkii.* I. Furanoid fatty acids. *Chem. Pharm. Bull.* 32(8):3281–3286.

Ota, T., and Takagi, T. 1983. Furan fatty acids in the lipids of kokanee, *Oncorhynchus nerka f. adonis. Bull. Fac. Fish. Hokkaido Univ.* 34(2):88–92.

Pfordt, J., Thoma, H., and Spiteller, G. 1981. Identification, structure elucidation, and synthesis of previously unknown urofuranic acids in human blood (in German). *Liebigs Ann. Chem.* 1981:2298–2308.

Privett, O. S. 1956. Determination of structure and analysis of highly unsaturated and saturated acids of fish oils. *Annual Reprt. Hormel Inst.* 1955–1956:59–61.

Puchta, V., and Spiteller, G. 1988. Structure of F-acid-containing plasmalipids (in German). *Liebigs Ann. Chem.* 1988:1145–1147.

Puchta, V., Spiteller, G., and Weidinger, H. 1988. F acids: A new component of the phospholipids of human blood (in German). *Liebigs Ann. Chem.* 1988:25–28.

Rahn, C. H., Sand, D. M., Krick, T. P., Glass, R. L., and Schlenk, H. 1981. Syntheses of radioactive furan fatty acids. *Lipids* 16(5):360–364.

Rahn, C. H., Sand, D. M., Wedmid, Y., Schlenk, H., Krick, T. P., and Glass, R. L. 1979. Synthesis of naturally occurring furan fatty acids. *J. Org. Chem.* 44:3420–3424.

Reiser, R., Stevenson, B., Kayama, M., Choudhury, R. B. R., and Hood, D. W. 1963. The influence of dietary fatty acids and environmental temperature on the fatty acid composition of teleost fish. *J. Am. Oil Chemists' Soc.* 40:507–513.

Rodegker, W., and Nevenzel, J. C. 1964. The fatty acid composition of three marine invertebrates. *Comp. Biochem. Physiol.* 11:53–60.

Sand, D. M., Glass, R. L., Olson, D. L., Pike, H. M., and Schlenk, H. 1984. Metabolism of furan fatty acids in fish. *Biochim. Biophys. Acta.* 793:429–434.

Sand, D. M., Schlenk, H., Thoma, H., and Spiteller, G. 1983. Catabolism of fish furan fatty acids to urofuran acids in the rat. *Biochim. Biophys. Acta* 751:455–461.

Schoedel, R., Dietel, P., and Spiteller, G. 1986. F-acids—precursors of urofuranic acids. *Liebigs Ann. Chem.* 1986:127–131.

Schoedel, R., and Spiteller, G. 1985. Structure elucidation of (hydroxy-oxo-cyclopentenyl) alkanoic acids, the aldol-condensation products of dioxoene acids from cattle liver (in German). *Helv. Chim. Acta* 68:1624–1634.

Schoedel, R., and Spiteller, G. 1987. On the occurrence of F acids in cattle liver and their enzymatic degradation during tissue damage (in German). *Liebigs Ann. Chem.* 1987:459–462.

Schuster, C. V., Froines, J. R., and Olcott, H. S. 1964. Phospholipids of tuna white muscle. *J. Am. Oil Chemists' Soc.* 41:36–41.

Scrimgeour, C. M. 1977. Quantitative analysis of furanoid fatty acids in crude and refined cod liver oil. *J. Am. Oil Chemists' Soc.* 54:210–211.

Sen, N., and Schlenk, H. 1964. The structure of polyenoic odd- and even-numbered fatty acids of mullet (*Mugil cehalus*). *J. Am. Oil Chemists' Soc.* 41:241–247.

Silk, M. H., and Hahn, H. H. 1954. South African pilchard oil. 4. The isolation and structure of a hexadecatetraenoic acid from South African pilchard oil. *Biochem. J.* 57:582–587.

Skoda, J., Ernest, I., Stanek, J., and Habermann, V. 1961. The relationship between structure and antibacterial effect of unsaturated δ-diketones. *Coll. Czech. Chem. Commun.* 26:874–880.

Spiteller, G. 1987. Furanoid fatty acids (in German). *Nachr. Chem. Tech. Lab.* 35:1241–1243.

Spiteller, M., Spiteller, G., and Hoyer, G. A. 1980. Urofuranic acids—a hitherto unknown class of metabolic compounds (in German). *Chem. Ber.* 113:699–709.

Stansby, M. E. 1952. Refractive index of free oil in canned salmon—Technical Note #17. Commercial Fisheries Review 14(2):31–33.

Stansby, M. E. 1967. *Fish Oils.* Westport, Conn.: Avi Publishing Co.

Stansby, M. E. 1981. Reliability of fatty acid values purporting to represent composition of oil from different species of fish. *J. Am. Oil Chemists' Soc.* 58:13–16.

Stansby, M. E. 1986. Fatty acids in fish. In *Health Effects of Polyunsaturated Fatty Acids in Seafoods*, ed. A. P. Simopolous, R. R. Kifer, and R. E. Martin, pp. 389–411. Orlando, Fla.: Academic Press.

Stansby, M. E., and Lemon, J. M. 1941. *Studies on the Handling of Mackerel.* Washington, D. C.: U.S. Department of Interior, Fish and Wildlife Service, Research Report #1.

Swain, L. A. 1953. Fatty acid composition of fish oils. III. Sockeye salmon offal oil. *Fisheries Res. Board Can. Progr. Repts. Pacific Coast Stats.,* 94:24–26.

Toyama, Y., Iwata, Y., and Fujimura, K. 1959. On the occurrence of eicosatetraenoic, docosapentaenoic and docosahexaenoic acids in fish oils. *Fette-Seifen-Anstrichmittel* 61:846–849.

Toyomizu, M., Kawasaki, K., and Tomiyasu, Y. 1963. Effect of dietary oil on the fatty acid composition of rainbow trout oil. *Bull. Japan. Soc. Sci. Fish.* 29:957–961.

Whitcutt, J. M. 1957. South African pilchard oil. 6. The isolation and structure of a docosahexaenoic acid from South African pilchard oil. *Biochem. J.* 67:60–64.

Whitcutt, J. M., and Sutton, D. A. 1956. South African pilchard oil. 5. The isolation and structure of an eicosapentaenoic acid from South African pilchard oil. *Biochem. J.* 63:469–475.

Yoshioka, M. 1981. The occurrence and distribution of furan fatty acids in marine organisms. *Kagaku Kenkyusho Kenkyu Hokoku* 14:10–13.

Chapter 3
THE ANALYSIS OF MARINE FATTY ACIDS

Jeanne D. Joseph and Gloria T. Seaborn

INTRODUCTION

Since Stansby edited an extraordinarily informative book on fish oils (Stansby 1967), major technological advances have been made in the analysis of marine fatty acids, particularly in gas-liquid chromatographic (GLC) technology. These advances include the development of sensitive flame ionization detectors and stable polar liquid phases such as the cyanosilicones. Among other improvements, bonded Carbowax-20M has replaced polyester liquid phases of lower polarity such as butanediol succinate (BDS). Most important of all, perhaps, are recent developments in wall-coated open-tubular (WCOT or capillary) columns. These GLC columns, generally 10–60 m in length and 0.25–0.32 mn in internal diameter, contain the liquid phase deposited in a thin film on the interior wall of the column. Initially, many of these columns were fabricated from stainless steel and, originally, stock columns were available commercially from the Perkin-Elmer Corp. (Norwalk, Connecticut) in a length of 47 m with 0.25 mm internal diameter. However, substantial losses of long-chain polyunsaturated fatty acids (PUFA), such as are prominent in marine fish oils, were commonly observed in these columns, particularly when the carrier gas contained traces of oxygen. This required additional work for the analyst in determining and applying empirically derived "column correction factors" (Ackman et al. 1967; Ackman and Eaton 1978). The next step in the evolution of the modern WCOT column was fabrication of the column from glass and, finally, the development of the flexible fused silica column, coated externally with a polyamide to prevent scratching and crystallization of the column wall and coated internally with cross-linked (or "bonded") liquid phases, especially polyglycols. These columns will be discussed in somewhat more detail below.

Although high-performance liquid chromatography (HPLC) is perhaps the most rapidly growing technology in lipid analysis, its application to *analytical* separation of fatty acids or esters has been limited. In fact, Aitzetmuller (1982) suggests that since most fatty acids and esters can be easily analyzed by GLC, that technology is, perhaps, superior to HPLC for these classes of lipids. Nevertheless, Ozcimder and Hammers (1980) explored the utility of argentation/HPLC and reverse phase/HPLC in the fractionation of fish oil fatty acid methyl esters (FAME). Christie et al. (1988) used argentation/HPLC in the isolation of FAME, according to their degree of unsaturation, from molluscan lipids. The fractions were then further separated and identified by gas chromatography/mass spectrometry (GC/MS).

It is not the objective of this chapter to present detailed descriptions of equipment or procedures, nor to conduct a critical evaluation of the pertinent literature. Our goal is to provide an overview of the most important elements of marine fatty acid analysis along with references that provide the details omitted herein. Methods and procedures described in this chapter are equally applicable to the lipids of most human and animal tissues.

FATTY ACID NOMENCLATURE

The nomenclature employed in this chapter for monoenoic and methylene-interrupted PUFA and esters has been suggested by the IUPAC-IUB Commission on Biochemical Nomenclature (1977) as a replacement of the "ωx" (omega) system, used extensively for many years. The only difference in the two systems is that the end-carbon chain designation is "n-x" in the recommended nomenclature, that is, $18:2n$-6 rather than $18:2\omega 6$, for example. Both specify (1) the number of carbon atoms, (2) the number of double bonds, and (3) the position of the terminal double bond relative to the nonpolar end of the molecule. Either system is appropriate in discussions of fatty acid biosynthesis by chain elongation and desaturation since, in this process, the end-carbon chain length is unchanged. Both systems also provide the basis for semilogarithmic plotting techniques and calculations of equivalent chain length (ECL) values that are widely used in the identification of FAME separated by GLC.

For those unsaturated FAMEs having non-methylene-interrupted double-bond systems, the number of carbon atoms in the chain and the number of double bonds are followed by the symbol Δ and the positions of the double bonds, relative to the carboxyl group of the molecule. Non-methylene-interrupted dienes (NMID), with chain lengths of 20 and 22 carbons, are common and prominent in sponges (Joseph 1979), oysters and clams (Joseph 1982), and some echinoderms (Takagi et al. 1980).

LIPID EXTRACTION

Lipids may be extracted from marine organisms through a variety of procedures. One of the oldest, and one that is still acceptable, is the method of Folch et al. (1957). Another method, that of Bligh and Dyer (1959), was developed specifically for extraction of low-fat fish such as cod (*Gadus morhua*) and has been widely used since its publication. This method has been used routinely at the Charleston Laboratory, but with the total volumes of solvents adjusted to suit the anticipated (if unknown) fat content of the tissue. The tissue to be extracted is first frozen, then cut into small chunks or slices, and then comminuted in a domestic food processor. It is important that the tissue remain frozen during this preparation. A Virtis[1] homogenizer is used to blend the solvent with the finely macerated sample using the proportions of solvents ($CHCl_3$, CH_3OH, and H_2O) called for in the Bligh and Dyer method. Lipids of some materials are more easily extracted if a filter aid such as Celite 545 AW (Supelco, Inc.), or equivalent product, is added prior to homogenization; oyster tissues and fish roe are two examples. After homogenization and lipid extraction, the mixture is filtered through a Buchner funnel and centrifuged to effect phase separation. The $CHCl_3$ phase is recovered, dried over anhydrous Na_2SO_4, and reduced in volume to less than 10 ml using a rotary evaporator. This residual $CHCl_3$, containing the lipids, is transferred to a 10-ml volumetric flask and made to volume with $CHCl_3$. The lipid content of aliquots of this solution may be determined gravimetrically.

It should be noted that H_2O is an important component of the Bligh and Dyer (1959) monophasic solvent system. If lyophilized tissues are to be extracted, it is necessary to add the appropriate quantity of water before extraction.

We, and others, have observed that the Bligh and Dyer (1959) method is not suitable for recovering all of the lipids from fish that have been subjected to frozen storage over long periods of time, such as in storage studies. Hardy et al. (1979) observed a decrease in phospholipid content of cod (*Gadus morhua*), freezer-stored for 200 days. This was accompanied by an increase in free fatty acids, but this fraction was lost in the upper CH_3OH/H_2O phase when the lipids were extracted by the original Bligh and Dyer method. This fraction could be recovered if a monophasic extraction procedure was used. In a number of freezer storage studies carried out on underutilized species of fish at the Charleston Laboratory,

---

[1]The use of trade names, commercial firms, or specific products is for identification purposes only and does not constitute endorsement by the National Marine Fisheries Service.

we found it impossible to effect complete separation of the two phases even after prolonged centrifugation (Joseph and Seaborn 1982). If the cloudy upper phase was removed and discarded, the lower $CHCl_3$ phase contained less lipid than did extracts from control samples. This difficulty was overcome by extraction of lipids using a solution of hexane and isopropanol (3 : 2, v : v) (Hara and Radin 1978; Radin 1981).

LIPID CLASS ISOLATION

In some studies it may be desirable or necessary to separate the total lipids into their component classes before fatty acid analysis, depending on the purpose of the study. Additionally, it is good practice to purify methyl esters before GLC analysis. Both tasks are easily accomplished by preparative thin-layer chromatography (TLC) on silica gel, although HPLC has also been used. For best results, commercial plates with a preadsorbant spotting/streaking zone at the bottom of the plate should be used, since this band concentrates the diffuse sample spots applied to the plate into narrow bands. A TLC sample streaker is convenient for sample application on these plates and essential for critical separations on standard analytical plates. After development, a nondestructive indicator spray such as 2',7'-dichlorofluorescein should be used to locate the bands of the separated lipid classes. Mangold's chapter (1969) in *Thin Layer Chromatography. A Laboratory Handbook,* edited by Stahl (1969), contains a wealth of information on TLC of lipids.

GLC INSTRUMENTATION

All modern GLC equipment suitable for WCOT analysis of FAME includes a column oven with plumbing for regulation and delivery of carrier gas; a flame ionization detector (FID) and ancillary supply lines for air, hydrogen, and makeup gas if detector design requires it; an injection port allowing split or splitless injection; and an electronic integrator. Controls for setting isothermal temperatures, temperature programming rates, times, and other parameters may be located on the oven module or the integrator chassis. For laboratories analyzing large numbers of samples on a routine basis, an autosampler might be considered a necessity since this allows the equipment to be kept in operation around the clock.

Two critically important elements of the gas chromatograph are the injection port and the detector, since poor design or improper operation of these components will impact severely on sample quantitation. A third factor of importance is the polarity of the column liquid phase.

Injection Port

Marine FAME are frequently analyzed using a heated injection port in the split mode, but care must be taken that there is no chain length discrimination in the port. Freeman (1981) has presented a number of suggestions for optimizing the inlet system so as to minimize splitter discrimination. Splitless injection is also used but requires very dilute samples to avoid column or detector overload. On-column injection of the sample through a cold injection port into a cold column is also a suitable technique for marine FAME. With this technique, elution of analytes only begins after initiation of a column temperature program. Traitler (1987) has noted that, when using this technique, discrimination of low-volatility compounds is much less pronounced than in heated port systems, and it gives accurate quantitation over a wide range of molecular weights. Injection port discrimination can be evaluated by analysis of a quantitative saturated hydrocarbon mixture, C19 to C40 in chain length, since no detector correction factors are required for hydrocarbons and the area percentages of the component peaks are equal to the weight percentages (Perkins et al. 1963).

Detectors

Flame ionization detectors are almost universally used for the analysis of FAME. These detectors require an optimized flow of gases in order to operate correctly, and generally, the low flow of the carrier gas (high purity helium or hydrogen) through a WCOT column must be supplemented by a makeup gas, usually less expensive nitrogen. For optimum performance, dead volume in the detector must be kept to a minimum. This is achieved by inserting the outlet of the column through the detector jet so that the effluent from the column is swept into the flame directly from the column by the hydrogen that feeds the flame.

Since the introduction and evolution of capillary columns, GC/MS has developed to the degree that the MS, itself, may be considered a very specific detector (Traitler 1987). The low flow rates, typical of capillary columns, permit direct connection to the ion source chamber of the mass spectrometer, eliminating the need for the interfacing devices required for packed GLC columns. This detector may be operated in "scan" mode, detecting all components in the sample, to produce a total ion chromatogram (TIC). Alternatively, only selected ions may be monitored (SIM mode), dramatically increasing the sensitivity for these ions. This mode of operation is particularly useful for obtaining structural evidence for the identification of minor components and to distinguish coeluting components.

Column Polarity

The importance of the polarity of the column liquid phase cannot be overemphasized in marine FAME analyses. Unlike vegetable oils that contain, at most, 15–20 different fatty acids, it is not uncommon to find 60–80 or more fatty acids in a marine oil. Consequently, the problem of even-carbon chain length overlap, discussed a number of years ago by Ackman (1967) with regard to packed columns, may create difficulties both in FAME identification and single-component quantitation. Additional discussions of this problem have been published more recently (Ackman 1986; Ackman 1987).

For a number of reasons, the most suitable column currently available for marine FAME analysis is a flexible fused silica WCOT column containing a cross-linked polyglycol liquid phase based upon Carbowax-20M. Currently, several companies offer such columns: SUPELCOWAX 10 (Supelco, Inc.), DB-Wax (J & W Scientific), Superox (Alltech Associates), HP-20M (Hewlett Packard), and CP Wax-52 (Chrompack, Inc.) are examples. When used in conjunction with an oxygen scavenger in the carrier gas line, these columns exhibit excellent stability and long life. Because of the thermal stability of bonded Carbowax-20M, marine FAME may be analyzed by temperature programming to accelerate the analysis, with little baseline drift. A second advantage provided by these polyglycol columns is that the equivalent chain length (ECL) values of eluted FAME vary little from column to column or between specific commercial liquid phase formulations. This is due to the fact that this liquid phase is a single entity, polyethylene glycol with a narrow molecular weight range, rather than composites of liquid phases such as the mixed diphenyl and dimethyl siloxanes. Consequently, the polarity of Carbowax-20M based columns changes little with use over time. This is well illustrated in Tables 4.3A and 4.3B of Ackman's chapter (1986) on WCOT GLC. The footnotes to these tables show that the data have been compiled from numerous worldwide publications of research carried out over a period of approximately six years. Thus, interlaboratory comparisons of data are possible. Finally, when performance of these columns deteriorates, they may be flushed with suitable solvents to restore performance. For these reasons, a recently completed collaborative study of marine fatty acid analysis required the use of these columns (Ackman and Joseph 1989).

SYSTEM OPTIMIZATION

The importance of system optimization in yielding accurate and reliable GLC data has been addressed at length (Bannon et al. 1985, 1986; Craske and Bannon 1987, 1988). In these publications, the authors confirmed the validity of the theoretical response factors (TRF) first proposed by Ackman and Sipos (1964). The TRF can be calculated for each individual FAME and is based on the number of carbon atoms not bonded to oxygen atoms in the molecule, relative to that in 18 : 0. Craske and Bannon (1988) have recently proposed that the term *empirical correction factor* (ECF) be introduced for use when a quantitative standard is analyzed and correction factors are calculated from the results obtained. The ECFs will then include the TRFs as well as factors whose magnitude reflects the extent to which the equipment has not been optimized. These workers also note that the nature of the analysis may be such that it is not practical to optimize according to theoretical principles. The application of these correction factors is described in the section on quantitation.

PREPARATION AND ANALYSIS OF METHYL ESTERS

Generally, marine fatty acids are derivatized directly from lipids to methyl esters by transesterification before their analysis by GLC. However, saponification followed by extraction for removal of nonsaponifiable materials before derivatization of the recovered free fatty acids may be more appropriate in some investigations. Christie (1982) has provided, in some detail, a variety of methylation procedures using both acidic and alkaline reagents, and Sheppard and Iverson (1975) have presented an excellent review of methylation procedures gleaned from published literature. More recently, Bannon et al. have reviewed methoxide-catalyzed methanolysis (1982A) and boron trifluoride (BF_3-CH_3OH) methylation (1982B). Unlike alkaline reagents, many of the acidic reagents have unwanted effects on fatty acids and other structures. In particular, acidic reagents should not be used if the presence of plasmalogens, common in bivalves (Joseph 1982), is suspected. Under acidic conditions, plasmalogens yield long-chain aldehydes that are converted to dimethyl acetals which, in turn, may be degraded to *cis* and *trans* methyl vinyl ethers in the injection port (Ackman 1972). Both dimethyl acetals and methyl vinyl ethers coelute with the FAME during GLC. Alkaline reagents must also be used for the methylation of cyclopropanoic and cyclopropenoic (Bianchini et al. 1981), and furanoid (Scrimgeour 1977) fatty acids. On the other hand, if substantial hydrolysis of the lipids has occurred, as may happen in storage stability studies, or if the free acid is the specific lipid species to be analyzed, then an acidic reagent must be used.

The appendix to this chapter describes, in detail, procedures for methylation and gas chromatographic analysis of soft-gelatin encapsulated fish oils that have been tested successfully in a collaborative study under the auspices of the Association of Official Analytical Chemists (AOAC) (Ack-

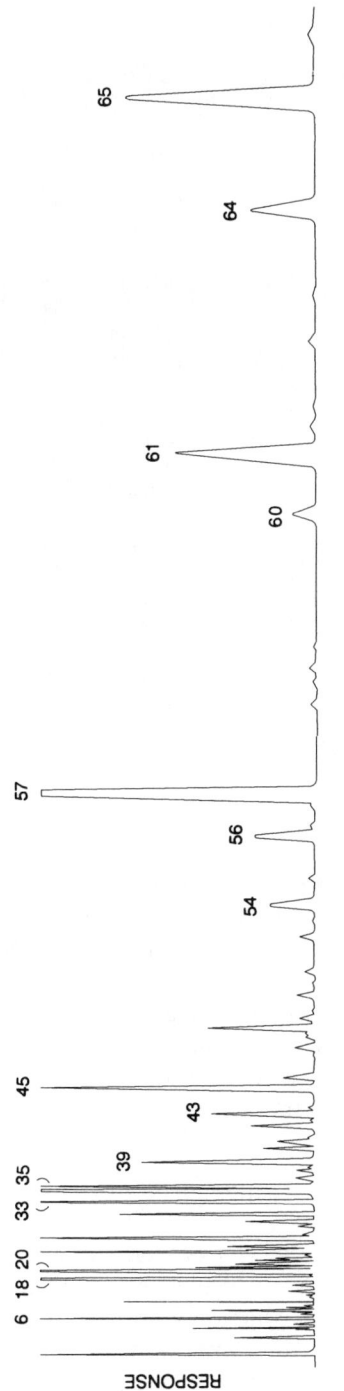

Fig. 3-1. Isothermal analysis of menhaden oil FAME on a flexible fused silica SUPELCOWAX 10 column, 30 m × 0.32 mm, at 185°C. Helium carrier gas. Figure generated from chromatogram by application of a CAD program.

Table 3-1.   Equivalent Chain Length Values from an Isothermal Analysis of Menhaden Oil FAME, Illustrated in Fig. 3-1

NO.	ECL	ID	NO.	ECL	ID	NO.	ECL	ID
1	12.00	12:0	23	16.58	16:2n-7	45	19.58	18:4n-3
2	12.45	iso 13:0	24	16.62	16:2n-6	46	19.70	18:4n-1
3	12.90	unknown	25	16.74	ai 17:0	47	20.00	20:0
4	13.03	13:0	26	16.81	16:2n-4	48	20.10	20:1n-11
5	13.45	iso 14:0	27	16.95	17:0	49	20.18	20:1n-9
6	14.00	14:0	28	17.15	16:3n-4	50	20.26	20:1n-7
7	14.15	TMTD[a]	29	17.26	16:3n-3	51	20.46	20:NMID?
8	14.25	14:1n-7	30	17.45	iso 18:0	52	20.63	20:2n-6
9	14.36	14:1n-5	31	17.56	16:4n-3	53	20.89	20:3n-6
10	14.46	iso 15:0	32	17.73	16:4n-1	54	21.10	20:4n-6
11	14.61	unknown	33	18.00	18:0	55	21.27	20:3n-3
12	14.68	ai 15:0	34	18.20	18:1n-9	56	21.53	20:4n-3
13	14.92	15:0	35	18.26	18:1n-7	57	21.76	20:5n-3
14	15.18	15:1?	36	18.38	18:1n-5	58	22.00	22:0
15	15.27	15:1?	37	18.51	18:2n-9	59	22.16	22:1n-11[b]
16	15.45	iso 16:0	38	18.56	18:2n-7	60	22.77	21:5n-3
17	15.71	unknown	39	18.64	18:2n-6	61	22.98	23:0 (IS)
18	16.00	16:0	40	18.84	18:2n-4	62	23.06	22:4n-6
19	16.12	16:1n-11?	41	18.93	18:3n-6?	63	23.32	22:5n-6
20	16.26	16:1n-7	42	19.13	18:3n-4	64	23.69	22:5n-3
21	16.36	16:n-5	43	19.27	18:3n-3	65	23.96	22:6n-3
22	16.47	iso 17:0	44	19.36	unknown	66	24.00	24:0

[a]Trimethyltridecanoate.
[b]Includes the n-13 isomer.

man and Joseph 1989). These procedures have been used in the Canadian Institute of Fisheries Technology of the Technical University of Nova Scotia and the Charlestown Laboratory of the National Marine Fisheries Service for some extended periods of time. In addition to the instructions, participants in the study were provided an annotated chromatogram similar to that shown in Fig. 3-1, since a number of them were inexperienced in marine fatty acid analysis. Table 3-1 lists the ECL values and provisional identities of the component peaks in Fig. 3-1.

FATTY ACID IDENTIFICATION PROCEDURES

The numerous components typically obtained in high-resolution GLC analysis of marine FAME provide a challenge to the chromatographer in assigning identities. Techniques commonly utilized for FAME identification are retention time comparisons with known primary and secondary standards, ECL value calculations, bromination, hydrogenation, argentation thin-layer chromatography ($AgNO_3$/TLC), and, more recently, GC/ MS and Fourier transform infrared spectrometry (FTIR). Nuclear magnetic resonance spectrometry (NMR) is a valuable tool, but if only minute quantities of unknown compounds are available for analysis; sufficiently sensitive instrumentation may not be readily accessible.

Comparison with Primary and Secondary Standards

Fatty acid methyl esters may be identified provisionally by comparison of their retention times with those of standards chromatographed on the same column under the same conditions. Commercially available standard mixtures are convenient for this purpose. Primary standards can include GLC Mixtures 87 and 68, available from Nu Chek Prep, Inc. (Elysian, Minnesota 52028) that contain both saturated and unsaturated FAME, ranging from 14 to 24 carbons in chain length. Spiking of the analytical sample with individual pure standards or a standard mixture and reanalysis is a more definitive approach. Comparisons should be made on two columns with liquid phases of different polarity.

Marine lipids include a large number of fatty acids for which no pure standards are available. Natural oils with well-established compositions are useful as secondary standards for these identifications. Cod-liver oil, recommended for use since it contains most of the fatty acids commonly encountered in marine lipids (Ackman and Burgher 1965), is widely utilized as a secondary standard. An excellent description of the use of the secondary standard PUFA-1 (Supelco, Inc.), in conjunction with canola oil, to identify marine FAME has been published recently (Ackman 1986).

Equivalent Chain Length Values

The linear relationship between the logarithm of retention time and the number of carbon atoms in the fatty acid chain has been accepted for many years. This relationship is the basis for the calculation of ECL values utilizing the following equation:

$$ECL_x = 2[(\log R_x - \log R_n)/(\log R_{n+2} - \log R_n)] + n$$

where R_x, R_n, and R_{n+2} are the retention times of the unknown ester and of the saturated esters of chain lengths n and $n + 2$, respectively (Jamieson 1970). Extensive tables of ECL values have been published (Jamieson 1970; Ackman 1984, 1986).

Equivalent chain length values of the commonly occurring unsaturated FAME consist of a cardinal even number, generally 14 to 24, corresponding to the saturated FAME whose retention times are used to calculate ECLs of the unsaturated FAME, and a decimal value, 0.01 to 1.99, known as the fractional chain length (FCL) value. Unsaturated FAME of different chain lengths with the same number of double bonds located in the same position in the molecule with respect to the end-carbon chain have very similar FCLs. The FCLs of unsaturated FAME of known structure can thus be used to tentatively identify unknown peaks of other chain lengths in the chromatogram.

Jamieson (1975) found that the ECL of 18:3n-3 gives a measure of the polarity of the column on which it is analyzed. He selected this FAME as the reference ester because: (1) it is readily available in high purity to give reliable retention data; (2) it is present in most FAME mixtures of biological origin; and (3) its ECL value shows acceptable changes with differences in liquid phase polarity. Using published data combined with data generated in his laboratory, Jamieson constructed graphs of the ECLs of the various FAME esters, plotted against the ECL values of 18:3n-3 in each of the analyses. A linear relationship with little data scatter was observed. The equation for this relationship was found to be:

$$ECL_x = a_x(ECL_{18:3n-3}) + b_x$$

where a_x and b_x are computer-derived constants for $FAME_x$. Using this equation, tables of ECL values for methylene-interrupted FAME corresponding to $ECL_{18:3n-3}$ values from 18.50 to 21.00, in increments of 0.01, were generated by computer. Jamieson suggests that these tables are useful for: (1) provisional identification of methylene-interrupted FAME using retention data from any polyester column operating in the normal temperature range; (2) prediction of the best column for a specific separation; (3) tentative identification of FAME of unusual structure; and (4) determination of the degree of unsaturation of unusual FAME using the slope value, a_x.

Ackman (1984) has emphasized that the chromatographic behavior of a methyl ester on one or several liquid phases is not ultimate proof of its identity. Complimentary spectrometric techniques such as ultraviolet (UV), infrared (IR), NMR, and MS are suggested. In addition, a variety of ancillary chemical and chromatographic procedures are frequently used (*vide infra*).

Gas chromatography coupled with MS is recommended as the method of choice for the identification of methyl esters in complex mixtures such as those encountered in marine lipids. With technological advances in instrumentation and resulting cost reductions, the use of GC/MS for FAME analysis has become more common.

Mass spectra found in the literature are commonly those of fatty acids analyzed as their methyl esters (Odham and Stenhagen 1972). Although much structural information may be gained from the analysis of methyl esters, geometric and positional isomers are not distinguished. Pyrrolidide (Andersson et al. 1975; Shukla et al. 1980), picolinyl (Christie et al. 1986, 1987), and oxazoline (Yu et al. 1989) derivatives have been suggested for double bond or methyl branch (Andersson and Holman 1975) location. However, the additional mass of such derivatives degrades the GLC resolution relative to that of FAME.

Recently, instruments have been developed that combine the techniques of GC, MS, and FTIR. These allow simultaneous MS and IR analysis of the individual fatty acid derivatives separated by GLC. Computer software compares spectra from the two analyses with those of known compounds stored in a computer library to predict identities of the separated components.

ANCILLARY IDENTIFICATION METHODS

For those lacking sophisticated spectrometric instruments described in the previous section, a number of ancillary methods are available, which, when used in conjunction with GLC, will strengthen a provisional identification. Some of these methods are also useful for isolation of unknown FAME for more rigorous structural identification by IR and NMR.

Bromination

Bromination is a simple way of distinguishing between saturated and unsaturated FAME (Walker 1975). A portion of the FAME sample may be streaked on a silica gel plate along with a saturated FAME standard and developed in a solvent containing a few drops of Br_2. After development of the plate and visualization with 2',7'-dichlorofluorescein under UV light, the saturated FAME band is scraped from the plate, eluted from the silica gel, and analyzed by GLC. Reaction with Br_2 produces nonvolatile bromo-derivatives of unsaturated FAME; the GLC analysis reveals only the saturated components originally present in the sample.

This is a particularly useful technique in marine FAME analysis because the numerous C16 PUFA can obscure the presence of *iso-* and *anteiso-*17 : 0. Depending on the column liquid phase, the esters of pristanic and phytanic acids may also be more easily identified and quantitated.

Hydrogenation

After GLC analysis, the FAME may be completely hydrogenated over platinum catalyst and reanalyzed; only saturated fatty acids are observed in the second analysis. The sums of the saturated and unsaturated components for each chain length in the unhydrogenated sample should agree closely with amounts of the saturates in the hydrogenated sample if proper identities have been assigned. If there is substantial disagreement, an error in identification has been made *or* losses of polyunsaturates have occurred, either in the column during analysis of the unhydrogenated sample (Ackman et al. 1967; Ackman and Eaton 1978) or during sample manipulation. Thus, sample hydrogenation can also be a valuable aid in system optimization. In addition, like bromination, this technique frequently reveals minor saturated branched-chain components that coelute with, or are obscured by, unsaturated components.

Hydrogenation is easily carried out in the laboratory and requires no specialized equipment. About 4 ml CH_3OH is added to a screw-capped culture tube containing about 25 mg of sample that has been freed of solvent under a flow of nitrogen. Approximately 30 mg of Adam's catalyst (PtO_2) is added and hydrogen that has passed through a CaO column is bubbled through a glass capillary tube into the solution. The reaction is completed in about 15 min at 37°C. The solution is then filtered through a Pasteur pipette containing a plug of glass wool. The hydrogenated esters are transferred to hexane, concentrated in a stream of nitrogen if necessary, and analyzed by GLC.

Argentation Thin-Layer Chromatography of *Cis* FAME

Since its introduction (Morris 1962), $AgNO_3$/TLC has been a valuable technique for the lipid analyst. The FAME are separated on $AgNO_3$-impregnated silica gel-coated TLC plates. The separation is based, primarily, on degree of FAME unsaturation. Recovered fractions are then analyzed by GLC. Although $AgNO_3$-impregnated silica gel plates are commercially available, the best separations are usually obtained on commercial plates freshly impregnated in the laboratory. Improved manufacturing techniques have provided "hard" coatings that are well bonded to the glass surface. These plates may be submerged in a solution of $AgNO_3$ in acetonitrile for impregnation without damage to the analytical layer. At the Charleston Laboratory, the best separations have been achieved using plates with a preadsorbent streaking/spotting zone at the bottom of the plate. The applied sample moves with the solvent front through this zone and is concentrated into a narrow band just below the analytical layer, resulting in less band diffusion and improved separations. Chromatograms of FAME bands from a typical AgNO₃/TLC separation are shown in Fig. 3-2. In this analysis, the TLC plate, with preadsorbent spotting area, was submerged for 30 min in a solution of 10% $AgNO_3$ in acetonitrile. After drying, the plate was streaked with the sample and developed full length in benzene/hexane (1 : 1, v : v), followed by full-length development in hexane/diethyl ether (peroxide-free)/acetic acid (90 : 10 : 1, v : v : v). The separated bands were visualized by spraying the plate with 2′,7′-dichlorofluorescein and viewing under long-wave UV light. The bands were scraped from the plate and the FAME extracted from the silica gel with hexane followed by $CHCl_3$. The FAME eluted from each of the bands were analyzed and their chromatograms compared with that of the original sample as an aid in identification.

Due to the bonding between Ag^+ and double bonds (Morris 1966), saturated FAME are the more mobile compounds, and polyunsaturates the least. In interpretation of results, however, care must be taken if more than one positional isomer (20 : 4n-6 and 20 : 4n-3, for example) is present in the sample since the end-carbon chain length affects the mobility. In addition, FAME of longer chain length (22 : 1) are more mobile than those of shorter chain length (18 : 1).

While AgNO₃/TLC is usually carried out on FAME, separations have also been carried out on methoxy-bromomercuri- (MBM) adducts of fatty acids. These adducts were derived from partially hydrogenated menhaden oil (PHMO) (Sebedio and Ackman 1981) and depot fat of cynomolgus monkeys fed a diet containing a partially hydrogenated herring oil (Sebedio et al. 1982). In the in-depth investigation of the fatty acid composition of PHMO (Sebedio and Ackman 1981), a clean AgNO₃/TLC separation of FAME could not be achieved due to the complexity of the matrix. This separation was successful with the MBM adducts because, unlike FAME, the geometry of the double bonds in MBM adducts does not influence their migration. As an added benefit, the double bonds of MBM adducts are not attacked by oxygen, a distinct advantage in the analysis of highly unsaturated fatty acids. Additionally, regeneration of FAME from MBM adducts is easy and complete.

Urea Adduction

Branch-chained, cyclic, and unsaturated FAME or nonesterified acids may be concentrated by urea crystallization. When a hot solution of urea, alcohol, and FAME is cooled to 5°–0°C, the urea crystallizes as a hexagonal crystal with a central channel sufficiently large to accommodate

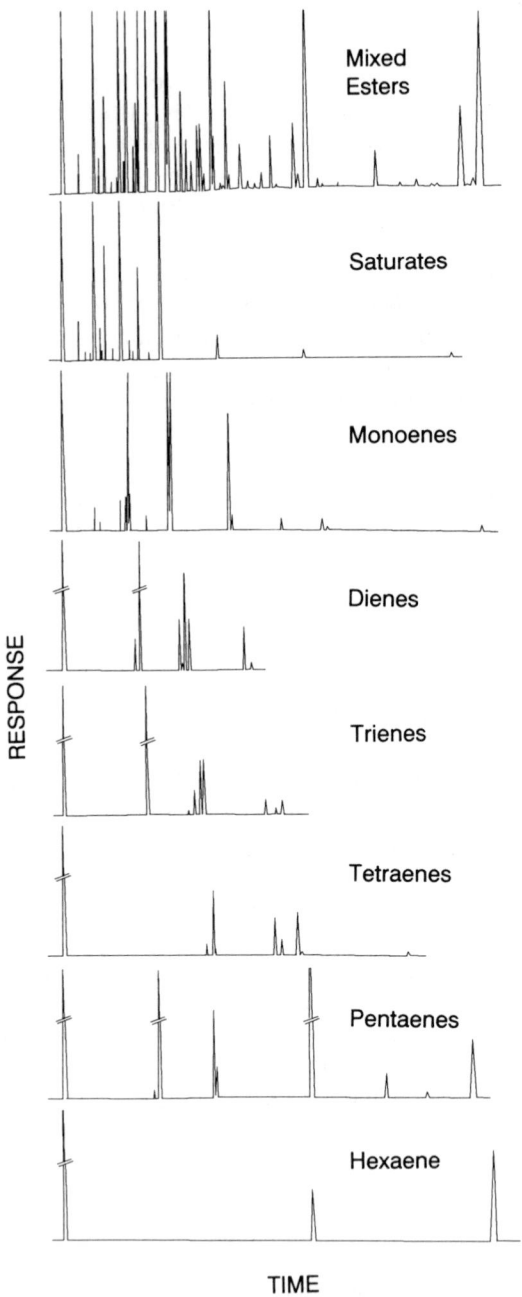

Fig. 3-2. Separation of menhaden oil FAME by AgNO₃/TLC. Temperature-programmed GLC analysis on a Silar 5-CP WCOT column. Figure generated from chromatogram by application of a CAD program.

aliphatic chains (Schlenk 1954). While straight-chained saturated FAME and free acids, six carbons or more in chain length, are readily adducted, the presence of double bonds in the carbon chain increases the bulk of the molecule and reduces the likelihood of adduction. Monoenes are more readily complexed than dienes which, in turn, are more readily complexed than trienes. After removal of the solid urea inclusion complexes by filtration or centrifugation, polyunsaturates are concentrated in the liquor and can be extracted into hexane by addition of water. The more saturated adducted components can be recovered from the solid complex by adding dilute HCl, heating gently, and extracting the solution with hexane.

Many publications have described the application of urea adduction as both an analytical and a preparative tool in fatty acid chemistry. Reviews include those of Schlenk (1954), Swern (1964), and Privett (1968). Two interesting papers correlate fatty acid structure with the preferential order of urea complex formation (Iverson and Weik 1967; Strocchi and Bonaga, 1975). More recent publications describe application of the technique to concentrate specific fatty acids: furanoid fatty acids (Gunstone et al. 1978); isoprenoid acids (Ackman et al. 1977); cis-trans isomers (Piconneaux et al. 1985); an unusual fatty acid bearing a methyl branch and a double bond on the same carbon atom, 7-methyl-7-hexadecenoic acid (Ackman et al. 1973); and a bench scale preparation of an n-3 fatty acid concentrate from cod-liver oil (Haagsma et al. 1982).

Exploration of the published literature reveals that both FAME and nonesterified acids have served as substrates for the reaction. Either ethanol or methanol may be used as the solvent, and the weight ratio of urea to substrate has varied from about 5:1 to 23:1. For the past two years, the Charleston Laboratory has used urea adduction as one step in pilot scale production of n-3 concentrates. For each kilogram of menhaden oil ethyl esters, 2.75 kg urea and 9.85 L of 95 wt% ethanol are used. After dissolving the esters in the hot solution of urea and ethanol under nitrogen, the mixture is chilled overnight to 5°C with stirring. The solid complex is allowed to settle before the liquid phase is siphoned from the crystallizer. This process increases the percentages of ethyl eicosapentaenoate from 14% to 47% and ethyl docosahexaenoate from 10% to 25%. The procedure can be easily reduced to analytical scale.

Ozonolysis

Ozonolysis is one of the older degradative chemical methods for determining the structure of unsaturated fatty acids and esters. Ozonolysis is initiated by passing ozone through the sample, dissolved in a suitable solvent, to yield ozonides (Privett 1968; Ackman, Sebedio, and Ratnayake 1981). The ozonides are then fragmented by chemical reduction or oxidation.

Reductive Ozonolysis. During the 1960s and 1970s, Privett and his colleagues at the Hormel Institute carried out a number of investigations, focusing on reductive ozonolysis (Privett and Nickell 1962, 1966; Nickell and Privett 1966; Nickell et al. 1976). Reductive fission of the ozonides has usually been brought about by reaction with triphenylphosphine (Stein and Nicolaides 1962; Beroza and Bierl 1966) although Nickell and Privett (1966) have described pyrolysis and fission of the ozonides of $18:1n$-9, $18:2n$-6, $18:3n$-3, and $20:4n$-6 within the injection port of the GC in the presence of Lindlar catalyst. Based on the same principal of pyrolysis, a microreactor, constructed from an electric soldering gun and supplied with ozone, has been used for structure determination of monoenoic fatty acids (Johnston and Dutton 1972; Bitner et al. 1970). Nickell and Privett (1966) and Cronin and Gilbert (1973) describe structural characterization of microgram quantities of esters by reductive ozonolysis.

When a mild, though toxic, reducing agent such as triphenylphosphine is used to decompose the ozonides of monoenoic esters, the terminal (hydrocarbon) end of the molecule yields aldehydes and the proximal end, aldesters. A third product, malondialdehyde, is produced in cleavage of methylene-interrupted polyunsaturated ozonides; longer-chained dialdehydes are produced in cleavage of ozonides of non-methylene-interrupted polyunsaturates. Aldesters and dialdehydes are unstable and may not be commercially available for use as standards for GLC analysis of the reduction products. Malondialdehyde is relatively volatile and water soluble, as compared with the aldehydes and aldesters, and it is unlikely that it would be recovered quantitatively for analysis by GLC from an "open" system such as triphenylphosphine reduction. Thus, only the proximal and terminal double bonds of a PUFA can be located by reductive ozonolysis. A strong reducing agent such as $LiAlH_4$ produces alcohols and alcohol esters that may be derivatized to acetates for GLC analysis (Ackman et al. 1981).

In the absence of a hydrogenation catalyst (Lindlar catalyst), pyrolytic decomposition of ozonides can produce artifacts such as acids, hydrocarbons, and esters; these artifacts increase in amount with increasing unsaturation of the parent substrate (Nickell and Privett 1966). Privett (1966) has reviewed the employment of degradative methods, with emphasis on reductive ozonolysis, in the structural analysis of fatty acids and esters. A more recent review, primarily focused on oxidative cleavage of ozonides, also provides a useful summary on the technology of reductive ozonolysis (Ackman et al. 1981).

Oxidative Ozonolysis.   Over the past few years, Ackman and co-workers have carried out a series of studies on oxidative fission of ozonides. In oxidative cleavage, a monocarboxylic acid is formed from the terminal end of the molecule and a dicarboxylic acid from the proximal end; internal fragments of polyunsaturates also give rise to dicarboxylic acids. The simplest and most efficient procedure devised (Ackman 1977) was to carry out the ozonolysis reaction itself on monoenes in 7% BF_3-CH_3OH at room temperature, then cleave the ozonides to acids with simultaneous conversion of acids to monomethyl and dimethyl esters at 100°C. The products were analyzed by GLC. In a study of ozonolysis and oxidative fission of 18 : 2n-6, only difunctional products were investigated (Sebedio and Ackman 1978).

When the effectiveness of BCl_3-, HCl-, and BF_3-CH_3OH were examined, only BF_3-CH_3OH gave consistently good yields (98%) of the principal reaction products of 18 : 1n-9; the other two reagents gave poor yields of 45–54%. In addition, both BCl_3- and HCl-CH_3OH gave rise to chlorinated derivatives in substantial quantity (Sebedio et al. 1984).

Oxidative fission with BF_3-CH_3OH was used to define the monoethylenic fatty acid composition of depot fat lipids from cynomolgus monkeys (*Macaca fascicularis*) fed a partially hydrogenated fish oil (Sebedio et al. 1982). Both *cis* and *trans* isomers of the C18, C20, and C22 chain lengths were determined. For both isomers and all three chain lengths, double bonds were located in the Δ4 through Δ16 positions of the monoenes.

Since oxidative cleavage of polyunsaturated ozonides produces dimethyl esters from both the proximal end of the molecule and the internal fragments, the position of the proximal double bond cannot be located directly by this technology. Ratnayake and Ackman (1979) overcame this difficulty by first reducing a mixture of dienoic fatty acids of unknown structure from seaweed, *Cladophora rupestris,* with a strong reducing agent ($LiAlH_4$) prior to ozonolysis in BF_3-CH_3OH. Oxidative fission then gave three products from each isomer in the mixture: methyl esters from the terminal ends, alcohol esters from the proximal ends, and dimethyl esters from the internal fragments. The alcohol esters were recovered by TLC, silylated with HMDS-TMCS, and all three reaction products analyzed by GLC. This led to the identification of 18 : 2n-4, 18 : 2n-7, and the unusual non-methylene-interrupted diene, 18 : 2Δ5,11. Sebedio and Ackman (1983) used essentially the same technique to identify the C20 dienes in partially hydrogenated menhaden oil. The only difference in this latter investigation was that the alcohol esters were derivatized to acetates for GLC analysis.

Hydrazine Reduction

Partial hydrazine reduction of polyunsaturates is a very useful technique for locating double-bond position, particularly when used in conjunction with ozonolysis. Hydrazine is a mild reducing agent and reduces double bonds randomly without geometric or positional isomerization of the double bonds not reduced (Privett and Nickell 1966; Scholfield et al. 1969). In practice, the unsaturated acid or ester is stirred with hydrazine hydrate dissolved in an alcohol and in the presence of an oxidizing agent, generally oxygen, or even air. Ratnayake (1980) recommends that the reaction be preferably carried out on the free acid form since a weak acid is required for generation of a protonated diimide, an intermediate in the reduction reaction. The reaction may be monitored by AgNO$_3$/TLC and stopped when a substantial amount of monoenes (ideally about 50%) has been formed. The monoenes, isolated by preparative AgNO$_3$/TLC, may then be subjected to ozonolysis or WCOT GLC.

In general, the approach is to carry out a preliminary purification of the sample by AgNO$_3$/TLC followed by hydrazine reduction and GLC analysis of the fractions of interest (Napolitano et al. 1988). Occasionally, the amount of lipid available for study may not permit any preliminary ester purification. In this case, the entire ester mixture may be reduced (Ackman et al. 1974). This produces an extremely complex GLC profile that can be interpreted by calculation of FCL values for products expected from the reaction (Ackman and Hooper 1973; Ackman et al. 1974).

An excellent review of the chemistry of hydrazine reduction and its application in structure determination of a number of novel marine fatty acids is available (Ratnayake 1980).

QUANTITATION IN GLC ANALYSIS

The flame ionization detector (FID), with a high degree of sensitivity and wide linear response, is ideally suited for the detection and quantitation of FAME. Albertyn et al. (1982) reported an increase in the effective linear range of the FID when operating at hydrogen flow rates greater than that required for optimum sensitivity. The detector response is directly proportional to the number of carbon atoms not bearing oxygen atoms in the FAME molecule, and theoretical response factors (TRF) based on these "active" carbons are well documented (Craske and Bannon 1988; Bannon et al. 1986; Ackman and Sipos 1964). The newer electronic integrators replace recorders and eliminate many of the problems of accurate measurement of peak areas associated with signal attenuation.

Determination of Correction Factors

Quantitative standards are used to assess instrument performance; to provide a criterion for optimization; and, if necessary, to establish empirical correction factors. Standards should also be used to verify the linear range for the components to be analyzed. All standards, regardless of source, should be examined for purity before use, by the most stringent means available, minimally, by TLC and GLC (Einig and Ackman 1987).

The difficulty in obtaining and maintaining pure quantitative standards of PUFA has been noted (Bannon et al. 1986; Craske and Bannon 1988). For this reason, these authors suggest that the GLC system be optimized so that only TCFs need be used. When this approach is not practical, empirical response factors (ECF) should be employed. Slover and Lanza (1979) have described, in detail, the determination and use of ECFs in an 11-month investigation to characterize the complex fatty acid compositions of foods. Typical ECFs for a wide range of FAME were listed. Correction factors plotted against chain length, for different degrees of unsaturation, gave a fairly smooth curve from which ECFs for unavailable fatty acids were predicted. If this approach is taken, purity should be suspected for those standards that significantly deviate from this pattern.

Reference standards should be used to monitor sample preparation and the performance of the GLC system. The instability and cost of pure polyunsaturated standards makes them highly impractical for this purpose. A natural oil with a composition similar to the sample to be analyzed may be used. The reference oil is thoroughly analyzed immediately following the verification of the TCFs or, if necessary, the calculation of EFCs, to establish reference sample composition. This reference sample is then reanalyzed with each group of samples. Significant deviation from the originally determined reference composition is an indication of problems in either sample preparation or instrumentation. A soft-gelatin encapsulated fish oil has been employed for this purpose at the Charleston Laboratory for several years. Over the past year, for 27 analyses of this reference sample, the coefficient of variation (CV) for 20:5n-3 is 1.66% and that for 22:6n-3, 1.57%, with no trend toward increasing or decreasing values.

Relative Composition

Depending on the information desired, quantitative data may be reported as normalized area percent, normalized weight percent, or in absolute amounts per weight of sample. Normalized area percentages are obtained by dividing the individual peak areas by the total area of the chromatogram. To determine weight percent composition, the individual peak areas are first multiplied by the appropriate correction factor (TCF or ECF) to account for differences in detector response and possible losses during sample preparation or analysis. Disadvantages of these methods are: (1) all fatty acids must be chromatographed, identified, and quantified; (2) the percentages of each component is affected by the amounts of all other fatty acids present; and (3) the method does not account for artifacts or components other than fatty acids that may be present in the sample. Einig and Ackman (1987) have suggested that effective reporting of normalized data requires considerable experience and is not well suited for the measurement of a few specific components (i.e., n-3 fatty acids in marine oil dietary supplements). They recommend use of an internal standard.

Absolute Composition

Absolute composition is determined through the use of internal or external standards. Since the use of an external standard requires the establishment of a calibration curve and injection of precise amounts, this method is less reproducible than other quantitation methods. As a result, and also because of the additional disadvantages of cost and instability, external FAME standards are used only when the composition of the sample is such that there is no suitable internal standard.

The internal-standard technique has been applied successfully to many gas chromatographic analyses to determine absolute quantities of one or more of the sample components. A known amount of an appropriate internal standard is added to the sample as early in the analysis as is practical. The amount of any or all components may then be calculated by relating peak areas of the components of interest to that of the internal standard. Compensation for differences in detector response is achieved by the application of appropriate correction factors. If ECFs are to be used, standards should be analyzed in the same manner as the samples.

The internal standard should be chemically similar to the components to be measured, should not be present in the sample, and should not coelute with any other component. Odd-carbon chain saturated fatty acids, particularly $21:0$ and $23:0$, have been used as internal standards

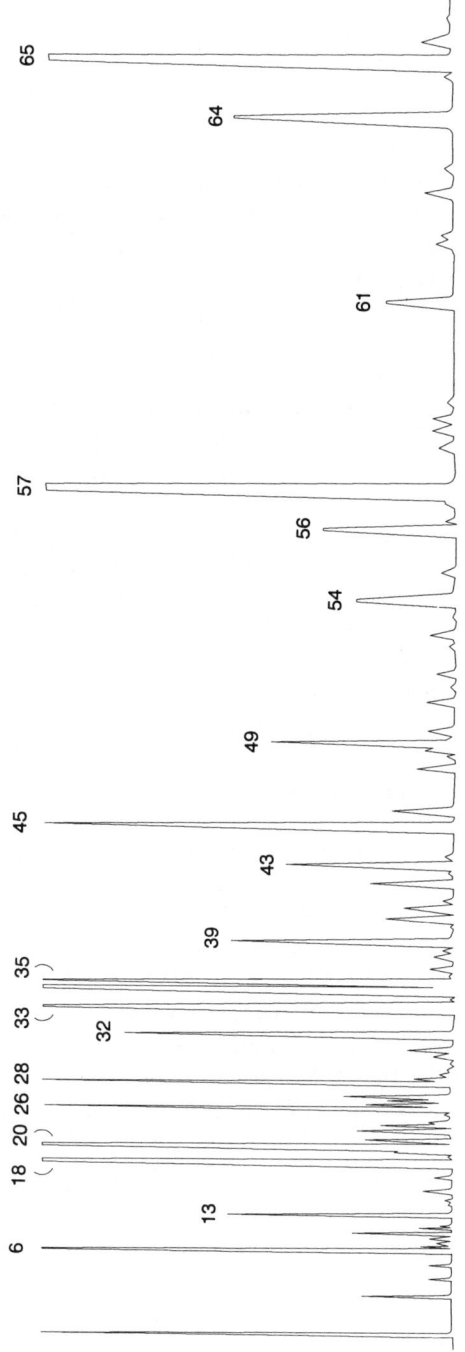

Fig. 3-3. GLC analysis of menhaden oil FAME on a flexible fused silica SUPELCOWAX 10 column, 30 m × 0.32 mm. Initial temperature, 170°C; rate, 1°C/min; final temperature, 220°C. Helium carrier gas. Figure generated from chromatogram by application of a CAD program.

for the analysis of FAME. If $20:5n$-3 and $22:6n$-3 are components of primary interest, $23:0$ is a good internal standard since it elutes between these two esters (Einig and Ackman 1987). Dihomo-γ-linolenic acid ($20:3n$-6) has been suggested as a better choice for the quantitation of PUFA since it is more similar in structure and solubility (Gerber et al. 1979). However, $20:3n$-6 is present in small quantities in most, if not all, marine oils. Regardless of the internal standard chosen, the best results are achieved with a $1:1$ ratio of internal standard to component of interest, although satisfactory results have been obtained with the amount of internal standard as low as 10% of the compound to be measured (Kuksis 1984).

The suitability of the $23:0$ ester as an internal standard for the quantitation of $20:5n$-3 and $22:6n$-3 was tested in an AOAC international collaborative study (Ackman and Joseph 1989). In order to encourage participation in the study, analysis time and expense were kept to a minimum by requiring only the use of theoretical correction factors. The detailed methodology used in the study is included in the Appendix. Equations are given for calculations of both normalized area percentages and absolute weights of $20:5n$-3 and $22:6n$-3 in milligrams per gram of sample.

Except for the purpose of calculating ECL values, most GLC separations of marine FAME are carried out by GLC temperature programming. Temperatures, initially, are lower than required for isothermal runs and are increased at a constant rate, or in discrete steps, to obtain optimum resolution over the entire range of FAME. In addition, improved quantitation has been demonstrated for temperature-programmed analysis. Iverson and Sheppard (1975) have observed relatively smaller and less erratic correction factors that closely agree with the "active" carbon concept as compared with an isothermal analysis. Moreover, a significantly greater number of fatty acids in complex marine lipids are resolved than by isothermal analysis; the detection of PUFA with 24–30 carbons has been reported in marine oils using this technique (Linko and Karinkanta 1970). Figures 3-1 and 3-3 illustrate the differences in peak resolution and detection of minor components for the temperature programmed run (Fig. 3-3) as compared to an isothermal analysis (Fig. 3-1). Although it is not evident in these figures, the temperature-programmed analysis was completed in about three-quarters of the time required for the isothermal analysis.

SUMMARY

Beyond doubt, GLC is the most commonly used single technique in lipid analysis. While it may appear to the uninitiated to be a relatively simple technique to apply, there are many "pitfalls for the unwary" (Ackman 1972). Both accurate identification and satisfactory quantitation require care and attention to detail. A variety of chemical procedures are available to assist in assigning accurate identity to GLC peaks, but reviews of these procedures (Dutton 1983; Walker 1975; Privett 1968) and numerous research publications cited in this chapter make it clear that no one single approach is sufficient for structural identification of unknown FAME. However, when used in concert, much valuable data on chemical structure can be obtained, even when sophisticated spectrometric instrumentation is not available.

ACKNOWLEDGMENTS

We thank Dr. R. G. Ackman and our colleagues, Dr. Sylvia B. Galloway, Ms. Frances VanDolah, and Mr. Malcolm B. Hale for reviewing the manuscript and providing many valuable suggestions. The assistance of Mr. Carl Kinerd in converting the manuscript to WordPerfect (WordPerfect Corp., Orem, Utah) is very much appreciated.

REFERENCES

Ackman, R. G. 1967. The chain length overlap problem in gas-liquid chromatography with polyester liquid phases. *Lipids* 2:502–505.

Ackman, R. G. 1972. The analysis of fatty acids and related materials by gas-liquid chromatography. In *Progress in the Chemistry of Fats and Other Lipids*, ed. R. T. Holman, pp. 165–248. New York: Pergamon Press.

Ackman, R. G. 1977. BF$_3$-MeOH: A single reagent for ozonolysis of monoethylenic unsaturation. *Lipids* 12:293–296.

Ackman, R. G. 1984. Straight chain fatty acids. In *CRC Handbook of Chromatography: Lipids*, vol. 1, ed. H. K. Mangold, pp. 95–240. Boca Raton, Fla.: CRC Press.

Ackman, R. G. 1986. WCOT (capillary) gas-liquid chromatography. In *Analysis Of Oils And Fats*, ed. R. J. Hamilton and J. B. Rossell, pp. 137–206. New York: Elsevier Applied Science.

Ackman, R. G. 1987. Simplification of analyses of fatty acids in fish lipids and related lipid samples. *Acta Medica Scandinavica* 222:99–103.

Ackman, R. G., and Burgher, R. D. 1965. Cod liver oil fatty acids as secondary reference standards in the GLC of polyunsaturated fatty acids of animal origin. Analysis of a dermal oil of the Atlantic leatherback turtle. *J. Am. Oil Chemists' Soc.* 41:39–42.

Ackman, R. G., and Eaton, C. A. 1978. Some contemporary applications of open-tubular gas-liquid chromatography in analyses of methyl esters of longer-chain fatty acids. *Fette, Seifen, Anstrichmittel* 80:21–37.

Ackman, R. G., and Hooper, S. N. 1973. Additivity of retention data for ethylenic functions in aliphatic fatty acids. 2. Polar liquid phases. *J. Chromatogr.* 86:83–88.

Ackman, R. G., and Joseph, J. D. 1989. Recent progress in lipid analysis: The omega-3 problem. *Proceedings of the 1988 International Society for Fat Research—Japan Oil Chemists' Society World Congress.* In press.

Ackman, R. G., Manzer, A., and Joseph, J. 1974. Tentative identification of an unusual naturally-occurring polyenoic fatty acid by calculations from precision open-tubular GLC and structural element retention data. *Chromatographia* 7:107–114.

Ackman, R. G., Safe, L., Hooper, S. N., and Paradis, M. 1973. 7-Methyl-7-hexadecenoic acid: Isolation from lipids of the ocean sunfish *Mola mola* (Linnaeus) 1758. *Lipids* 8:21–24.

Ackman, R. G., Sebedio, J. L., and Ratnayake, W. N. 1981. Structure determinations of unsaturated fatty acids by oxidative fission. *Methods in Enzymol.* 72:253–276.

Ackman, R. G., and Sipos, J. C. 1964. Application of specific response factors in the gas chromatographic analysis of methyl esters of fatty acids with flame ionization detectors. *J. Am. Oil Chemists' Soc.* 41:377–378.

Ackman, R. G., Sipos, J. C., Hooper, S. N., and Dube, G. 1977. Selection of internal standards for determining quantitative recovery of isoprenoid acids after urea complexing. *J. Am. Oil Chemists' Soc.* 54:199–201.

Ackman, R. G., Sipos, J. C., and Jangaard, P. M. 1967. A quantitation problem in the open tubular gas chromatography of fatty acid esters from cod liver lipids. *Lipids* 2:251–257.

Aitzetmuller, K. 1982. Recent progress in the high performance liquid chromatography of lipids. *Prog. Lipid Res.* 21:171–193.

Albertyn, D. E., Bannon, C. D., Craske, J. D., Hai, N. T., O'Rourke, N. L., and Szonyi, C. 1982. Analysis of fatty acid methyl esters with high accuracy and reliability. I. Optimization of flame-ionization detectors with respect to linearity. *J. Chromatogr.* 247:47–61.

Andersson, B. A., Christie, W. W., and Holman, R. T. 1975. Mass spectrometric determination of positions of double bonds in polyunsaturated fatty acid pyrrolidines. *Lipids* 10:215–219.

Andersson, B. A., and Holman, R. T. 1975. Mass spectrometric localization of methyl branching in fatty acids using acylpyrrolidines. *Lipids* 10:716–718.

Bannon, C. D., Breen, G. J., Craske, J. D., Hai, N. T., Harper, N. L., and O'Rourke, K. L. 1982A. Analysis of fatty acid methyl esters with high accuracy and reliability. Part 3. Literature review of and investigations into the development of rapid procedures for the methoxide-catalysed methanolysis of fats and oils. *J. Chromatogr.* 247:71–89.

Bannon, C. D., Craske, J. D., Hai, N. T., Harper, N. L., and O'Rourke, K. L. 1982B. Analysis of fatty acid methyl esters with high accuracy and reliability. Part 2. Methylation of fats and oils with boron trifluoride-methanol. *J. Chromatogr.* 247:63–69.

Bannon, C. D., Craske, J. D., and Hilliker, A. E. 1985. Analysis of fatty acid methyl esters with high accuracy and reliability. Part 4. Fats with fatty acids containing four or more carbon atoms. *J. Am. Oil Chemists' Soc.* 62:1501–1507.

Bannon, C. D., Craske, J. D., and Hilliker, A. E. 1986. Analysis of fatty acid methyl esters with high accuracy and reliability. Part 5. Validation of theoretical relative response factors of unsaturated esters in the flame ionization detector. *J. Am. Oil Chemists' Soc.* 63:105–110.

Beroza, M., and Bierl, B. A. 1966. Apparatus for ozonolysis of microgram to milligram amounts of compound. *Anal. Chem.* 38:1976–1977.

Bianchini, J. P., Ralaimanarivo, A., and Gaydou, E. M. 1981. Determination of cyclopropenoic and cyclopropanoic fatty acids in cottenseed and kaypok seed oils by gas-liquid chromatography. *J. Am. Chemical Soc.* 53:2194–2201.

Bitner, E. D., Lanser, A. C., and Dutton, H. J. 1970. MRA microreactions for lipid analysis. *Lipids* 5:707–712.

Bligh, E. G., and Dyer, W. J. 1959. A rapid method for total lipid extraction and purification. *Can. J. Biochem. Physiol.* 37:911–917.

Christie, W. W. 1982. *Lipid Analysis: Isolation, Separation, Identification and Structural Analysis of Lipids,* 2nd ed. Oxford: Pergamon Press.

Christie, W. W., Brechany, E. Y., and Holman, R. T. 1987. Mass spectra of the picolinyl esters of isomeric mono- and dienoic fatty acids. *Lipids* 22:224–228.

Christie, W. W., Brechany, E. Y., Johnson, S. B., and Holman, R. T. 1986. A comparison of pyrrolidide and picolinyl ester derivatives for the identification of fatty acids in natural samples by gas chromatography–mass spectrometry. *Lipids* 21:657–661.

Christie, W. W., Brechany, E. Y., and Stefanov, K. 1988. Silver ion high-performance liquid chromatography and gas chromatography–mass spectrometry in the analysis of complex fatty acid mixtures: Application to marine invertebrates. *Chem. Phys. Lipids* 46:127–135.

Craske, J. D., and Bannon, C. D. 1987. Gas liquid chromatography analysis of the fatty acid composition of fats and oils: A total system for high accuracy. *J. Am. Oil Chemists' Soc.* 64:1413–1417.

Craske, J. D., and Bannon, C. D. 1988. Analyzing fatty acid methyl esters by gas chromatography. Letter to the editor. *J. Am. Oil Chemists' Soc.* 65:1190–1191.

Cronin, D. A., and Gilbert, J. 1973. Hydrogenation and ozonolysis of submicrogram quantities of unsaturated organic compounds eluted from gas chromatographic columns. *J. Chromatogr.* 87:387–400.

Dutton, H. J. 1983. Chemical methods for today's lipid laboratory. In *Dietary Fats and Health*, ed. E. G. Perkins and W. J. Visek, pp. 209–219. Champaign, Ill.: American Oil Chemists' Society.

Einig, R. G., and Ackman, R. G. 1987. Omega-3 PUFA in marine oil products. *J. Am. Oil Chemists' Soc.* 64:499–502.

Folch, J., Lees, M., and Sloane-Stanley, G. H. 1957. A simple method for the isolation and purification of total lipids from animal tissues. *J. Biol. Chem.* 226:497–509.

Freeman, R. R., ed. 1981. *High Resolution Gas Chromatography*, 2nd ed. Palo Alto, Calif.: Hewlett-Packard Co.

Gerber, J. G., Barnes, J. S., and Nies, A. S. 1979. Measurement of arachidonic acid in the plasma by gas-liquid chromatography–flame ionization using dihomo-γ-linolenic acid as an internal standard. *J. Lipid Res.* 20:912–914.

Gunstone, F. D., Wijesundera, R. C., and Schrimgeour, C. M. 1978. The component acids of lipids from marine and freshwater species with special reference to furan-containing acids. *J. Sci. Food Agric.* 29:539–550.

Haagsma, N., van Gent, C. M., Luten, J. B., de Jong, R. W., and van Doorn, E. (1982. Preparation of an omega-3 fatty acid concentrate from cod liver oil. *J. Am. Oil Chemists' Soc.* 59:117–118.

Hara, A., and Radin, N. S. 1978. Lipid extraction of tissues with a low-toxicity solvent. *Anal. Biochem.* 90:420–426.

Hardy, R., McGill, A. S., and Gunstone, F. D. 1979. Lipid and autoxidative changes in cold stored cod (*Gadus morhua*). *J. Sci. Food Agric.* 30:999–1006.

International Union of Pure and Applied Chemistry. 1977. The nomenclature of lipids. *Lipids* 12:455–468.

Iverson, J. L., and Sheppard, A. J. 1975. Programmed temperature gas chromatographic analysis of esters of fatty acids. *J. Chromatogr. Sci.* 13:505–508.

Iverson, J. L., and Weik, R. W. 1967. Correlation of fatty acid structure with preferential order of urea complex formation. *J. Assoc. Off. Anal. Chem.* 50:1111–1118.

Jamieson, G. R. 1970. Structure determination of fatty esters by gas liquid chromatography. In *Topics in Lipid Chemistry*, vol. 1, ed. F. D. Gunstone, pp. 107–159. London: Logos Press.

Jamieson, G. R. 1975. GLC identification techniques for long-chain unsaturated fatty acids. *J. Chromatogr. Sci.* 13:491–497.

Johnston, A. E., and Dutton, H. J. 1972. Reductive ozonolysis for monoenoic fatty acid structure determination in the microreactor apparatus. *J. Am. Oil Chemists' Soc.* 49:98–100.

Joseph, J. D. 1979. Lipid composition of marine and estuarine invertebrates: Porifera and Cnidaria. *Prog. Lipid Res.* 18:1–30.

Joseph, J. D. 1982. Lipid composition of marine and estuarine invertebrates. 2. Mollusca. *Prog. Lipid Res.* 21:109–153.

Joseph, J. D., and Seaborn, G. T. 1982. Preliminary studies in marine lipid oxidation. *NOAA Technical Memorandum*, NMFS SEFC-95. 92 pp.

Kuksis, A. 1984. Quantitative and positional analysis of fatty acids. In *Lipid Research Methodology*, ed. J. A. Story, pp. 77–131. New York: A. R. Liss, Inc.

Linko, R. R., and Karinkanta, H. 1970. Fifty acids of long chain length in Baltic herring lipids. *J. Am. Oil Chemists' Soc.* 47:42–46.

Mangold, H. K. 1969. Aliphatic lipids. In *Thin Layer Chromatography. A Laboratory Handbook*, ed. E. Stahl, pp. 363–421. London: Springer-Verlag.

Morris, L. J. 1962. Separation of higher fatty acid isomers and vinylogues by thin layer chromatography. *Chem. Ind. (London)* July 7:1238–1240.

Morris, L. J. 1966. Separations of lipids by silver ion chromatography. *J. Lipid Res.* 7:717–732.

Napolitano, G. E., Ratnayake, W. M. N., and Ackman, R. G. 1988. All-*cis*-3,6,9,12,15-octadecapentaenoic acid: A problem of resolution in the GLC analysis of marine fatty acids. *Phytochemistry* 27:1751–1755.

Nickell, E. C., Albi, M., and Privett, O. S. 1976. Ozonization products of unsaturated fatty acid methyl esters. *Chem. Phys. Lipids* 17:378–388.

Nickell, E. C., and Privett, O. S. 1966. A simple, rapid micromethod for the determination of the structure of unsaturated fatty acids via ozonolysis. *Lipids* 1:166–170.

Odham, G., and Stenhagen, E. 1972. Fatty acids. In *Biochemical Applications of Mass Spectrometry*, ed. G. R. Waller, pp. 211–228. New York: Wiley-Interscience.

Ozcimder, M. and Hammers, W. E. 1980. Fractionation of fish oil fatty acid methyl esters by means of argentation and reversed-phase high-performance liquid chromatography, and its utility in total fatty acid analysis. *J. Chromatogr.* 187:307–317.

Perkins, G., Laramy, R. E., and Lively, L. D. 1963. Flame response in the quantitative determination of high molecular weight paraffins and alcohols by gas chromatography. *Anal. Chem.* 35:360–362.

Piconneaux, A., Grandgirard, A., and Sebedio, J. 1985. Identification of an unusual polyunsaturated fatty acid in liver of rats fed with heated linseed oil. *Comptes Rendus de l'Academie des Sciences, Serie 3. Sciences de la Vie* 300:353–358.

Privett, O. S. 1966. Determination of the structure of unsaturated fatty acids via degradative methods. In *Progress in the Chemistry of Fats and Other Lipids*, vol. 9, part 1, ed. R. T. Holman, pp. 93–117. New York: Pergamon Press.

Privett, O. S. 1968. Preparation of polyunsaturated fatty acids from natural sources. In *Progress in the Chemistry of Fats and Other Lipids*, vol. 9, part 3, ed. R. T. Holman, pp. 407–452. New York: Pergamon Press.

Privett, O. S., and Nickell, E. C. 1962. Determination of structure of unsaturated fatty acids via reductive ozonolysis. *J. Am. Oil Chemists' Soc.* 39:414–419.

Privett, O. S., and Nickell, E. C. 1966. Determination of the specific positions of *cis* and *trans* double bonds in polyenes. *Lipids* 1:98–103.

Radin, N. S. 1981. Extraction of tissue lipids with a solvent of low toxicity. *Methods Enzymol.* 72:5–7.

Ratnayake, W. M. N. 1980. Studies on fatty acids from Nova Scotian seaweeds and on the specificity of hydrazine reduction of unsaturated fatty acids. Ph. D. Thesis. Dalhousie University, Halifax, Nova Scotia, 232 pp.

Ratnayake, W. N., and Ackman, R. G. 1979. Identification of novel octadecadienoic fatty acids in the seaweed *Cladophora rupestris* through oxidative ozonolysis of the alcohols prepared from the acids. *Lipids* 14:580–584.

Schlenk, H. 1954. Urea inclusion compounds of fatty acids. In *Progress in the Chemistry of Fats and Other Lipids*, vol. 2, ed. R. T. Holman, W. O. Lundberg, and T. Malkin, pp. 243–267. New York: Pergamon Press.

Scholfield, C. R., Butterfield, R. O., Mounts, T. L., and Dutton, H. J. 1969. Relative reduction rates of fatty acid isomers by hydrazine. *J. Am. Oil Chemists' Soc.* 46:323–326.

Scrimgeour, C. M. 1977. Quantitative analysis of furanoid fatty acids in crude and refined cod liver oil. *J. Am. Oil Chemists' Soc.* 54:210–211.

Sebedio, J. L., and Ackman, R. G. 1978. Oxidative ozonolysis of a polyunsaturated fatty acid in BF₃-MeOH medium. *Can. J. Chem.* 56:2480–2485.

Sebedio, J. L., and Ackman, R. G. 1981. Application of methoxy-bromomercuri-adduct fractionation to the analysis of fatty acids of partially hydrogenated marine oils. *Lipids* 16:461–467.

Sebedio, J. L., and Ackman, R. G. 1983. Hydrogenation of a menhaden oil: 2. Formation and evolution of the C-20 dienoic and trienoic fatty acids as a function of the degree of hydrogenation. *J. Am. Oil Chemists' Soc.* 60:1992–1996.

Sebedio, J. L., Farquharson, T. E., and Ackman, R. G. 1982. Improved methods for the isolation and study of the C-18, C-20 and C-22 monoethylenic fatty acid isomers of biological samples: Hg adducts, HPLC, AgNO₃-TLC/FID, and ozonolysis. *Lipids* 17:469–475.

Sebedio, J. L., Ratnayake, W. M. N., and Ackman, R. G. 1984. Comparison of the reaction products of oleic acid ozonized in BCl₃-, HCl- and BF₃-MeOH media. *Chem. Phys. Lipids* 35:21–28.

Sheppard, A. J., and Iverson, J. L. 1975. Esterification of fatty acids for gas-liquid chromatographic analysis. *J. Chromatogr. Sci.* 13:448–452.

Shukla, V. K. S., Clausen, J., Egsgaard, H., and Larsen, E. 1980. The content of fat and polyenoic acids in the major food sources of the arctic diet. Localization of double bonds in fatty acids by means of mass spectrometry of fatty acid pyrrolidides. *Fette, Seifen, Anstrichmittel* 82:193–199.

Slover, H. T., and Lanza, E. 1979. Quantitative analysis of food fatty acids by capillary gas chromatography. *J. Am. Oil Chemists' Soc.* 56:933–943.

Stahl, E., ed. 1969. *Thin-Layer Chromatography: A Laboratory Handbook*. New York: Springer-Verlag.

Stansby, M. E., ed. 1967. *Fish Oils*. Westport, Conn.: Avi Publishing Co.

Stein, R. A., and Nicolaides, N. 1962. Structure determination of methyl esters of unsaturated fatty acids by gas-liquid chromatography of the aldehydes formed by triphenyl phosphine reduction of the ozonides. *J. Lipid Res.* 3:476–478.

Strocchi, A., and Bonaga, G. 1975. Correlation between urea inclusion compounds and conformational structure of unsaturated C-18 fatty acid methyl esters. *Chem. Phys. Lipids* 15:87–94.

Swern, D. 1964. Techniques of separation. Part E. Urea complexes. In *Fatty Acids; Their Chemistry, Properties, Production, and Uses*, 2nd ed., part 3, ed. K. S. Markley, pp. 2309–2358. New York: Interscience.

Takagi, T., Eaton, C. A., and Ackman, R. G. 1980. Distribution of fatty acids in lipids of the common Atlantic sea urchin *Strongylocentrotus droebachiensis*. *Can. J. Fisheries and Aquatic Sci.* 37:195–202.

Traitler, H. 1987. Recent advances in capillary gas chromatography applied to lipid analysis. *Prog. Lipid Res.* 26:257–280.

Walker, B. L. 1975. Structural determination of lipids by chemical means. In *Analysis of*

Lipids and Lipoproteins, ed. E. G. Perkins, pp. 108–122. Champaign, Ill.: American Oil Chemists' Society.

Yu, Q. T., Kiu, B. N., Zhang, J. Y., and Huang, Z. H. 1989. Location of double bonds in fatty acids of fish oil and rat testis lipids. Gas chromatography-mass spectrometry of the oxazoline derivatives. *Lipids* 24:79–83.

APPENDIX

Collaborative Study on Analysis of Fish Oils and Fish Oil Ethyl Esters by Wall-Coated Open Tubular Gas-liquid Chromatography

Purpose of the Study

To develop an AOAC-approved method for gas chromatographic analysis of marine oils and ethyl esters of polyunsaturated fatty acids derived therefrom, using a polyglycol liquid phase bonded to a flexible fused silica capillary column.

Column

The columns should be of flexible fused silica, 25 m or more in length and 0.20–0.35 mm ID. The liquid phase must be *bonded* Carbowax-20M or an equivalent polyglycol. An example of the latter is SUPERCOWAX-10, 30 m × 0.25 mm (or 0.32 mm) with 0.25-μm coating (Supelco, Inc. catalog 2-4079 or 2-4080). No constraints are placed on the column supplier provided it is accurately reported. Please report the manufacturer's claim for upper temperature limit of the column.

Injection System

A split-type injector is preferred (there is usually sufficient sample in marine oil analysis) operated at a split ratio of about 1 : 100. Record whether any uncoated tubing is used to connect the injection system with the column.

Carrier Gas

Hydrogen or helium, 99.99% pure or better, is required. Note that an oxygen scrubber is *mandatory* with Carbowax-20M and similar columns.

Detector

A flame ionization detector is required. Record whether the column end is inserted directly into the detector jet or whether there is a connection at the base of the jet, with or without makeup gas. Nitrogen is satisfactory for use as a makeup gas.

Amplifier/Recorder/Integrator/Data Processor

Record the make of all data acquisition equipment by manufacturer and model number. If the equipment is that supplied with the gas chromatograph itself, simply report that fact.

Operating Temperatures

Record the temperatures of the injection port, oven, and detector. Report the details of temperature programming if used.

Sample Injection

Manual injection with a microsyringe is preferred. However, there is no objection to autoinjection as long as only one random injection per sample is reported.

Detector Correction Factors

Theoretical detector correction factors relative to $23:0$ (the internal standard) for $20:5n$-3 (0.99) and $22:6n$-3 (0.97) should be applied to the analytic data for optimal accuracy.

Suggested Chromatographic Conditions for a 30-M Column

Injection port: 250°C
Detector: 270°C
Temperature program
— Initial temperature: 170°C
— Hold time: 0 min
— Rate: 1°C/min
— Final temperature: 225°C
— Final time: 55 min

Report

Use enclosed forms to report analytic conditions and results. Note that while each sample consists of three capsules, two are to be used, if necessary, to establish suitable operating parameters. Submit the results of a single analysis on the contents of *one* capsule. Authentic standards of saturated fatty acid esters, if needed for peak identification, are widely available.

Sample Preparation:

Reagents:

— Sodium hydroxide (reagent grade)
— Methyl alcohol
— 12% BF_3 in methanol (2-ml ampules, Supelco Cat. No. 3-3020 or equivalent)
— Iso-octane (reagent grade)
— Sodium chloride (reagent grade)
— 23 : 0 methyl ester (supplied with fish oil capsules)
— 23 : 0 ethyl ester (supplied with ethyl ester capsules)

Solutions:

— 0.5N alcoholic NaOH: Dissolve 2.0 g NaOH in methanol and make to 100 ml with methanol.
— Saturated solution NaCl: Dissolve 36 g NaCl in 100 ml distilled water.

Equipment:

— Constant temperature water bath or dry heating block, maintained at 100°C
— Screw-cap culture tubes (16 × 125 mm) with leaktight Teflon-lined caps
— Screw-cap or crimp-cap 2-ml vials
— 1- and 2-ml volumetric pipettes
— Pasteur-type pipettes
— Volumetric flasks (25 ml)
— Analytical balance
— Source of dry N_2

Procedure—Oils

Accurately weigh (*xx.x* mg) approximately 25 mg of 23 : 0 methyl ester internal standard (IS) into a 25-ml volumetric flask and make to volume with iso-octane.

Pipette 1.0 ml aliquots of the IS into culture tubes and evaporate the solvent.[1] Store the tubes in a freezer if they will not be used immediately.

Cut open capsule and accurately weight (*xx.x* mg) approximately 25 mg of the oil into a culture tube containing the IS.

Add 1.5 ml 0.5N NaOH. Blanket with N_2, cap tightly, mix, and heat at 100°C for 2 min.

Cool, add 2 ml BF_3/MeOH, blanket with N_2, cap tightly, mix, and heat at 100°C for 20 min.

Cool to 30–40°C, add 1 ml of iso-octane, blanket with N_2, cap, and vortex or shake vigorously for 30 sec, while tepid.

---

[1] If the peak height of the IS is less than or equal to one-half that of the EPA or DHA peaks, repeat the analysis using 2.0 ml of IS.

Immediately add 5 ml of saturated NaCl solution, blanket with N_2, cap, and agitate thoroughly.

Allow iso-octane to separate and transfer to a second tube.

Extract the MeOH/water phase again with an additional 1 ml of iso-octane.

Combine iso-octane extracts[2] and concentrate to approximately 1 ml with a stream of dry N_2.

Inject 1–2 μl under appropriate gas chromatographic conditions.

Procedure—Ethyl Esters

Accurately weigh (*xx.x* mg) approximately 25 mg of 23 : 0 ethyl ester internal standard (IS) into a 25-ml volumetric flask and make to volume with iso-octane.

Pipette a 1.0-ml aliquot of the IS into a culture tube and evaporate the solvent.[3]

Cut open one capsule of the ethyl ester unknown and accurately weigh (*xx.x* mg) no more than 15 mg of the esters into the tube containing the IS, add 1.0 ml iso-octane, blanket with N_2, cap, and mix thoroughly.

Inject 1–2 μl under appropriate gas chromatographic conditions.

Calculations

I. Area Percentages. Calculate the area percent for each of the 24 fatty acids listed by the formula:

$$\text{Area \% fatty acid}_x = \frac{100(A_x)}{A_t - A_{is}}$$

where

A_x = area counts of fatty acid x
A_t = total area counts for the chromatogram
A_{is} = area counts of the IS

II. Calculations of mg of EPA and DHA per g of Sample

A. For Fish Oil Capsules. Weight of EPA and DHA: express as mg of EPA/ DHA *fatty acid* per gram of oil.

$$\text{EPA/DHA (mg/g)} = \frac{(A_x)(W_{is})(CF_x)}{(A_{is}(W_s)(1.04)} \times 1000$$

---

[2] Optional: wash iso-octane with 2 ml of water and dry over anhydrous sodium sulfate.
[3] If the peak height of the IS is less than or equal to one-half that of the EPA or DHA peaks, repeat the analysis using 2.0 ml of IS.

B. For Ethyl Ester Capsules.   Weight of EPA and DHA: express as mg of EPA/ DHA *fatty acid* per gram of oil.

$$\text{EPA/DHA (mg/g)} = \frac{(A_x)(W_{is})(CF_x)}{(A_{is}(W_s)(1.08)} \times 1000$$

where

A_x = area counts of EPA or DHA
A_{is} = area counts of internal standard
CF_x = theoretical correction factor for EPA or DHA
W_{is} = weight of IS added to the sample (in mg)
W_s = sample weight (in mg)

Chapter 4
FRACTIONATION OF FISH OILS AND THEIR FATTY ACIDS[1]

Virginia F. Stout, William B. Nilsson, Judith Krzynowek, and Hermann Schlenk

INTRODUCTION

Crystallization, distillation, supercritical fluid extraction, and chromatographic procedures are major preparative methods for fractionation of fish oils and their constituent fatty acids. Fish oils consist primarily of triacylglycerols, commonly called triglycerides. They contain fatty acids in much greater variety than found elsewhere, for example, in vegetable oils. Although some degree of order does occur in the distribution of fatty acids (Brockerhoff and Hoyle 1963; Takahashi et al. 1988), the mixture of triglycerides from fish oils is too complex for efficient isolation of individual components. At best, modest enrichments can be expected from their fractionation. Therefore, most efforts are directed toward fractionating the acids or their methyl or ethyl esters, which are easily obtained from the oils. The principal advantage is that in dealing with those simpler, single-chain compounds, differences in chain length or degree of unsaturation can effectively be addressed. In triglycerides, such differences may be minimized or fully compensated for by the two other acids in the molecules being separated. A practical advantage is the greater volatility of the acids and their simple esters compared to that of the triglycerides. After separation of individual esters, specific triglycerides or free acids

---

[1] Abbreviations and definitions used in this chapter: C_{16}, C_{18} . . . , acids or esters of that chain length without specified degree of unsaturation. $16:1$, $18:3$ . . . , hexadecenoic, octadecatrienoic acid or ester, without specified position of double bonds. $9\text{-}16:1$; $9, 12, 15\text{-}18:3$ . . . ; 9-hexadecenoic (palmitoleic); 9, 12, 15-octadecatrienoic (linolenic) acid or ester, with specified position of double bonds. "Vinylogous compounds" differ by number of double bonds, but not by chain length, e.g., $18:0$, $18:1$, $18:2$. "Homologous vinylogous compounds" differ by one double bond and two carbon atoms, e.g., $16:0$ and $18:1$, $16:1$ and $18:2$ and $20:3$, $17:1$ and $19:2$. EPA: All-*cis*-5,8,11,14,17-eicosapentaenoic acid, often referred to as $20:5\omega3$, to connote that the first double bond begins at the third carbon from the methyl end of the chain. DHA: All-*cis*-4,7,10,13,16,19-docosahexaenoic acid or $22:6\omega3$. $\omega3$: Omega-3 compounds (see under EPA). Solvent mixtures in chromatography are specified as volume/volume.

can be reconstituted as needed (Lehman and Gauglitz 1964; Nilsson et al. 1989A).

In the following discussion, the principles of several fractionation methods will be outlined, examples given, and modifications pointed out as they may be useful in work with fish oil acids and esters. The discussion will concern mainly preparative scale separations. Analytical techniques such as gas-liquid chromatography (GLC) are covered in Chapter 3. The present chapter, taken extensively from the original version by Schlenk and Sand (1967), also contains recent references to older topics as well as a new section on supercritical fluid extraction (SFE) and the addition of two new chromatographic techniques: high-performance (pressure) liquid chromatography (HPLC) and supercritical fluid chromatography (SFC).

Fatty acid mixtures derived from fish oils are distinct from those of other sources in variety of chain length, degree of unsaturation, and multitude of isomeric compounds. Isolation of individual components is difficult even on microscale. Generally, separation efficiency of a procedure and apparatus decreases with increased amount of sample, volume of solvent used for crystallization, dimensions of a column for distillation or chromatography, or rate at which a process is carried out. There are practical limits to expanding such parameters proportionately with the amount treated, though less so with SFE. When applied to fish oil acids, most methods yield only group fractionations and two or more procedures are necessary to afford individual components in high purity.

Crystallizations can be carried out on milligram to kilogram quantities. For efficient fractionation, distillation requires a minimum of several grams. Liquid-liquid (partition) and liquid-solid (absorption) chromatography (LLC, LSC) were originally performed on a somewhat smaller scale until HPLC expanded the scale to 60 g or more. Normally GLC is applied to not more than a fraction of a gram. The recent techniques of SFC and SFE together cover the gamut from analytical to, potentially, kilogram-scale operation.

Obviously, the choice of methods and their sequence depends on the size and composition of the sample and required degree of fractionation. The patterns of fractionation by different methods are outlined in Fig. 4-1. For simplicity, the scheme lists only even-numbered straight-chain acids and the number of double bonds; odd-numbered acids and isomerism are disregarded. Of course, fractionations of real mixtures are not achieved as precisely as the separating lines in Fig. 4-1 would indicate.

Fractionation principles are: by crystallization and LSC in the presence of silver nitrate, according to unsaturation rather than chain length (vertical lines in Fig. 4-1); by distillation and SFE, according to chain length rather than unsaturation (horizontal lines in Fig. 4-1); by countercurrent

Fractionation principles

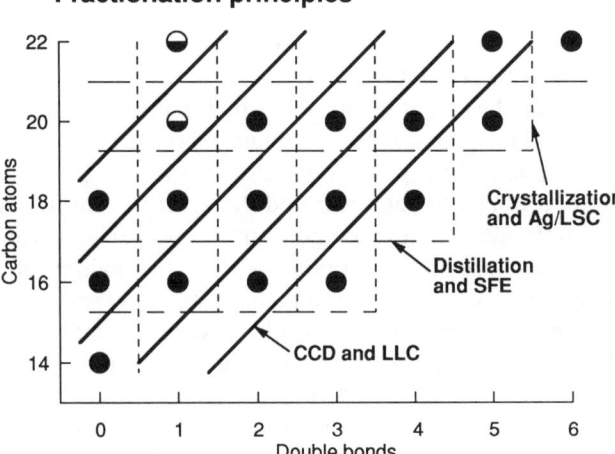

Fig. 4-1. Patterns of fractionation by different methods. Crystallization and LSC in the presence of AgNO$_3$ separate according to unsaturation (vertical lines), distillation and SFE according to chain length (horizontal lines), CCD and LLC according to a combination of both chain length and unsaturation (diagonal lines). Filled circles indicate fatty acids commonly occurring in fish oils. Half-filled circles are for monoenoic acids present in higher concentrations in some species.

distribution (CCD) and LLC, according to a certain combination of chain length and unsaturation (diagonal lines in Fig. 4-1); by GLC on nonpolar or polar phases according to chain length and unsaturation. Similarly, LSC on the most commonly used material, silicic acid, responds to chain length and degree of unsaturation, although not as distinctly as does GLC. Evidence to be discussed later suggests that SFE has the potential for accomplishing separation according to both chain length and degree of unsaturation. The problem of separating isomers remains a challenge.

Figure 4-1 illustrates the earlier statement that individual components are separated only by a combination of several methods. Intersecting lines indicate suitable combinations to achieve this separation. Knowledge of the composition, now routinely available by analytical GLC, guides the exact design of separation procedures.

The methods described in this chapter are exemplified, whenever possible, by applications to fish oil fatty acids and esters. Early examples reflect the research interests of Schlenk and Sand (1967). Later examples come from recent literature and research at the Seattle, Washington; Gloucester, Massachusetts; and Charleston, South Carolina, Utilization Research Laboratories of the National Marine Fisheries Service.

CRYSTALLIZATION

Fractionation of a mixture by crystallization is based on the difference in composition of the equilibrated solid and liquid phases, depending on the solubilities of the components. Except for the industrial process of melting and partial solidification to obtain "pressed fatty acids," fractional crystallization of fatty acids or esters always employs solvents.

Brown and Kolb (1955) demonstrated the efficiency of fractional crystallization of fatty acids at low temperature by preparing several acids in higher purity than previously obtainable. The solubilites of numerous acids and esters in a variety of solvents have been determined (Singleton 1960). These investigations were also of physical chemical interest since the homologous (C_{16}, C_{18}, C_{20}, C_{22}) or vinylogous (20:1, 20:3, 20:4, 20:5) series of acids offered materials for comparative study that were not easily accessible from any other sources (Skau and Boucher 1954). Figure 4-2 illustrates such data.

A comparison of solubilities reveals the following rules: when the acids are saturated, long-chain are less soluble than short-chain; saturated are less soluble than monoenoic and dienoic acids of equal chain length; *trans* isomers are less soluble than *cis*, and normal acids are less soluble than

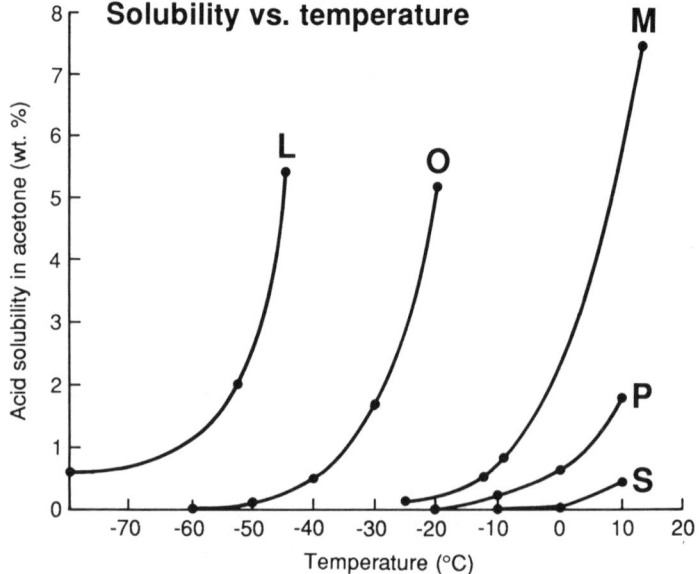

Fig. 4-2. Solubilities of fatty acids in acetone. L = linoleic (18:2ω6), O = oleic (18:1ω9), M = myristic (14:0), P = palmitic (16:0), and S = stearic (18:0).

Solubility vs. chain length

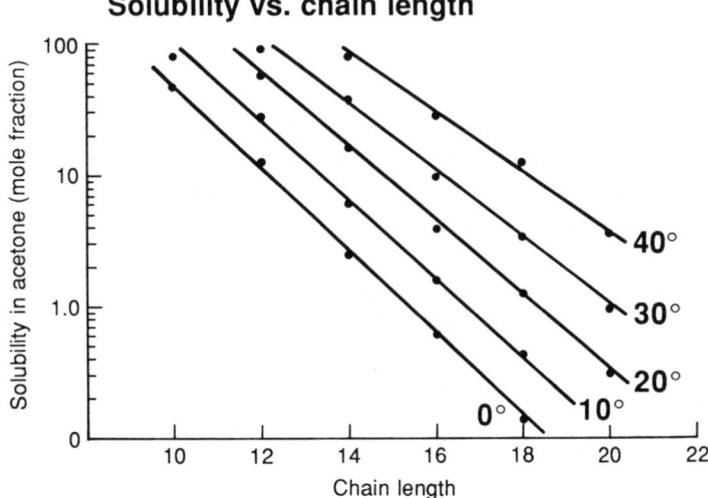

Fig. 4-3. Solubility of saturated acids versus chain length in acetone. Note that only even-numbered acids are included; temperatures are in degrees centigrade.

branched acids; acids are always less soluble than their methyl esters. These widely valid features show quantitative differences with different solvents. In a series of structurally related compounds, those with higher melting points are less soluble, behavior suggesting a correlation between the heat of fusion and solubility.

Skau and Boucher (1954) derived the formula $\log N = a + bn$ for the solubility of homologs, where N is the mole fraction of solute in the solution; a and b are constants which depend on the temperature and the system; n is the number of carbon atoms of the solute. The semilog function of N versus n is confirmed for acids with even numbers of carbons (Fig. 4-3). However, regular increments in the heat of fusion of homologs implies their having comparable crystal structure. This is not the case for odd-numbered acids compared to even-numbered ones. Just as the melting points of odd- and even-numbered acids are not interpolative, so neither are their solubilities.

Little is known about the mechanism of crystallization of fatty acids. As with all other organic compounds, their crystals cannot be overheated but the melted products and solutions are easily undercooled. Again in reference to crystallization from the melt, one has to assume that an optimal temperature exists for the growth of crystals from solution and that cosolutes lower the growth rate.

Intersolubilization effects are pronounced with fatty acids, particularly in solvents like benzene or chloroform. Although association phenomena common in acids are much reduced in the methyl esters, the practical advantage is limited by the greater solubility of the esters. Furthermore, eutectics are often formed. They prevent attainment of the degree of separation one would predict from solubility data alone. Mixtures of oleic, stearic, and palmitic acids were studied extensively in this regard (Singleton 1948, 1949). The complexities of crystallization phenomena of C_{16}, C_{17}, and C_{18} mixtures have been described (Aurousseau and Bauchart 1980).

In spite of factors adverse to separation, crystallization is an indispensable method for preparing pure fatty acids (Markely 1964). It requires the least equipment, and simple apparatus for crystallization of fatty acids have been described (Brown and Kolb 1955; Singleton 1960; Schlenk 1961). Furthermore, until the introduction of SFE and HPLC, crystallization at low temperature was the method least destructive to highly unsaturated acids.

Common solvents for crystallization are methanol, acetone, or petroleum ether with concentrations of solute between 5 and 15%. Acetonitrile is preferred for small amounts. Nitromethane was particularly useful for enriching $16:4$ and $18:4$ from fish oil ester mixtures (Jangaard 1965). Liquid propane was used on an industrial scale (Hixson and Bockelman 1942; Drew and Hixson 1944).

Examples

1. Separation of C_{14}–C_{16} from C_{18}–C_{20}. Mullet fatty esters, obtained by alkaline interesterification of the oil, were subjected to successive crystallizations from a 10% solution in acetone at $-30°C$ and $-60°C$ (Schlenk and Sand unpublished). The characteristic pattern in fish acids of saturated chains occurring predominantly as C_{14} and C_{16}, and more unsaturated ones as longer chains, is reflected by the data in Table 4-1 showing C_{14}–C_{16} depleted and C_{18}–C_{22} enriched in the final mother liquor. The obvious exception is the major C_{16} component $16:1$, which largely accounts for the 30.8% C_{16} in the $-60°C$ mother liquor; $16:1$ is notoriously more difficult to crystallize from mixtures than $18:1$. The unsaponifiables, present at low levels initially, were enriched in the final mother liquor. The mullet fatty acids discussed above and in subsequent examples are distinguished by an unusually high percentage of odd-numbered acids. Fractionation of such a mixture does not present a novel problem but requires refined application of the usual methods (Sen and Schlenk 1964).

Table 4-1. Crystallization of Mullet Fatty Acid Esters

		AT −30°C		AT −60°C	
	ORIGINAL	PREC.[a]	M.L.[b]	PREC.[c]	M.L.[b]
Grams	2435	388		535	1512
IV[d]	151.2	19.6	180.7	47.9	224.6
CHAIN LENGTH[e]	%	%	%	%	%
14	5.3	2.4	5.8	19.1	1.8
15	13.7	17.2	10.1	22.3	2.5
16	33.8	64.1	31.4	35.6	30.8
17	11.1	5.6	11.6	6.6	13.9
18	10.6	6.2	11.4	6.3	13.6
19	2.6	0.6	2.9	1.1	3.7
20	13.1	2.1	15.9	5.0	19.7
21	1.8	0.4	1.6	0.8	2.3
22	7.9	1.3	9.2	3.5	11.7

[a] Precipitate from first crystallization.
[b] M.L. = mother liquor.
[c] Precipitate from second crystallization.
[d] Iodine value.
[e] Percentages determined by hydrogenation followed by GLC.

2. Isolation of 17:1 Esters. A distilled fraction of mullet esters, consisting of 51% 17:1 and 49% C_{17} polyunsaturated esters, was crystallized at −62°C. The 10% solution of 46 g in methanol yielded 21 g precipitate. The solid material contained 96.4% 17:1 and 3.6% polyunsaturated esters, while the mother liquor contained 13.6% 17:1 and 86.4% polyunsaturated esters (Schlenk and Sand unpublished). Thus, a preliminary chain length separation by distillation reduced the isolation of >96% 17:1 to one crystallization step in comparison to the laborious 21-step process required without distillation (Bauchart and Aurousseau 1980).

Modified Crystallization Methods

Crystallization Compounds with Urea.

Bengen's discovery (1940, 1953) that urea crystallizes with straight-chain compounds but not with branched or cyclic ones led to a new technique for fractionation of fatty acids or esters (Schlenk 1954; Moreno and Roncero 1964). Studies of the crystal structure of the complexes showed that while urea alone crystallizes in a tightly packed tetragonal structure, in the presence of long straight-chain molecules it crystallizes in a hexagonal structure (W. Schlenk, Jr. 1949; Smith 1952). In this form, the hexagonal openings are wide enough to adapt molecules with a diameter of 5 Å, but they do not easily accept molecules with larger diameters, for example, branched ones.

Although both saturated and *cis*-unsaturated fatty acids are straight-chain compounds, they are quite different in shape. Saturated acids can completely adjust to the straight axis of the hexagonal urea channel, whereas *cis*-double bonds produce irregularities in the chain. The methylene-interrupted polyunsaturated fatty acids from fish are crooked enough that they can be separated in stages somewhat according to chain length and more by number of double bonds.

The extent of crystallization depends on the concentration of urea and the temperature of crystallization. Wille et al. (1987) reported that 18:4ω3 and docosahexaenoic acid (DHA or 22:6ω3) are concentrated more efficiently in the filtrate when crystallizaton occurs at −5°C, whereas eicosapentaenoic acid (EPA or 20:5ω3) and total omega-3 (ω3) content maximize at 15° and 10°C, respectively. Traitler et al. (1988) noted that 18:3ω3 separated from 18:3ω6, which cofractionated with 18:4ω3. Haagsma et al. (1982) and Ratnayake et al. (1988) noted that EPA complexes to a greater extent than 18:4ω3 or DHA. Both these groups confirmed as optimal the long-known factor of 3:1 urea to fatty acid or ester. By segregating Baltic herring oil into nine fractions, Linko and Karinkanta (1970A, B) isolated 24:5, 26:5, 24:6, and 28:7 polyenoic acids.

Qualitatively, the solubilities of fatty acids in the presence of urea parallel but are much lower than their solubilities alone. Without urea, polyenoic compounds do not normally crystallize even at the temperature of dry ice, but will do so in high concentrations of urea above 0°C. Thus, approximately 90% DHA (iodine value, IV, of the methyl ester 421, pure DHA 445), was obtained from a concentrate of polyunsaturated fatty acids (IV 315) prepared by molecular distillation (Stout 1963). Successive crystallization with increasing concentrations of fatty acids and urea at decreasing temperatures down to 13°C allowed separation of DHA from the other compounds. Interestingly, urea complexing protects these polyunsaturated molecules from autoxidation (Schlenk and Holman 1950). The application of urea crystallization to analysis of fatty acid mixtures was discussed already in Chapter 3.

Complex formation is exothermic but requires solution of both urea and the long-chain compound. Methanol and ethanol are preferred solvents for small-scale fractionation. A slurry procedure can be employed when working on a kilogram scale since complete solution of the components is not necessary for the reaction to proceed. Benzene has been used with small amounts of methanol, acetone, or other polar solvents added to promote transformation of the solid tetragonal urea into the hexagonal complex. In conventional solvents, the acids or esters are recovered by dissolving the complexes in acidified water and extracting with ether, trimethylpentane, or similar lipophilic solvent. Quite recently, carbon dioxide at high pressures has been used as a solvent for urea complexing (Saito 1986; Suzuki 1988). Uncomplexed polyunsaturates are easily recovered solvent-free by expanding CO_2 to atmospheric pressure. Other processes using CO_2 will be described in the section on SFE.

Swern (1964) reviewed urea fractionation of acids from many natural oils. More recently, Patokina et al. (1988) have studied the thermodynamics and other aspects of the formation of urea adducts.

Lead and Lithium Soaps.   Fractionation of acids in the form of their soaps has been replaced by newer methods. Recently, however, they were used to prepare pure DHA (Wright et al. 1987). Lead salts were mostly used to separate unsaturated from saturated acids. Recovery of the free acids is rather inconvenient, and acids outside the range of $C_{16}-C_{18}$ and *trans* unsaturated acids interfere with the separation (Mehlenbacher 1960). However, such procedures were prominent in the earlier research on fish oil acids, and selected references for such applications have been compiled (Markley 1964).

The properties of lead soaps are supplemented, to some extent, by lithium soaps. For the latter, the major difference in solubilities is between monoenoic and dienoic compounds (Silk et al. 1954; Silk and Hahn 1954A, B).

Examples

1. Comparative Fractionation of Acids from Menhaden, Herring, Tuna Body, and Other Marine Oils.   Domart et al. (1955) crystallized 50-g samples in 100 ml ethanol with 600 ml of methanol containing about 100 g urea (saturated at room temperature) successively at $+25°$, $+1°$, $-18°$, and $-30°$C. From starting materials with IV of 120 and 160, the first precipitates had IV 20–50 and the mother liquors of the last precipitates 210–250. Salmon egg acids with initial IV 207 yielded a final filtrate with IV 290.

2. Incremental Addition of Urea After Each Filtration.   Stepwise addition of urea yielded fractions with increasing numbers of double bonds, as indicated by the IV. Figure 4-4 gives results from cod-liver fatty acid ethyl esters (Abu-Nasr et al. 1954). Comparative fractionations of esters and acids from cod-liver oil, shark liver oil, and similar materials suggested that urea binds polyenoic esters more easily than the analogous acids.

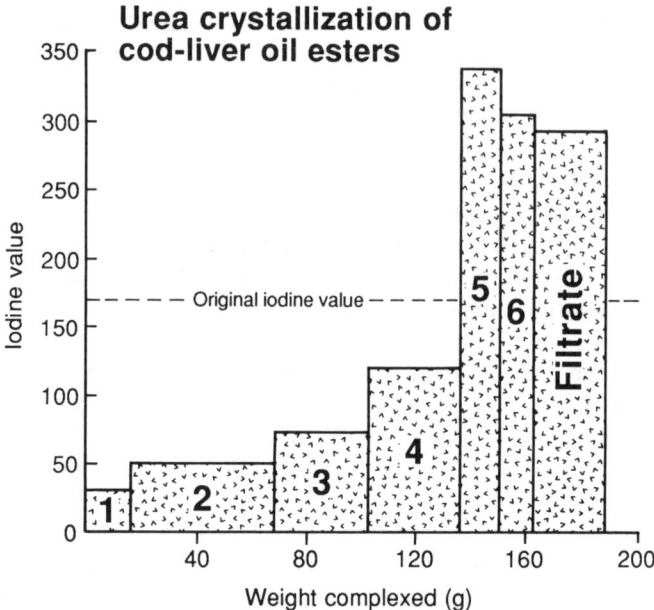

Fig. 4-4. Fractionation of cod-liver oil fatty acid ethyl esters by successive additions of urea for stepwise complexation.

3. Fractionation of South African Pilchard Acids.   Silk et al. (1954) and Silk and Hahn (1954A) compared urea and lithium soap-acetone methods and combined the two to isolate 16 : 4 acid (Silk and Hahn 1954B).

4. Four-Step Preparation of Pure DHA Without Distillation or Chromatography.   Recently, the old lithium soap method was combined with a chemical derivatization in a process unique to DHA (Wright et al. 1987). After saponification of 200 g of cod-liver oil to fatty acids, the saturated and monounsaturated acids were precipitated as lithium soaps. Next, DHA was preferentially converted to its iodolactone derivative, from which all the remaining acids were extracted with potassium carbonate. The final step was recovery of ~14 g DHA from its derivative. EPA also forms an iodolactone, but the reaction can be controlled to allow selective formation with DHA (Corey et al. 1983).

5. Production of Biomedical Test Materials.   Urea fractionation is now being performed in 80-kg batches (J. Joseph, NMFS Charleston, South Carolina, Utilization Research Laboratory, unpublished data). Ethyl esters obtained from refined menhaden oil are mixed with a hot solution of urea and 95% ethanol. Complexes form by cooling to 5°C overnight. After filtration and evaporation of the filtrate by passage through a scraped wall film evaporator, the concentrate of polyenes is washed with dilute HCl and deionized water. The process yields ~16 kg of neat $\omega 3$ esters (46% EPA, 24% DHA). Distillation in a glass, two-stage wiped film molecular still (see below) removes ~50% of the 16-carbon polyenes ($16:3\omega 4$ and $16:4\omega 1$) and some $18:4\omega 3$ in the first stage. The second stage distillate amounts to ~10 kg esters (49% EPA, 27% DHA).

DISTILLATION

Fractional distillation exploits differences in the vapor pressure of the components of a mixture. Assuming ideality, the total vapor pressure of a mixture is the sum of the partial pressures of its components (Dalton's law) while the partial pressure of each component is equal to its vapor pressure in the pure state multiplied by its mole fraction in the liquid mixture (Raoult's law). Since fatty acid methyl esters approximate the requirement of ideality (Monick et al. 1946) while free fatty acids deviate markedly, esters are preferred for distillation. In addition, the lower boiling point of esters is an important factor for thermally unstable $\omega 3$ components.

The progress of a distillation can be described using Fig. 4-5, which shows a generalized vapor-liquid composition diagram for a binary mixture of A and B. The enrichment achieved by evaporating and separately condensing a small portion of this mixture depends on the ratio of individual vapor pressures, p_A and p_B. The factor $\alpha = p_A/p_B$ indicates the separation that theoretically might be accomplished by evaporating a small portion of a mixture and condensing it. Conventionally, the higher-vapor-pressure (lower-boiling) compound is placed in the numerator. Assume, for example, that A is the more volatile, that is, $\alpha = p_A/p_B > 1$. In the figure, the concentration of A in the liquid is represented by X while that of A in the vapor is represented by Y, both in units of mole percent. Consider a starting (liquid) material having a mole percent of A of X_s. The vapor-liquid composition curve predicts that the vapor above the liquid will have a mole percent of A of Y_s, which is enhanced over that in the liquid by virtue of its greater volatility. If this vapor is condensed, the resulting liquid will have the same concentration with respect to A as Y_s, that is, $X_1 = Y_s$ (indicated by the horizontal line drawn between the vapor-liquid equilibrium curve and the auxiliary line of 45° slant followed by projection to the abscissa). In the same manner, the vapor in equilibrium with the liquid of composition X_1 will have a composition Y_1, which

Enrichment by fractional distillation

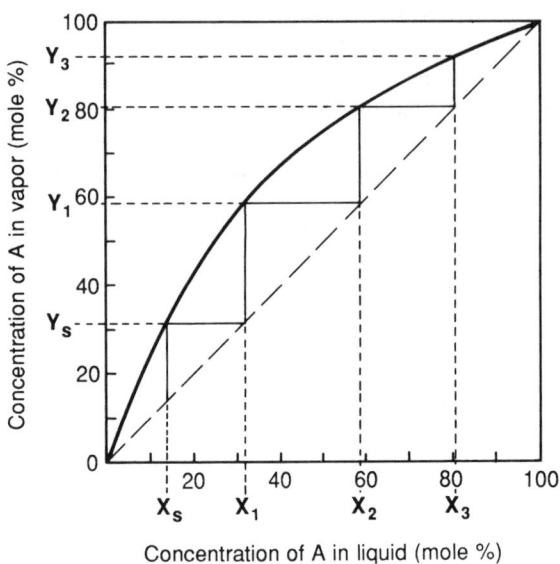

Concentration of A in liquid (mole %)

Fig. 4-5. Principles of enrichment by repeated evaporation and condensation. The concentration at the start is X_s.

is further enhanced with respect to A, again because of relative volatility considerations. If this vapor is then condensed, the resulting liquid has the same enhanced mole percent of A ($X_2 = Y_1$) and so on. This "stepping off" procedure can be further applied to permit the estimation of the number of vaporization-condensation cycles necessary to obtain a distillate of any desired purity with respect to A. Note that if the relative volatilities of A and B are very nearly equal (i.e., α approaches unity), the vapor-liquid equilibrium curve approaches the auxiliary line, and the stepping-off procedure predicts that an increasing number of evaporation-condensation steps are necessary to obtain a desired product.

Difficulties in fractionation of marine oil esters are aggravated by their high content of C_{20} and longer-chain esters because separation factors decrease with increasing molecular weight (Weitkamp 1955). Distillation processes developed by the petroleum industry utilized slow withdrawal of volatile low-molecular-weight fractions at conditions near equilibrium. While useful for only slightly volatile, predominantly monoenoic herring oil, the effect of long-lasting distillation on polyunsaturated esters is particularly detrimental. For instance, Privett et al. (1959) and Privett and Nickell (1963) found marked decomposition of 20:4ω6 (arachidonate) when it was distilled slowly in a spinning band column. Even when the catalytic effects of metal parts were eliminated in an all-glass apparatus, high temperature and exposure to oxygen caused major losses of ω3 components (Ackman et al. 1973).

Various packing materials facilitate contact of liquid and vapor but cause holdup of material as well as a pressure drop and temperature differential (50–100°C) between the pot and takeoff (Rose 1936). Spinning band-type concentric tube columns (Jantzen and Wieckhorst 1954) were designed to minimize the holdup and the pressure drop in packed columns. Unfortunately, the fractionation efficiency of a column at atmospheric pressure is lowered to about one-half when the pressure is reduced to 1–10 mm, and to one-quarter below 1 mm. Fractional distillation of fatty esters requires insulated or heated mantles around the columns, as well as devices for regulating takeoff and reflux rate, temperature, and constant vacuum. Many such accessories have been described and they simplify operation (Murray 1955; Markley 1964).

Boiling points of unsaturated esters are slightly lower than those of saturated ones. Therefore, unsaturated esters are enriched in the early fractions of a specific chain length. Conversely, the saturated component is enriched in the end of fractions of the same chain length. In the transition from one chain length to the next, the distillate consists essentially of the saturated lower and the unsaturated higher chain length components, for example, of 16:0 + 18:3, 18:2.

Examples

1. Mullet Oil Esters Versus Hydrogenated Menhaden Oil Methyl Esters (Schlenk et al. Unpublished). Hydrogenation of highly unsaturated materials prevents polymerization and isomerization in high-temperature processes by saturating the readily oxidized double bonds. Distillation of the hydrogenated menhaden esters in a 90 × 2.5 cm column (Semical High Temperature Unit, Podbielniak, Inc.) lasted 30 hours; the highest pot temperature was 255°C with 1 mm pressure and a maximum value of ~203°C at the takeoff (Fig. 4-6). The fractionation of unhydrogenated mullet esters was more difficult because the sensitive polyunsaturated double bonds were intact. Lower temperatures were necessary to avoid thermal degradation. The process lasted 50 hours at a maximum pot temperature of 225°C with 0.5 mm pressure and a maximum of ~135°C at the takeoff. Nonetheless, the residue, nearly 30% of the charge, contained 37% *trans* double bonds formed during the extended distillation procedure. Indications of isomerization began with the C_{17} components (frac-

Chain length enrichment by distillation

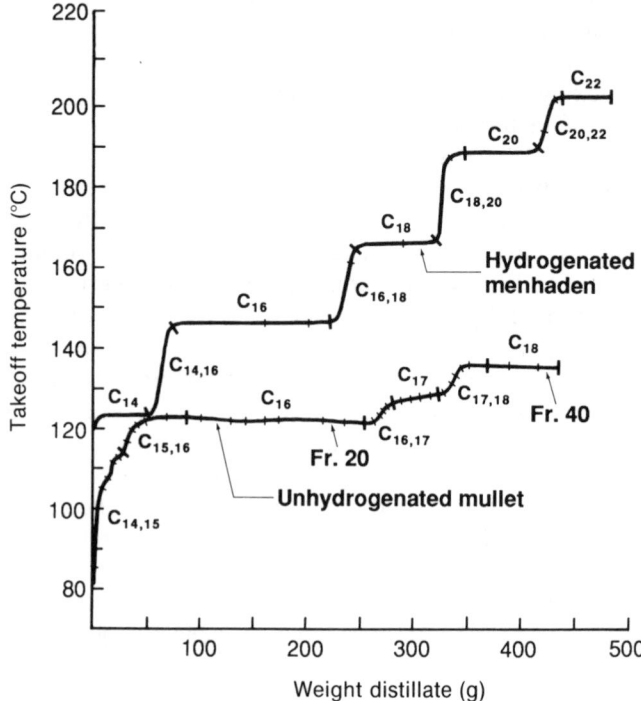

Fig. 4-6. Distillation of hydrogenated versus unhydrogenated esters. Distillation of the unhydrogenated mullet esters was stopped after 70% of the material had distilled because of degradation of the long-chain and polyunsaturated components. (Fr. indicates fraction number.)

tions 26-32), but were still less than 5% in the C_{18} components (fraction 38 of the 40-fraction process) (Fig. 4-6).

2. EPA from Herring Oil Esters. Distillation in a concentric tube column (Klenk et al. 1961) did not produce *trans* isomers, in contrast to results from packed columns such as Example 1 above.

Modified Distillation Methods

Amplified Distillation. Amplified distillation "spaced" the fractions of esters by distilling the sample together with a mixture of petroleum hydrocarbons that had the same boiling range as the esters. The method is particularly advantageous when only a few grams of material are available. It has been applied mainly to saturated and monounsaturated fatty esters and to fatty alcohol acetates (Weitkamp 1947, 1955).

Molecular Distillation.   In this technique, the molecules at very low pressure travel only a short distance between the evaporating and condensing surfaces, essentially without collisions that return them back to the pot. The principle is based on considerations developed by Langmuir (1916) and Markely (1964). Under the assumption of complete absence of extraneous gas molecules, the rate of evaporation depends on the molecular weight of the substance and its vapor pressure. For example, triolein, having a vapor pressure of 0.0043 mm at 250°C, evaporates at a theoretical rate of 2 g/min/100 cm² surface. In practice, however, the rate ranges from 90% of this value at about 0.1 μ to only 10% at 10 μ. In binary mixtures, the separation is proportional to the ratio, partial pressure/ $\sqrt{\text{mol. weight}}$ of the components.

The development of molecular stills received major impetus from the market for vitamins A and D available from fish oils (Hickman 1944; Markley 1964). Here the differences in molecular weight were large. The narrower range of molecular weights of fatty esters permits only crude enrichment, mainly by chain length rather than with respect to individual compounds. Centrifugal as well as falling film stills are commercially available; some designs also provide for several distillation stages or for recycling. Thin-film molecular stills that continuously renew the source of esters are preferred to batch operation in pot stills since heat exposure is much shorter. At a vacuum between 1 and 10 μ, the distillation temperature is 50–100°C lower than for the same substances at 1–2 mm. As already mentioned, because of the multitude of triesters (triglycerides) present in fish oils, the isolation of individual compounds is more efficient from the monoester (methyl or ethyl) derivatives than from the original triglycerides.

Examples

1. Enrichment of C_{14}–C_{16} and C_{20}–C_{22} Esters from Mullet Oil.   As the first step in the isolation of individual compounds, ~530 g of esters were distilled twice to give a volatile fraction of 350 g containing 88, 77, and 75% of the C_{14}, C_{15}, and C_{16} esters. The residue contained 56, 78, and 85% of the C_{20}, C_{21}, and C_{22} esters (Utzinger 1943, 1954). The intermediate chain lengths were distributed about evenly between the two fractions. During distillation, the esters were exposed to temperatures of <100°C for about 10 sec at a pressure of <50 μ.

2. Refinement of Menhaden Oil. Distillation through a two-stage wiped film molecular still removed nontriglyceride entities, organic contaminants, and cholesterol (Jeanne Joseph, Charleston, South Carolina, Utilization Research Laboratory of NOAA Fisheries, unpublished). The charge was specially processed menhaden oil, which had been winterized, alkali refined, and cold bleached by the producer. The first stage, operated at 150°C, with a wiper speed of 150 rpm, and under 400-μ vacuum, served to degas, dehydrate, and preheat the oil. The second stage at 260°C, 250 rpm, and 200 μ reduced chlorinated hydrocarbons and polychlorinated biphenyls (PCBs) to below detectable levels and cholesterol from ~5 mg/g to ~2 mg/g. The yield was ~95% of feed at a production rate of 8–10 kg/hr.

3. Removal of Cholesterol from Salmon Head Oil with a Codistillate. Linoleic acid added to the charge facilitated removal of cholesterol during processing in a 19-L centrifugal still (Gauglitz and Hunter, Northwest Fisheries Center, unpublished data). One of the practical difficulties in removing cholesterol from salmon head oil by molecular distillation is that the oil contains so much cholesterol that it solidifies on the condenser and clogs the feed lines. Addition of a liquid that codistills with and dissolves cholesterol reduces operating problems. Linoleic acid was selected because it is readily available in purity suitable for food-grade production. In this way, by the addition of 200 ml linoleic acid to ~19 L of raw salmon head oil, the cholesterol content was reduced from 4.7 mg/g in the charge to <0.7 mg/g, in 79% yield of product.

4. Large-Scale Fractionation of Triglycerides Versus Esters. Comparison of Northwest Fisheries Center data (Gauglitz and Hunter, unpublished data) from a 19-L centrifugal molecular still emphasizes the practical difficulty of concentrating only ω3 fatty acid from fish oil in the natural triglyceride form. The distillation of menhaden oil itself (triglycerides) effected a concentration of EPA from 16.0% originally to 19.5% in the pot residue. The distillation of ethyl esters increased the EPA content from 15.9 to 28.4%. The concentration of DHA was even more dramatic. While DHA doubled from 8.4 to 17.3% in the triglycerides, in the esters, it approached a fivefold increase from 9 to 43.9%. The changes in EPA and DHA composition over the course of molecular distillation are shown in Fig. 4-7.

FRACTIONATION USING SUPERCRITICAL FLUIDS

Several studies over the last decade have investigated supercritical fluids as both extracting and fractionating media for processing complex

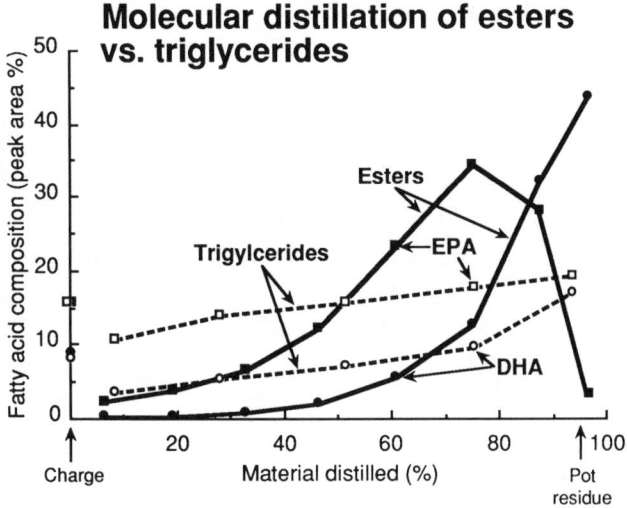

Fig. 4-7. Effectiveness of molecular distillation for concentrating ω3 components from triglycerides as compared to monoesters.

lipid mixtures. The region in which a substance exists as a supercritical fluid (SF) is defined by the critical pressure (P_c) and critical temperature (T_c) of the substance. The single-component pressure-temperature phase diagram shown in Fig. 4-8 defines the critical region for the specific case of CO_2. The physicochemical properties of supercritical fluids tend to be intermediate between those typically associated with gases and liquids (McHugh 1986). For example, supercritical fluids are generally found to have values of transport properties such as viscosity and diffusivity that are more gaslike than those typical of liquids. On the other hand, under a range of conditions the density of a SF tends to be on the order of 0.2 to 0.9 g/cc, that is, similar to liquids. This unique combination of properties makes supercritical fluids attractive for extraction and fractionation applications. The higher density of supercritical fluids results in greatly enhanced solvent power relative to gases while gaslike transport properties are favorable for many processes dependent on efficient mass transfer (McHugh and Krukonis 1986). In addition, many of the common, inexpensive substances often considered as solvents in SFE processes, for example, light hydrocarbons and carbon dioxide, have normal boiling (or in the case of CO_2, sublimation) points that are well below room temperature. Therefore, the extracted product can be obtained virtually free of solvent upon complete depressurization. For this reason, SFE processes using such solvents are of particular interest for applications in the food and pharmaceutical industries.

P-T phase diagram of CO₂

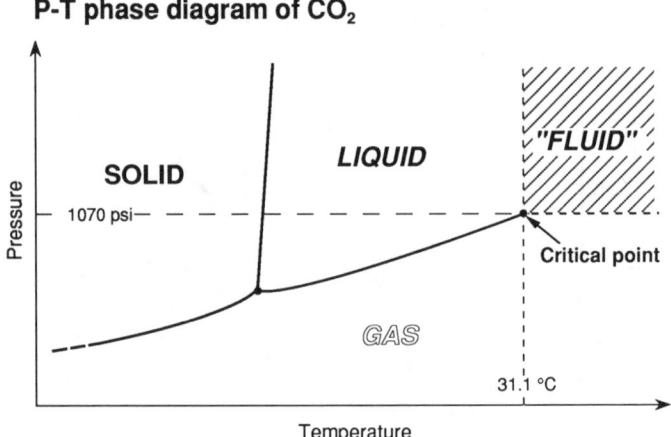

Fig. 4-8. Pressure-temperature phase diagram for CO_2. The cross-hatched area indicates the region in which CO_2 exists as a "supercritical fluid."

Carbon dioxide is among the most widely investigated solvents for food and pharmaceutical applications because it is nontoxic, nonflammable, and environmentally acceptable. Perhaps of greatest practical importance is the mild critical temperature of CO_2 (31.1°C). Consequently, SFE processing of thermally labile materials can be performed at moderate temperatures vis-à-vis more conventional methods such as fractional distillation.

Within a certain range of temperature and pressure, glycerides and glyceride derivatives dissolve to an appreciable extent in SF-CO_2. This finding, coupled with the possibility of fractionating lipid mixtures at temperatures below 100°C, has recently stimulated investigations of the fractionation of fish oils and fish oil derivatives by SFE. Most effort has been directed toward concentrating $\omega 3$ fatty acids, although some reports have shown that CO_2 SFE can effect purification of fish oil (Spinelli et al. 1987) and removal of PCBs (Krukonis 1989). Several groups have also reported fractionation of mixtures of mono-, di-, and triglycerides using various fluids (Peter and Brunner 1978; Brunner and Peter 1982; Nilsson et al. 1989A). Some enhancement of $\omega 3$ fatty acids present in fish oil triglycerides has been reported by Zosel (1978), but a significant concentration of an individual fatty acid such as $20:5\omega 3$ in triglycerides has not been clearly demonstrated, and if the goal is to produce significant quantities of highly concentrated samples of individual $\omega 3$ fatty acids, derivatization of the triglycerides to free fatty acids or alkyl esters is necessary. Early work showed that fish oil esters could be fractionated by SFE to produce DHA of 60–65% purity (Stout and Spinelli 1987). The fractionation of free fatty acids using SFE has also been demonstrated (Krukonis 1984; Rizvi et al. 1988). In each of these two studies, low recoveries of $\omega 3$ components were reported. The observed decomposition is possibly due to the formation of free radicals catalyzed by the carboxyl group of the free fatty acids (Mayashita and Takagi 1986). Decomposition was found to be especially extensive for EPA, with reported recoveries of less than 40%. Most other work has therefore been done with the less unstable ethyl esters.

Knowledge of the phase behavior of mixtures is necessary for a complete understanding of any SFE process. Sight glass experiments, which allow the visual observation of phase behavior, have established that under the conditions of pressure and temperature discussed here, the CO_2-ester system consists of two phases (Krukonis and Nilsson unpublished). The denser (lower) phase is primarily composed of fatty acid ethyl esters in which some CO_2 is dissolved. The upper phase is rich in SF-CO_2 but contains measurable quantities of esters. Fractionation of fish oil acids or esters using CO_2 SFE exploits differences in the solubility of individual components of the complex multicomponent mixture in the upper phase. As a measure of the relative solubility of a single component of a mixture in SF CO_2, we define the distribution coefficient (DC) of component A as:

$$DC(A) = \frac{(X_A)_F}{(X_A)_E} \qquad (4\text{-}1)$$

where

$(X_A)_F$ = the concentration of A in the fluid (CO_2-rich) phase
$(X_A)_E$ = the concentration of A in the ester-rich phase

Any consistent units may be used. In the following discussion, concentrations are on a weight/weight basis.

Table 4-2 shows the distribution coefficients for selected components of an ethyl ester mixture derived from menhaden oil at three sets of pressure and temperature (Nilsson and Hudson, unpublished). These DC values were obtained using the "dynamic flow" rather than the more rigorous static method (McHugh and Krukonis, 1986). Only the CO_2-rich phase was sampled directly; no information concerning CO_2 solubility in the ester-rich phase was obtained. Instead, the composition of the ester-rich phase was deduced from mass balance considerations on a CO_2-free basis. This and other errors inherent in the flow method are largely system-

Table 4-2. Distribution Coefficients (DC) for Selected Components of a Menhaden Oil Ethyl Ester Mixture in SF-CO_2 at Three Sets of T and P^a

P (psi)	T (°C)	14:0	16:0	18:1ω9	20:1ω9	20:4ω6	20:4ω3	20:5ω3	22:6ω3
		DISTRIBUTION COEFFICIENT × 10^3							
2000	70	17	9.6	6.0	3.0	3.7	3.3	3.6	1.9
2200	70	63	32	18	8.1	10	9.0	9.9	4.8
2200	90	21	11	5.5	2.2	2.9	2.5	2.8	1.1

[a]Since these values were obtained by dynamic rather than static sampling, they are accurate in a relative rather than an absolute sense. Each value represents the mean of 6–10 determinations.

atic in nature (Nilsson et al., 1987). The values shown in Table 4-2 therefore can only be considered correct in a relative sense but are nevertheless useful to illustrate a number of basic concepts.

First, at a given temperature and pressure, esters of longer chain length are less soluble, as reflected by a decrease in the DC with increasing chain length. Second, components of equal chain length but differing in degree of unsaturation have similar DC values, with those of the higher unsaturation having slightly higher solubilities. Both trends, incidentally, are qualitatively the same as those observed for ester solubility in organic solvents such as acetone at atmospheric pressure (Singleton 1960).

Table 4-2 also shows the dependence of the DC, and thus the relative solubility, on pressure and temperature. At a given temperature, a rise in pressure increases the DC and the solubility of a given component due to the increase in fluid density (and thus solvent power) with pressure. The dependence of solubility on temperature is generally not so straightforward. At 2200 psi, an increase of temperature from 70 to 90°C decreases the value of the DC for all components. This behavior, known as "retrograde condensation" (Brulé and Corbett 1984; Debenedetti and Kumar 1988), will not necessarily be observed under other sets of conditions. For example, Friedrich (1984) found that, in a certain range of temperatures at pressures above ~5000 psi, soybean oil triglyceride solubility increases with temperature, that is, exhibits nonretrograde behavior. However, at the conditions chosen for the data in Table 4-2, all components in the ester mixture exhibit retrograde behavior. The same is true of the processing conditions chosen for work discussed in the following examples.

Examples

1. Batch SF-CO_2 Fractionation of Fatty Acid Ethyl Esters Using a "Hot Finger."   Eisenbach (1984) reported results of a fractionation using an apparatus consisting of a packed column into the top of which was in-

serted a "hot finger." The process was operated at 2175 psi, with a column temperature of 50°C, a hot-finger temperature of 90°C, and a charge of 2350 g cod-liver ethyl esters. A portion of the charge that dissolved in CO_2 was driven up the column. When the solute-loaded fluid reached the top of the column, an increase in temperature brought about by the hot finger caused part of the dissolved esters to condense and fall back down as reflux due to a decrease in fluid density and associated solvent power. The rectification resulted in extract that was enriched with respect to the more soluble components present in the mixture at that point in the fractionation. As predicted by the data in Table 4-2, the extract was initially concentrated with respect to 14- and 16-carbon esters. In a like manner, the extract sequentially became enriched in 18-, 20-, and finally 22-carbon components. One fraction amounting to about 300 g contained C_{20} esters of ~96% purity. Several other fractions from this first fractionation containing only C_{18}, C_{20}, and C_{22} esters were combined to give 500 g of material for a second pass. Fractionation of this mixture yielded a second concentrate (purity 94.5%) of C_{20} esters weighing 122 g and 140 g of C_{22} esters of 98% purity. An important point that has occasionally been misunderstood is that those C_{20} concentrates were not 95+% with respect to 20:5ω3. Since the feed contained 11.4% C_{20} monoenes as well as 14.5% 20:5ω3, the 96% C_{20} fraction was about 55% 20:5ω3. Similarly, because of a relatively large C_{22} monoene content in the feed (8.6%) relative to DHA (5.7%), the 98% pure C_{22} esters could not have been more than ~40% 22:6ω3.

The distribution coefficient data in Table 4-2 for C_{20} esters provide an explanation for the failure of these fractionations to yield products of higher purity with respect to EPA. The conditions of 2200 psi and 90°C were selected to correspond closely to the pressure and hot-finger temperature used by Eisenbach. Esters differing by two carbons have DC values, and thus relative solubilities, which differ by a factor of about two or more. On the other hand, esters of equal carbon number, but differing degree and configuration of unsaturation, differ much less in their solubility and therefore are much more difficult to separate. Consequently, the technique of Eisenbach using a hot finger to effect rectification accomplished a very good separation by carbon number of feedstocks derived directly from cod-liver triglycerides, but it was limited in its ability to separate EPA from other C_{20} components. The same argument applies to DHA.

2. Batch Fractionation Using SF-CO2 with a Column Temperature Gradient.

Rectification was accomplished in a simpler apparatus by passing solute-loaded fluid through successively warmer column temperature "zones" (Nilsson et al. 1988). A schematic diagram of the apparatus is

SFE apparatus

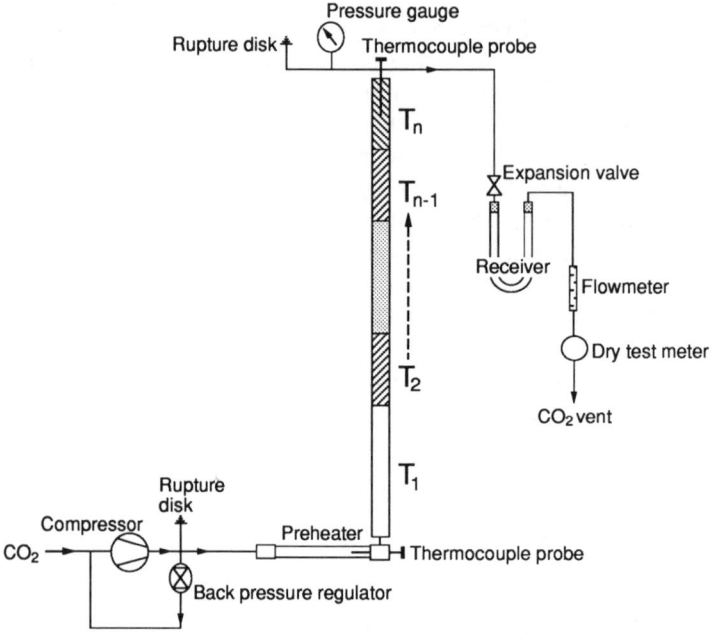

Fig. 4-9. Schematic diagram of a supercritical fluid extraction unit; T_n, T_{n-1}, . . . T_2 represent temperature "zones" maintained by $n - 1$ independently controlled heaters. T_1 was held at room temperature.

shown in Fig. 4-9: essentially, a 6' packed column was wrapped with a number of independently controlled silicon rubber heaters to establish a temperature gradient. Fractionations were carried out under conditions leading to retrograde condensation. For this reason, the temperatures increased from the bottom to the top of the column. Since the bottom was at room temperature, initially the CO_2 was actually a liquid rather than a supercritical fluid. Esters, 20–100 g, loaded into the bottom section of the vessel, dissolved in the CO_2 and were forced up the column through zones of increasing temperature. The heating in successive zones caused the condensation of a portion of the ester solute. Again, data in Table 4-2 indicate that there would be preferential condensation of longer-chain-length components. The temperature gradient thus served to sequentially enrich the rising fluid with respect to the shorter-chain-length components present in the mixture at a given point in the fractionation.

Figure 4-10 shows a set of curves for the fractionation of 20 g of whole ethyl esters derived from menhaden oil (Nilsson et al. 1987). In confirma-

SFE of whole menhaden oil esters

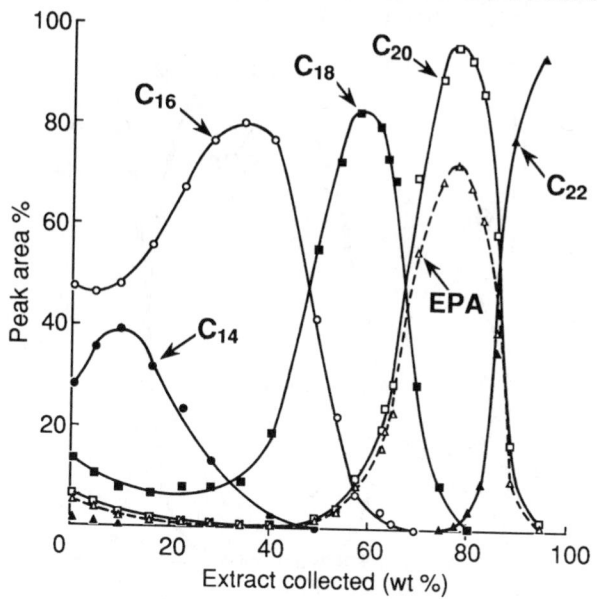

Fig. 4-10. Curves from the fractionation of whole menhaden oil esters using supercritical fluid CO_2. Solid curves represent the summation of esters of equal carbon number. Conditions: $P = 2200$ psi, $T_4 = 100°C$, $T_3 = 80°C$, $T_2 = 70°C$, $T_1 = 23°C$ (see Fig. 4-9).

tion of Eisenbach, shorter-chain-length components were recovered early in the fractionation while longer-chain-length esters were obtained in later stages. As in the previously discussed work, C_{20} and C_{22} esters were obtained in purities of ~95%. Superimposed on the fractionation curve for C_{20} esters is the single-component curve for EPA, which has a maximum at 75% purity. Eisenbach did not achieve this level of concentration of EPA from cod-liver oil, but menhaden oil typically contains a lower level of compounds that are equal in chain length to EPA, and therefore difficult to separate. The feedstock contained 17% EPA in a total of 23% C_{20}. Thus, if the process is only capable of separating by chain length, a pure C_{20} fraction could only be about 75% pure with respect to EPA, which is the maximum in the EPA curve of Fig. 4-10.

3. Batch SF-CO₂ Fractionation of Urea-Complexed Menhaden Esters. Since to a first approximation SFE, like distillation, separates by ester chain length, a second procedure that separates on the basis of degree of unsaturation is necessary either before or after fractionation using SF-

SFE of urea-complexed menhaden oil esters

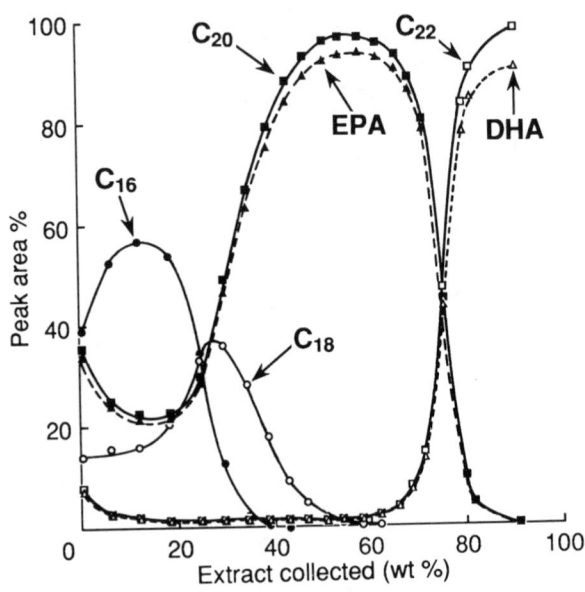

Fig. 4-11. Curves from the fractionation of urea-complexed menhaden oil esters using supercritical fluid CO_2. Solid curves represent the summation of esters of equal carbon number. Conditions: $P = 2200$ psi, $T_5 = 80°C$, $T_4 = 70°C$, $T_3 = 60°C$, $T_2 = 50°C$, $T_1 = 23°C$ (see Fig. 4-9).

CO_2 in order to obtain individual components in higher purity. Complexing with urea provides such a technique. Figure 4-11 shows the results of a fractionation of menhaden oil esters that had previously been urea complexed to remove saturated and less unsaturated components from the original mixture (Nilsson et al. 1987). The resulting feedstock prepared as described on page 82, example 5, of this chapter was more concentrated with respect to EPA (48%) and DHA (22%) and at the same time contained a smaller proportion of interfering C_{20} and C_{22} components. The fractionation was performed at 2200 psi using five distinct temperature zones. Both EPA and DHA were obtained in better than 90% purity at yields of 58% and 77%, respectively.

A number of modifications to the technique described above have recently been investigated (Nilsson et al. 1989B). Product yields can be improved by performing fractionations using incremental pressure programming rather than fractionating the mixture isobarically. As an example, consider a fractionation using column temperatures identical to those of Fig. 4-11, but instead of beginning the fractionation at 2200 psi, the initial pressure is 1900 psi. At this pressure, the short-chain C_{16} esters are appreciably soluble but those of higher carbon number are less so. Once the residual esters are depleted with respect to the C_{16} components, the pressure is raised to 2000 psi to extract the next most soluble components—in the present case C_{18} esters, and so on. Product yields are not only improved, but by the judicious selection of even lower processing pressures, successful fractionations can be carried out with maximum temperatures of 70°C and 60°C, thus further minimizing possible thermal degradation of highly unsaturated esters. The disadvantage of the use of incremental pressure programming is that for a given set of temperatures, minimization of the pressure decreases the solubility of all components (see Table 4-2). Consequently, the amount (weight) of CO_2 required to fractionate a unit weight of esters, called the solvent-to-feed ratio (S/F), will be higher than if the fractionation is performed isobarically at elevated pressures. Whereas the S/F was ~220 in the isobaric fractionation discussed initially in this example, with pressure programming, the S/F increased to 340.

4. Production Scale Continuous-Countercurrent SFE Process. Recent reports described the results of a preliminary design study for a continuous-countercurrent SFE process for the fractionation of fish oil esters (Krukonis et al. 1987; Krukonis 1988). In general terms, esters are continuously introduced into the side of a column to contact SF-CO_2 flowing in the opposite direction, that is, countercurrently. The direction of each stream depends on which is of higher density. Conditions selected for the design study were $T = 60°C$ and $P = 2200$ psi; visual observation of the ester-CO_2 system at these conditions revealed the presence of two phases, with the more dense being the ester-rich phase (Krukonis and Nilsson unpublished). Thus, the CO_2 stream would flow upward while the ester stream would flow downward.

The first step in the design of such a process is the experimental determination of distribution coefficients for all components in the starting material at the chosen process conditions. DCs are necessary for estimation of the solvent (CO_2) requirements, an important factor in evaluating the process economics. Also vital is determination of the selectivity, β, of CO_2 for extraction of a component A relative to component B, given by:

$$\beta = \left(\frac{X_A}{X_B}\right)_F \div \left(\frac{X_A}{X_B}\right)_E = \frac{DC(A)}{DC(B)} \tag{4-2}$$

where

$(X_A/X_B)_F$ = the ratio of the concentration of A to B in the fluid-rich (extract) phase

$(X_A/X_B)_E$ = the ratio of the concentration of A to B in the ester-rich phase

If $\beta > 1$, A will be preferentially extracted and the ratio of the concentration of A to B in the extract will be:

$$\left(\frac{X_A}{X_B}\right)_F = \beta\left(\frac{X_A}{X_B}\right)_E \tag{4-3}$$

If this extract is then brought into contact with an ester phase of the same composition in another stage, the extract leaving that stage will be further concentrated in A relative to B by, again, the value of β. This stagewise enhancement is the basis of countercurrent extraction.

One case studied by Krukonis et al. (1987) was the fractionation of urea-complexed menhaden oil esters. The basis of the design was production of 90% EPA in a yield of 90% at a rate of 10 lb/day. Because esters of equal carbon number have similar DCs (see Table 4-2), fatty acid ester components of equal chain length were treated as a single component and it was assumed that the feed contained only C_{16}, C_{18}, C_{20}, and C_{22} esters.

A simplified process flow sheet of a continuous-countercurrent operation for producing concentrated EPA and DHA products is shown in Fig. 4-12. For clarity, ester streams are accented and considerable detail has been omitted. The feed stream is introduced somewhere near the center of column 1 (C-1) at a location to be described below. Since the entering esters are more dense, they flow downward, contacting the upward-flowing CO_2 stream supplied from the bottom of C-1. The fluid "strips" the shorter-chain, more soluble components from the ester stream and concentrates C_{16} and C_{18} esters in the rising fluid. At the same time, the downflowing esters are enriched with respect to C_{20} and C_{22} components. The "bottoms" product, or raffinate, from C-1 is then fed into the side of column 2 (C-2) which, with the possible exception of height, is identical to C-1. Separation of C_{20} from C_{22} esters is accomplished in C-2, the more soluble C_{20} esters isolated as the overhead product while C_{22} components are obtained in the raffinate. Both columns would contain some kind of stages or "internals." The column internals are mass transfer and area-enhancing devices, for example, random or structured packing, sieve trays, or agitated components that bring about the transfer of esters between phases in order to effect the stagewise enhancement described above (Treybal 1951, 1980).

Countercurrent-continuous SFE plant for production of EPA and DHA

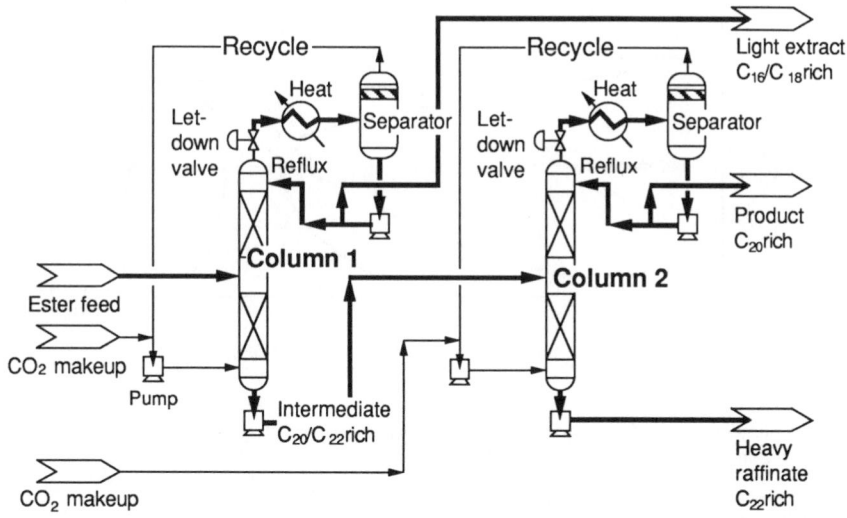

Fig. 4-12. Simplified flow diagram of a plant for continuous-countercurrent fractionation of urea-complexed menhaden oil ethyl esters using supercritical fluid carbon dioxide.

The "condenser" or "separator" isolates the extract at the top of each column by decreasing the pressure or, taking advantage of retrograde condensation, by increasing the temperature. This concomitantly serves two important purposes. First, a portion of the condensed extract is returned to the column, providing a downward-flowing stream above the feed stage. Second, the condenser accomplishes the necessary cleanup of the CO_2 before it is recycled to the bottom of the column.

Trial-and-error computational procedures were performed to determine the required number of separation stages, the composition of the esters at each stage of the column, and from these data, the best location for introduction of the feedstock. Feed is introduced at the stage at which the computed composition of the condensed esters is the same as that of the feedstock. A complete description of these procedures is beyond the scope of this discussion but is available in many mass transfer and distillation texts (Treybal 1951, 1980).

Figure 4-13 indicates the computed composition of the condensed esters by carbon numbers at each stage of C-1. An imaginary horizontal line at stage 1 (indicated as "raffinate") predicts that the condensed esters isolated at the bottom of C-1 would consist mainly of C_{20} and C_{22} components along with ~4.5% shorter-chain-length esters. Eleven stages are

Composition profiles--column 1

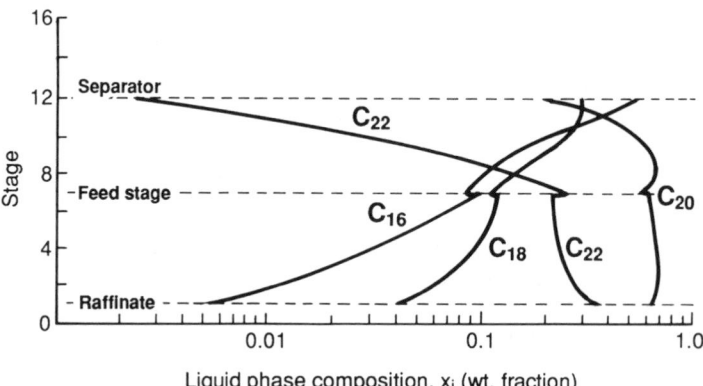

Liquid phase composition, x_i (wt. fraction)

Fig. 4-13. Concentration profiles of ethyl esters in C-1 of Fig. 4-12. A horizontal line drawn at any stage gives the CO_2-free composition of the liquid phase at that stage with respect to carbon number.

predicted to be necessary to obtain this bottoms product (the separator is not a true stage since its function is simply to condense esters leaving the highest stage). Figure 4-14 shows the analogous concentration profile for C-2. Computations predict that by use of 13 stages, the overhead product would contain EPA of 90% purity and the raffinate DHA of similar purity (Krukonis et al. 1987; Krukonis 1988).

The solvent-to-feed ratio (S/F) for the overall process was predicted to be ~30, much lower than the S/F for the batch process discussed above. This economically desirable reduction of the S/F is characteristically achieved when batch extraction is translated to continuous-countercurrent operation. The capital and operating costs were also studied, and the estimated cost of producing the 90% EPA product was ~$108/lb exclusive of the cost of producing the urea-complexed ester feedstock. This is an extremely low figure relative to current prices.

5. Feasibility of Producing EPA of High Purity from Menhaden Oil Esters Without Previous Urea-Complexing. Distribution coefficients for several of the C_{20} components typically present in menhaden oil were measured at 60°C and 2200 psi to determine whether their separation from EPA was practical (Krukonis et al. 1987). Only one of these components, 20 : 4ω6, had a DC greater than that of EPA. The selectivity of CO_2 for EPA relative to the remaining components was found to be on the order of 1.1. Although selectivity values between C_{20} components are not as large as those between components of different chain length, these data predict

Composition profiles--column 2

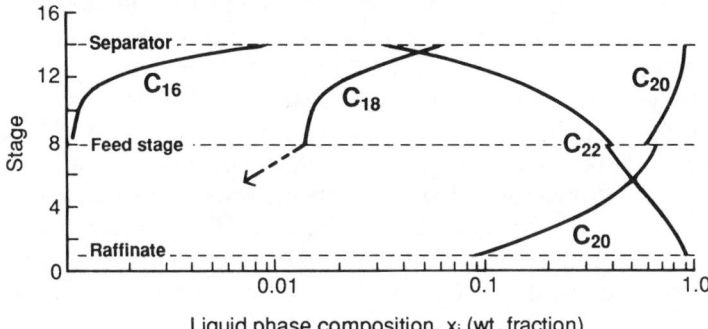

Fig. 4-14. Concentration profiles of ethyl esters in C-2 of Fig. 4-12. A horizontal line drawn at any stage gives the CO_2-free composition of the liquid phase at that stage with respect to carbon number.

that isolation of EPA in high purity using whole esters is theoretically possible using continuous-countercurrent extraction.

One possible configuration begins with the same two-column system discussed above, which again performs the separation by carbon number. As before, the overhead product of C-2 would primarily consist of C_{20} esters but would also contain about 6% C_{18} and 3% C_{22} components (see Fig. 4-14). This material would then be sent to a third column (C-3), where EPA, 20:4ω6, and the C_{18} components would constitute the overhead product while the remaining C_{20} components and the C_{22} esters would be obtained as raffinate. Finally, the EPA-rich overhead product from C-3 would be sent to yet a fourth column (C-4) to separate the C_{18} esters from the EPA and 20:4ω6, with the latter two compounds recovered as raffinate. Since the selectivity of EPA relative to the other C_{20} components is small compared to that for EPA relative to components of different chain length, many more stages would be required to carry out the separation in C-3. In practical terms, the height of C-3 would be considerably greater than that of C-1, C-2, or C-4. However, columns of 200 feet are not uncommon in the pharmaceutical and chemical process industries. The proposed four-column process is the sole example of one that could produce high-purity EPA from fish oil esters without the application of any other processes such as complexing with urea.

COUNTERCURRENT DISTRIBUTION

Separation by CCD, involving repeated distribution of solutes between two immiscible liquid phases, had a brief popularity with the advent of automatic equipment (Craig et al. 1951), but died out soon due to the complexity of the equipment. One application of CCD, liquid-solid CCD, is mentioned as an option for small-scale separations when more sophisticated equipment is unavailable. Sumerwell (1957) showed that urea, discussed under "Modified Crystallization Methods," can be used with advantage for liquid-solid CCD. Crystallizations were carried out in Erlenmeyer flasks and filtrations in Buchner funnels. Stearic, palmitic, and oleic acids were separated very satisfactorily by 24 transfers which were carried out in sequence as in a standard CCD apparatus. Figure 4-15 shows the separation of hydrogenated salmon egg fatty acids by chain length. Nonhydrogenated acids were fractionated into four distinct portions. Centrifugal partition chromatography is a recent modification of CCD that potentially can be scaled up (Murayama et al. 1988).

CHROMATOGRAPHY

Like CCD, chromatographic separations make use of the different rates of migration at which the components of a mixture move in a two-phase system. The phases may be liquid-liquid, liquid-solid, gas-liquid, or gas-solid, including SF-solid, the phases named second being the stationary ones. However, in contrast to CCD, the transport of mobile phase is by continuous flow rather than by batchwise transfers. The driving force for flow is gravity, capillarity, or pressure. The stationary phase must possess a very high surface area to provide for efficient equilibration of solute

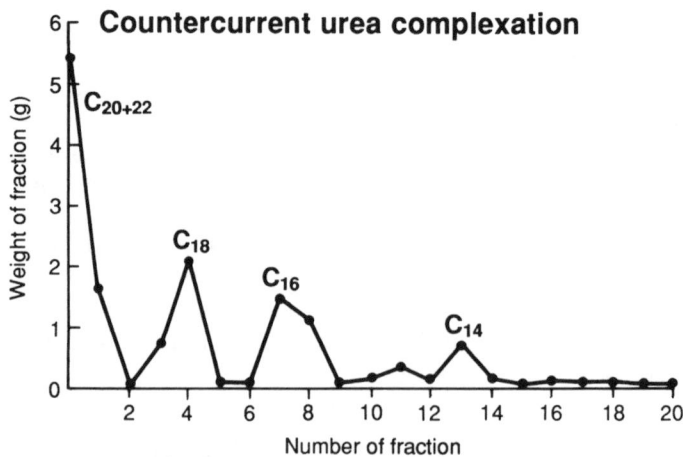

Fig. 4-15. Chain length separation of hydrogenated salmon egg oil fatty acids via liquid-solid countercurrent urea complex formation.

between the mobile and stationary phases. The advantages of very small particle size for the adsorbent or support for the stationary liquid phase must be balanced against the resistance to flow through finer materials. Over time, equipment capable of maintaining constant flow under elevated pressures has been developed along with the modern techniques of capillary GLC and HPLC.

The chromatographic separation can be visualized as follows. The sample is introduced into the stream of mobile phase and percolates with it through the stationary phase. Since a portion of the analyte is always in the stationary phase, transport of the sample is slower than the flow of the mobile solvent or gas. A compound will migrate more slowly when it is relatively more soluble in, or has an affinity for, the stationary phase; it will migrate more quickly when it is relatively more soluble in, or has an affinity for, the mobile phase. In this way, compounds are separated according to the rate at which they migrate.

Figure 4-16 describes this type of separation (Martin 1947). The horizontal arrows in the right part of the figure symbolize the chromatographic column and give the direction of flow; concentrations are indicated vertically above and below this axis. The left part of the figure represents distribution isotherms. A mixture of A and B was added at the origin with a small volume of solvent or gas. A has relatively more affinity for the mobile phase and migrates faster than B for which the distribution is more in favor of the stationary phase. Under ideal conditions (top diagram) distribution is instantaneous and independent of concentration. Actually, diffusion takes place and equilibrium is not instantaneous (center diagram), which brings about bell-shaped curves for the concentrations in the phases. Furthermore, distribution isotherms are never strictly linear (bottom diagram), and this results in tailing or skewing of the curves.

Theoretical treatment of chromatography (Martin and Synge 1941) commonly visualizes a chromatographic column as divided into a stack of plates each of which has such thickness that the sample leaving one plate is equilibrated between the two phases of this volume. The concept of plates derived for the theory of fractional distillation was later applied to chromatography. Common to both methods, and SFE as well, is the need for numerous equilibrations of the sample between two phases, but in distillation the system is made up solely by the sample, while in SFE and chromatography another component—gas, liquid, fluid, or solid—participates. Similarly, reference to CCD has been taken as a model for the chromatographic process. However, conditions are better defined in CCD than chromatography where the many factors affecting distribution, transport, and separation are difficult to evaluate (Craig 1950). Theory

Principles of chromatographic separation

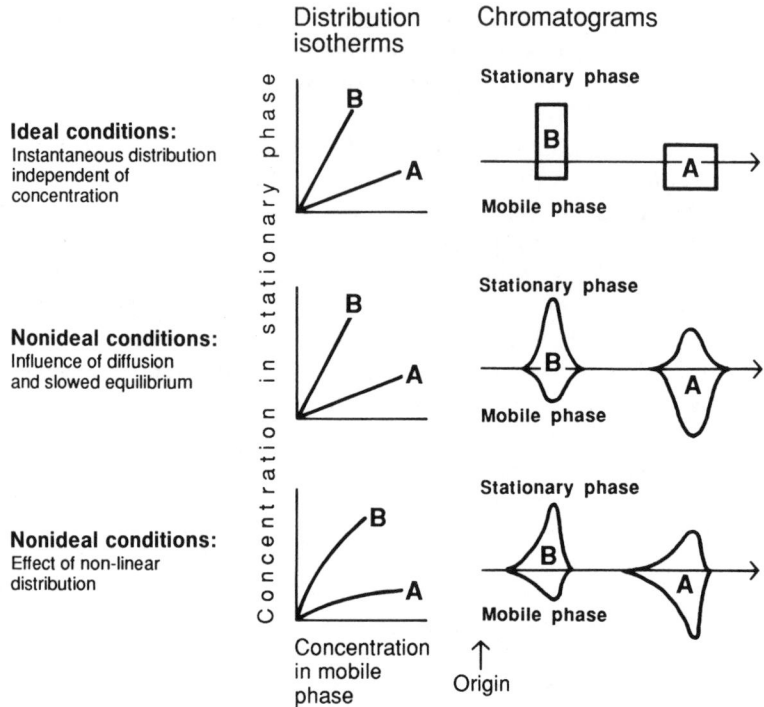

Fig. 4-16. Chromatographic separation of a two-component system under ideal and nonideal conditions.

and experimental data of chromatographic procedures meet best in GLC and HPLC.

LSC and LLC are often contrasted as absorption and partition chromatography. Both are of importance as column procedures for the sample sizes discussed here and still have merit today when expensive equipment is not available. Thin-layer chromatographic (TLC) separations on such a scale are mostly the result of multiple operations on a much smaller scale and, therefore, are not discussed here (see Chapter 3). Development of GLC was mainly toward analysis on microscale; nonetheless, some small-scale preparative work will be discussed here. HPLC has become the method of choice for large-scale, rapid separations and is discussed in detail.

Silicic acid is the preferred adsorbent for LSC. It was used in many early preparations of unsaturated acids (Herb et al. 1951A, B; Hammond and Lundberg 1953; Privett et al. 1959). Low-boiling petroleum ether with small percentages of diethyl ether is a typical solvent for adsorption chromatography.

Low-vulcanized latex powder was the first stationary phase that rendered good separation of homologous and of vinylogous fatty acids by LLC (Boldingh 1953). Paraffin oil on a carrier of water-repellent diatomaceous earth was used with fish oil acids (Silk and Hahn 1954A, B) and heptane with other polyunsaturated esters (Matic 1958; Privett et al. 1959; Privett and Nickell 1963). Silicone oil on untreated diatomaceous earth substituted for hydrocarbon phases in work on menhaden and mullet esters (Schlenk and Gellerman 1961; Sen and Schlenk 1964). Typical mobile phases for partition chromatography of fatty acids or esters are methanol, acetone, or acetonitrile, all containing 10–30% water.

The stationary phases of these systems are less polar than the mobile phases, in contrast to the chromatographic systems for amino acids or carbohydrates. There the stationary phase was always more polar than the mobile phase. Hydrophobic lipids require solvent pairs where the relative polarity of the phases is reversed. According to historical development, since stationary phases for lipids were developed later, the systems for lipids are called reversed-polarity or reversed-phase systems.

The reversed-polarity systems quoted above yield about equal separations. The choice is mainly determined by convenience in preparing the column, its stability, and potential reuse; by facile monitoring and analysis of the eluate; and by easy removal of solvents and of a stationary phase that is eluted with the sample. For subsequent GLC analysis of fractions and for increased detection sensitivity, it is more expedient to use esters instead of acids.

It was mentioned earlier that palmitic + oleic, and myristic + palmitoleic + linoleic, and other homologous-vinylogous combinations superimpose in LLC (see Fig. 4-1). Although this pattern can be slightly shifted under special conditions, it is often more expedient to attempt perfect superposition rather than improved resolution of single components. Further separations are then simplified. Figure 4-17 serves as an example where a rather complex mixture has been subjected to LLC (Gellerman and Schlenk 1965). In this experiment, 14 components have been separated into five portions and there is no overlapping from fraction to fraction. Subsequent separation by GLC was possible on a relatively large scale since each fraction contained only one component of each chain length.

Recently developed equipment which allows rapid pumping of the mobile phase with high pressure and small particle size column packing uses all the principles of LLC, but has the advantage of greater speed of

LLC separation pattern

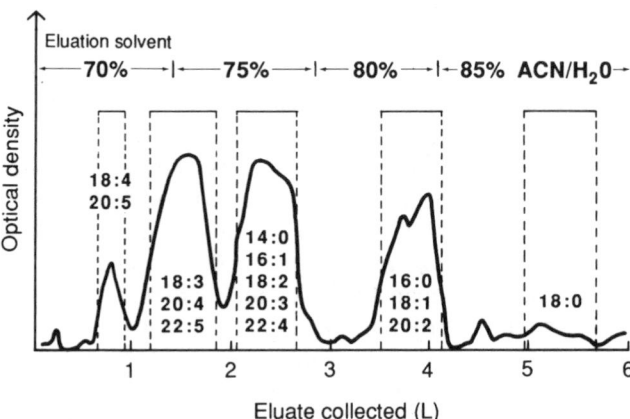

Fig. 4-17. Fractionation of methyl esters from lipids of the protozoan, *Ochromonas danica,* by liquid-liquid chromatography on silicone oil. (Positional isomerism of double bonds was ignored.)

separation. This technique has come to be called high-performance (or pressure) liquid chromatography (HPLC). As with LLC, reversed-phase (polarity) systems are chosen for maximum efficiency in separating fatty acid esters (Scholfield 1975; Bascetta et al. 1984). Typically, the stationary liquid phase is a C_8 or C_{18} hydrocarbon bonded to a solid support such as silica. Columns are commercially available in a wide variety of sizes and configurations to effect analytical as well as production-scale separation. The mobile phase is a more polar solvent. The choice of solvent depends on the desired separation, considerations of reuse or disposal of recovered solvent, and hazards of handling the solvent.

Fatty acid esters can be detected in the eluate with a refractive index detector only if the run is done isocratically. Alternatively, UV detectors set at wavelengths of 210, 212, 215, 223, 245, or 254 nm monitor the polyunsaturated double bonds. Fatty acids esterified with a fluorescent agent can be detected with a fluorometer (Ichinose et al. 1984). A mass detector is another approach to peak location (Christie 1987). Fatty acid identification is usually confirmed by capillary GLC.

Emphasis today is on the need for highly purified fractions of EPA and DHA to be used in biomedical research. Separations are done on fish oil acids or esters that have been concentrated in polyunsaturates by one or a combination of the enrichment techniques already mentioned, such as urea adduct complexation coupled with fractional distillation (Wille et al.

1987; Perrut 1988; Tokiwa et al. 1981). The enrichment eliminates coeluting saturates, monoenes, and dienes from the fractions shown in Fig. 4-17, and attention can be given to optimizing resolution of the remaining compounds or to enhancement techniques such as silver resin HPLC or supercritical fluid chromatography (SFC).

Solvent choice for the separation of fatty acid esters depends on the desired purity of the eluted fractions, end use of the eluted fractions, and production requirements. The following authors used C_{18} bonded columns and fish oil fatty acid esters enriched in polyunsaturates by urea fractionation. Tokiwa et al. (1981) separated 10 g of methyl esters using tetrahydrofuran : methanol : water (25 : 55 : 20) to yield fractions of EPA and DHA at 91% and 85.5% purity, respectively. Methanol : water (90 : 10) was used to separate 136 g of ethyl esters (Perrut 1988) and 90 g of methyl esters (Wille et al. 1987). Perrut (1988) obtained purities of 91–96% EPA and 75–85% DHA. Wille et al. (1987) obtained optimum purities of 86% EPA and 83% DHA. Purities of 98% EPA and 92% DHA were separated from 60 g of ethyl esters using ethanol : water (80 : 20) as the mobile phase (Krzynowek et al. 1988). Krzynowek et al. (1988) obtained higher-purity fractions of EPA and DHA using the THF system of Tokiwa et al. (1981) (Table 4-3). However, THF oxidizes readily and is potentially explosive. It requires special OSHA considerations that assure safe handling and waste disposal. THF is also undesirable because THF peroxides would initiate autoxidative decomposition of the polyunsaturated structure of the fatty acids. Methanol, the solvent used by the others cited, as well as THF, is toxic to humans. Ethanol and water would be the solvents of choice if the end product might be consumed by humans, because the solvents can be purchased as food grade materials, require no special OSHA handling or waste disposal measures, and do not oxidize.

Table 4-3. Purity of Eluted EPA/DHA Fractions from a Fish Oil Concentrate Containing 48% EPA and 24% DHA Comparing Two Mobile Phases on Two Analytical HPLC Columns of Differing Particle Size

MOBILE PHASE COMPOSITION	PACKING PARTICLE SIZE	PURITY OF ELUTED FRACTION[a]	
		% EPA	% DHA
THF : MeOH : H$_2$O	8 μm	99	95
15 : 65 : 20	20–30 μm	99	89
EtOH : H$_2$O	8 μm	98	92
80 : 20	20–30 μm	97	87

[a]Purities expressed as percent of total fatty acid ethyl esters.

Krzynowek et al. (1988) discussed other parameters that could be changed to obtain higher-purity fractions of EPA and DHA with the corresponding trade-offs in yields or in production rates. For instance, the smaller particle size solid supports of about 8 μm yielded higher-purity EPA and DHA than particle sizes of about 30 μm (Table 4-3), but the flow (production) rate was necessarily slower through the 8-μm column. Furthermore, the higher the purity of the starting material, the higher the purity of the resulting EPA and DHA in the eluate (Table 4-4). The starting materials labeled at 79% purities were obtained through urea fractionation of fish oil esters followed by SFE, a technique described above.

Preparative-scale separations by GLC specifically for lipids are discussed in older reviews (Horning et al. 1964; Henly 1965). Fulco and Mead (1959, 1960) isolated polyenoic acids from 100–300 mg of concentrate using GLC. Schlenk and Sand (1962) and Gellerman and Schlenk (1965) further separated *Ochromonas danica* methyl esters previously fractionated by LLC (Fig. 4-17) using GLC (Fig. 4-18). Jones (1988) points out in a recent review of preparative/production-scale chromatography that there are only two companies which supply preparative-scale GLC equipment today, showing the move to other techniques.

As in distillation, so in GLC, conditions suitable for gramwise separation of low-boiling mixtures cannot be extrapolated to high-boiling fatty esters. Major difficulties in preparative GLC of fatty esters are: the requirement for rapid evaporation of a large sample without decomposition; the size, in particular the diameter, of a column having an efficiency equivalent to that of an analytical column; instability of the sample and of the stationary phase during prolonged heating; and satisfactory recovery of the fractions. Nonetheless, samples of esters prefractionated by LLC (Fig. 4-17) were separated into individual compounds by preparative GLC as shown in Fig. 4-18 (Schlenk and Sand 1962; Gellerman and Schlenk

Table 4-4. Purity of Eluted EPA/DHA Fractions Using THF : MeOH : H$_2$O as the Solvent System on an Analytical HPLC Column with Differing Concentrations of EPA and DHA in the Starting Material

STARTING MATERIAL COMPOSITION[a]	PURITY OF ELUTED FRACTIONS[a]	
% EPA/% DHA	% EPA	% DHA
32/19	98	82
57/31	99	89
79% EPA	100	—
79% DHA	—	96

[a] Percent of total fatty acid ethyl esters.

GLC separation pattern of LLC fraction

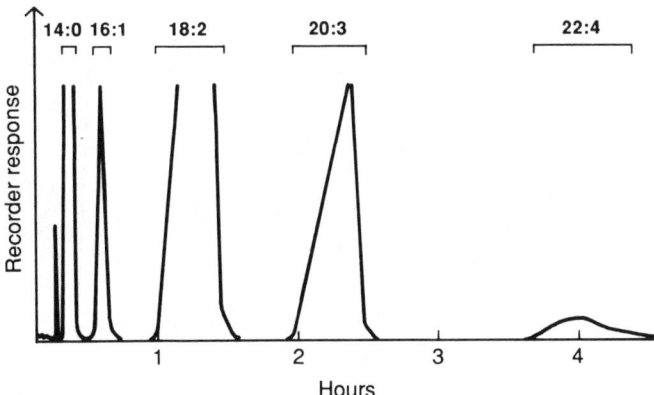

Fig. 4-18. Gas-liquid chromatographic separation of a 100-mg fraction of esters obtained by LLC (shown in Fig. 4-17).

1965). Despite exposure to a temperature of 300°C in the inlet and 236°C in the column, the process succeeded without alteration of the all-*cis,* methylene-interrupted structure of the polyunsaturated esters. With different systems, Fulco and Mead (1959, 1960) isolated pure polyenoic esters and Hardy and Keay (1967) separated a concentrate from cod-liver oil. For many separation problems, repeated operation on a relatively small scale may be preferable to expanding the capacity by considerable investment in large-scale equipment.

Examples

1. Isolation of Pure DHA and Methyl Arachidonate by LSC.   Hog brain fatty esters, enriched in 22 : 6, were further fractionated by adsorption chromatography on silicic acid (Hammond and Lundberg 1953). A column, 6 × 104 cm, was prepared with about 1300 g of a mixture of SiO_2 : celite, 4 : 1. A sample of 50 g of concentrate chromatographed in petroleum ether containing 1.75% diethyl ether yielded a recovery of about 85%. Rechromatography of the pertinent portion gave 22 : 6 ester in a purity of ~95%, with 22 : 5 being the probable chief contaminant. Further chromatography yielded 22 : 6, which satisfied all purity criteria.

This same method was used for the separation of methyl arachidonate from EPA (Privett and Nickell 1963). At low concentrations of diethyl ether in petroleum ether, the pentaenoate is held on the column while

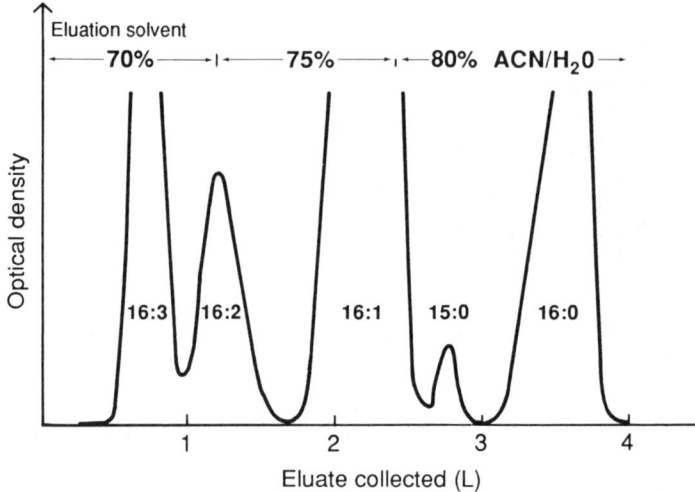

Fig. 4-19. Liquid-liquid chromatographic separation on silicone oil of the C_{16} fraction of methyl esters from mullet oil.

tetraenoate is eluted. Privett and Nickell (1963) used heptane as the stationary phase for a reversed-phase separation of 22 : 5 and 22 : 6.

2. Separation of C_{16} Mullet Oil Methyl Esters by Reversed-Phase LLC.   The 16 : 0, 16 : 1, 16 : 2, and 16 : 3 components were isolated with a high-boiling fraction of Dow Corning No. 200, 10 cs, silicone oil as the stationary phase. First a 300-g mixture of silicone oil and untreated celite, 1 : 1, was rinsed into the column with acetonitrile : water (70 : 30). Then 1 g of C_{16} mullet esters was applied. The concentration of water was lowered during the procedure, and pure compounds eluted as indicated in Fig. 4-19 (Sen and Schlenk 1964). The chromatogram of *O. danica* esters, which is shown in Fig. 4-17, was carried out under very similar conditions.

Peaks were located by adding water to an aliquot of the effluent and then measuring the optical density of the resultant emulsion. Esters were recovered by evaporation of part of the solvent and extraction with petroleum ether. They were purified from contaminating silicone oil, <1.5%, either by alembic distillation or saponification and extraction.

Celite as commercially received is used; the columns need not be thermostated and can be reused several times; monitoring is simple and rapid. On the other hand, molecular distillation of the commercial silicone oil is advisable, and the final purification from traces of this phase is a nuisance.

3. Separation of Menhaden Oil Fatty Acid Esters by HPLC. Menhaden oil ethyl esters, enriched in polyunsaturates by urea adduct fractionation and molecular distillation, have been separated on C_{18} bonded phase columns using ethanol : water (80 : 20) as the mobile phase (Krzynowek et al. 1988). Ten grams were separated on a column, 45 mm × 25 cm, at a flow rate of 50 ml/min, and 60 g were separated on a column, 10 cm × 60 cm, at 240 ml/min (Fig. 4-20). Final purities of 98% EPA and 92% DHA at 70% yields can be obtained with these columns.

Modified Chromatographic Methods

Argentation. Unsaturated fatty esters in solutions of silver nitrate form rather unstable complexes by interaction of the electrons of the double bond with the silver ion. Differences in the equilibria can be exploited for CCD and chromatographic separations (Winstein and Lucas 1938; Nichols 1952). When silver nitrate is added to the system of aqueous methanol: heptane, it dissolves in the polar portion. The stationary phase is thus modified to distinguish specifically by unsaturation. In this way, oleate, linoleate, and linolenate are easily separated. Isomeric dienes resulting from the reduction of linolenate with hydrazine were fractionated into 9,15–18 : 2 and 9,12–18 : 2 + 12,15–18 : 2. Separation of *cis* and *trans* isomers was also accomplished (Butterfield et al. 1964). Silver nitrate is inconvenient to handle when working with large volumes. Therefore, argentation is applied more often in chromatography than in CCD.

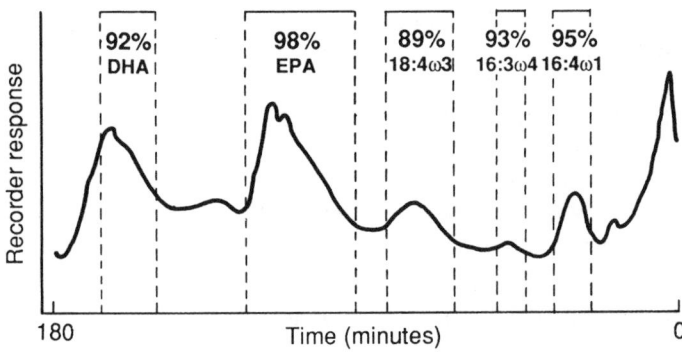

Preparative HPLC of omega-3 esters

Fig. 4-20. HPLC separation of 60 g of enriched fish oil ethyl esters on a C_{18} reversed-phase column using ethanol : water (80 : 20). (*Note:* This trace runs in the reverse direction from those in preceding figures.)

Although the method was applied mainly to TLC in the past, 2-g samples were separated according to unsaturation on columns of SiO_2 + $AgNO_3$ (Privett and Nickell 1963). The samples consisted of C_{18} + 20 : 4 or 22 : 5 + 22 : 6 esters. The eluent was petroleum ether : diethyl ether with a gradient of composition from 100 : 0 to 0 : 100.

Cation exchange resins saturated with silver were used for separation of 18 : 1, 18 : 2, and 18 : 3 esters on a milligram scale (Wurster et al. 1963), and for the separation of *cis* and *trans* monoenoic and dienoic isomers in amounts of 400 mg (Emken et al. 1964).

Argentation chromatography was initially adapted to HPLC by impregnating $AgNO_3$ onto silica gel HPLC columns (Mikes et al. 1973; Heath et al. 1977; Scholfield 1979; Battaglia and Frohlich 1980). The $AgNO_3$ bled from these columns under pressurized flows, however, coating the detection cells and contaminating the samples.

More recently, columns packed with cation exchange resins saturated with silver ions have been used successfully with HPLC in the separation of unsaturated esters. The Northern Regional Research Center, United States Department of Agriculture Laboratory in Peoria, Illinois, has done considerable research using silver resin chromatography for the separation of both vegetable and fish oil fatty acids or their methyl esters (Rakoff and Emken 1978; Adlof et al. 1980; Adlof and Emken 1980, 1981, 1985; DeJarlais et al. 1983). Optimally, they fractionated 100 mg of fish oil concentrate methyl esters containing 29.1% EPA and 20.5% DHA into fractions of 87.7% EPA and 95.4% DHA using solvent programming with increasing amounts of acetonitrile (0–30%) in methanol. They also fractionated 9 g and 8 g of nonenriched menhaden methyl esters and fatty acids, respectively, which contained about 12.5% EPA and 11.1% DHA. The separation was done isocratically using about 40% acetonitrile in acetone to yield one of the eluted fractions concentrated to about 69% EPA plus DHA.

Mercuration.   Olefinic double bonds form stable methoxy acetoxymercury compounds. These derivatives provide another alternative for fractionation of unsaturated esters by LLC or LSC in columns (Jantzen and Andreas 1961; White and Quackenbush 1962A, B). However, the argentation method appears more attractive for chromatographic procedures.

Preparative Supercritical Fluid Chromatography

Along with gases and liquids, supercritical fluids (see Fig. 4-8) can also be used as a mobile phase in chromatography. Since the first report (Klesper et al. 1962), interest in SFC has grown, in large part owing to the development of reliable HPLC pumping systems capable of operating at higher pressures which have in turn been adapted for SFC. Among the cited advantages of SFC (Lee and Markides 1987) are:

1. The relatively high density and low critical temperature of fluids such as CO_2 permit analysis of low vapor pressure and thermally sensitive materials without derivatization.
2. Separation efficiency per unit time is generally better than that observed in HPLC, since supercritical fluids have viscosities and densities that are intermediate between those of gases and liquids.
3. Solute retention times can be controlled using three programming methods. Like GC, temperature programming is available. Also, controlled addition of a second solvent to the mobile phase (often called a "modifier") offers a method of adjusting the mobile phase composition which is the basis for HPLC gradient programming methods. Finally, unique to SFC is the ability to pressure (or density) program, a technique first demonstrated by Jentoft and Gouw (1970). An excellent discussion of various SFC programming methods has been published recently (Klesper and Schmitz 1988).

Although to date SFC has been used primarily as an analytical tool, like HPLC it also shows some promise as a preparatory technique. In this regard, SFC offers another potential advantage; assuming the use of a pure fluid such as CO_2 or low-boiling short-chain hydrocarbons, the product(s) isolated by preparative SFC would be virtually free of solvent. To date, there is a single report (Berger et al. 1988) on the use of preparative SFC for producing concentrates of individual components from fish oil esters.

Example

Isolation of DHA by Preparatory SFC. A recent report (Berger et al. 1988) describes a preparative SFC method for isolating high-purity DHA from fish oils. The authors used a 6 cm × 60 cm column with reverse-phase C_{18} (45–60 μm) packing and UV detection. The methyl ester feed, which had been previously urea-complexed and further concentrated by SFE, contained 73% DHA and 15% EPA. An hourly injection rate of 17.5 g yielded 7.3 g/hr of DHA of 89.8% purity. The authors, who did not attempt isolation of high-purity EPA, performed over 100 runs to investigate the influence of pressure, temperature, feedstock composition, and mobile-phase flow rate on the purity of the final product. In one test, DHA of 95% purity was obtained from a feedstock containing 81% DHA. It was concluded that preparatory SFC holds promise for isolating EPA and DHA from fish oil esters and that the reported results could be greatly improved upon. Since the authors do not report utilizing any of the programming methods offered by SFC, this conclusion certainly appears warranted.

REFERENCES

Abu-Nasr, A. M., Potts, W. M., and Holman, R. T. 1954. Highly unsaturated fatty acids. II. Fractionation by urea inclusion compounds. *J. Am. Oil Chem. Soc.* 31:16–20.

Ackman, R. G., Ke, P. J., and Jangaard, P. M. 1973. Fractional vacuum distillation of herring oil methyl esters. *J. Am. Oil Chem. Soc.* 50:1–8.

Adlof, R. O., and Emken, E. A. 1980. Partial argentation resin chromatography (PARC): II. Separation of saturated and mono-, di-, tri- and tetraenoic fatty esters. *J. Am. Oil Chem. Soc.* 57:276–278.

Adlof, R. O., and Emken, E. A. 1981. Partial argentation resin chromatography (PARC): III. The effects of sodium ion incorporation and solvent on the separation of mixtures of fatty acids, of fatty esters, and of triglycerides. *J. Am. Oil Chem. Soc.* 58:99–101.

Adlof, R. O., and Emken, E. A. 1985. The isolation of omega-3 polyunsaturated fatty acids and methyl esters of fish oils by silver resin chromatography. *J. Am. Oil Chem. Soc.* 62:1592–1595.

Adlof, R. O., Rakoff, H., and Emken, E. A. 1980. Partial argentation resin chromatography (PARC): I. Effect of percent silver on elution and separation of methyl octadecadienoate isomers. *J. Am. Oil Chem. Soc.* 57:273–275.

Aurousseau, A., and Bauchart, D. 1980. Stepwise purification of fatty acids: compared fractional crystallization with urea or from acetone solutions of palmitoleic, heptadecaenoic, and oleic acids. *J. Am. Oil Chem. Soc.* 57:125–128.

Bascetta, E., Gunstone, F. D., and Scrimgeour, C. M. 1984. The purification of fatty acid methyl esters by high pressure liquid chromatography. *Lipids* 19:801–803.

Battaglia, R., and Frohlich, D. 1980. HPLC-separation of cis and trans monounsaturated fatty acids. *Chromatographia* 13:428–431.

Bauchart, D., and Aurousseau, B. 1980. Preparation of heptadecaenoic acid from *Candida tropicallis* yeast. *J. Am. Oil Chem. Soc.* 57:121–124.

Bengen, F. 1940; 1953. Decomposing mixtures of organic compounds. German Patent 869,070, appl. date March 18, 1940; granted March 2, 1953.

Berger, C., Jusforgues, P., and Perrut, M. 1988. Purification of unsaturated fatty acid esters by preparative supercritical fluid chromatography. Paper read at the 1st International Symposium on Supercritical Fluids, Oct. 17–19:1988, at Nice, France.

Boldingh, J. 1953. The separation of fatty acids by chromatography. *Int. Conf. Biochem. Probl. Lipids, Proc. 1st,* 1953, 64–81.

Brockerhoff, H., and Hoyle, R. J. 1963. On the structure of the depot fats of marine fish and mammals. *Arch. Biochem. Biophys.* 102:452–455.

Brown, J. B., and Kolb, D. K. 1955. Applications of low temperature crystallization in the separation of the fatty acids and their compounds. *Prog. Chem. Fats Other Lipids* 3:57–94.

Brulé, M. R., and Corbett, R. W. 1984. What makes critical-solvent processes work? *Hydrocarbon Process* 63(6):73–77.

Brunner, G., and Peter, S. 1982. On the solubility of glycerides and fatty acids in compressed gases in the presence of an entrainer. *Sep. Sci. Tech.* 17:199–214.

Butterfield, R. O., Scholfield, C. R., and Dutton, H. J. 1964. Preparation of 9,15-octadecadienenoate isomers. *J. Am. Oil Chem. Soc.* 41:397–400.

Christie, W. W. 1987. A stable silver-loaded column for separation of lipids by high performance liquid chromatography. *J. High Resolut. Chromatogr. Chromatogr. Commun.* 10:148–150.

Corey, E. J., Shih, C., and Chapman, J. R. 1983. Docosahexaenoic acid is a strong inhibitor of prostaglandin but not leukotriene biosynthesis. *Proc. Natl. Acad. Sci. U.S.A.* 80:3581–3584.

Craig, L. C. 1950. Partition chromatography and countercurrent distribution. *Anal. Chem.* 22:1346–1352.

Craig, L. C., Hausmann, W. H., Ahrens, E. H., Jr., and Harfenist, E. J. 1951. Automatic countercurrent distribution equipment. *Anal. Chem.* 23:1236–1244.

Debenedetti, P. G., and Kumar, S. K. 1988. The molecular basis of temperature effects in supercritical extraction. *AIChE J.* 34:645–657.

DeJarlais, W. J., Adlof, R. O., and Emken, E. A. 1983. Acetonitrile as eluent in silver resin column chromatography. *J. Am. Oil Chem. Soc.* 60:975–978.

Domart, C., Miyauchi, D. T., and Sumerwell, W. N. 1955. The fractionation of marine-oil fatty acids with urea. *J. Am. Oil Chem. Soc.* 32:481–483.

Drew, D. A., and Hixson, A. N. 1944. The solubility relations of high molecular weight fatty acids and their esters in propane near the critical temperature. *Trans. Am. Inst. Chem. Eng.* 40:675–694.

Eisenbach, W. O. 1984. Supercritical fluid extraction: A film demonstration. *Ber. Bunsenges. Phys. Chem.* 88:882–887.

Emken, E. A., Scholfield, C. R., and Dutton, H. J. 1964. Chromatographic separation of *cis* and *trans* fatty esters by argentation with a macroreticular exchange resin. *J. Am. Oil Chem. Soc.* 41:388–390.

Friedrich, J. P. 1984. Supercritical CO_2 extraction of lipids from lipid-containing material. U.S. Patent 4,466,923, Aug. 21, 8 pp.

Fulco, A. J., and Mead, J. F. 1959. Origin of 5,8,11-eicosatrienoic acid in the fat-deficient rat. *J. Biol. Chem.* 234:1411–1416.

Fulco, A. J., and Mead, J. F. 1960. The biosynthesis of the octadecadienoic acids in the rat. *J. Biol. Chem.* 235:3379–3384.

Gellerman, J. L., and Schlenk, H. 1965. Preparation of fatty acids labeled with ^{14}C from *Ochromonas danica*. *J. Protozool.* 12:178–189.

Haagsma, N., van Gent, C. M., Luten, J. B., de Jong, R. W., and van Doorn, E. 1982. Preparation of an ω3 fatty acid concentrate from cod liver oil. *J. Am. Oil Chem. Soc.* 59:117–118.

Hammond, E. G., and Lundberg, W. O. 1953. A methyl docosahexaenoate: Its isolation and characterization. *J. Am. Oil Chem. Soc.* 30:438–441.

Hardy, R., and Keay, J. N. 1967. The isolation of the polyunsaturated acids of the fish oils as their methyl esters by preparative scale gas chromatography. *J. Chromatogr.* 27:474–479.

Heath, R. R., Tumlinson, J. H., and Doolittle, R. E. 1977. Analytical and preparative separation of geometrical isomers by high efficiency silver nitrate liquid chromatography. *J. Chromatogr. Sci.* 15:10–13.

Henly, R. S. 1965. Preparative gas-liquid chromatography of lipids. *J. Am. Oil Chem. Soc.* 42:673–681.

Herb, S. F., Riemenschneider, R. W., and Donaldson, J. 1951A. Isolation of natural arachidonic acid as its methyl ester. *J. Am. Oil. Chem. Soc.* 28:55–58.

Herb, S. F., Witnauer, L. P., and Riemenschneider, R. W. 1951B. Isolation of eicosapentaenoic and docosahexaenoic acids from natural sources as their methyl esters by adsorption and distillation techniques. *J. Am. Oil Chem. Soc.* 28:505–507.

Hickman, K. C. D. 1944. High-vacuum short-path distillation. *Chem. Rev.* 34:51–106.

Hixson, A. W., and Bockelmann, J. B. 1942. Liquid-liquid extraction employing solvents in the region of their critical temperatures. *Trans. Am. Inst. Chem. Eng.* 38:891–930.

Horning, E. C., Karmen, A., and Sweeley, C. C. 1964. Gas chromatography of lipids. *Prog. Chem. Fats Other Lipids* 7(2):167–246.

Ichinose, N., Nakamura, K., Shimizu, C., Kurokura, H., and Okamoto, K. 1984. High-performance liquid chromatography of 5,8,11,14,17-eicosapentaenoic acid in fatty acids (C_{18} and C_{20}) by labeling with 9-anthryldiazomethane as a fluorescent agent. *J. Chromatogr.* 295:463–470.

Jangaard, P. M. 1965. A rapid method for concentrating highly unsaturated fatty acid methyl esters in marine lipids as an aid in their identification by GLC. *J. Am. Oil Chem. Soc.* 42:845–847.

Jantzen, E., and Andreas, H. 1961. Reaction of unsaturated fatty acids with mercury(II)-acetate. The use for preparative separation (in German). *Chem. Ber.* 94:628–633.

Jantzen, E., and Wieckhorst, O. 1954. Concentric tube columns for efficient distillation at low pressure (in German). *Chem. Ing. Tech.* 26:392–396.

Jentoft, R. E., and Gouw, T. H. 1970. Pressure-programmed supercritical fluid chromatography of wide molecular weight mixtures. *J. Chromatogr. Sci.* 8:138–142.

Jones, K. 1988. A review of very large scale chromatography. *Chromatographia* 25:547–559.

Klenk, E., Oette, K., Kohler, J., and Scholl, H. 1961. Metabolism of polyenoic fatty acids (in German). *Hoppe-Seyler's Z. Physiol. Chem.* 323:270–277.

Klesper, E., Corwin, A. H., and Turner, D. A. 1962. High pressure gas chromatography above critical temperatures. *J. Org. Chem.* 27:700–701.

Klesper, E., and Schmitz, F. P. 1988. Gradient methods in supercritical fluid chromatography. *J. Supercrit. Fluids* 1:45–69.

Krukonis, V. J. 1984. Supercritical fluid fractionation of fish oils—Concentration of eicosapentaenoic acid. Paper read at the 75th Annual Meeting of the American Oil Chemists' Society, Apr. 29–May 3, 1984, at Dallas, Tex.

Krukonis, V. J. 1988. Processing with supercritical fluids. Overview and applications. In *Supercritical Fluid Extraction and Chromatography.* ACS Sym. Ser. 366:26–43.

Krukonis, V. J. 1989. Supercritical fluid processing of fish oils: Extraction of polychlorinated biphenyls. *J. Am. Oil Chem. Soc.* 66:818–821.

Krukonis, V. J., Bambara, C. J., Vivian, J. E., Nilsson, W. B., and Martin, R. M. 1987. Concentration of eicosapentaenoic acid by supercritical fluid extraction: A design of a continuous production process. Paper read at the 194th ACS Meeting, Aug. 30–Sept. 4, 1987, at New Orleans, La.

Krzynowek, J., D'Entremont, D. L., Panunzio, L. J., and Maney, R. S. 1988. Purification of omega-3 fatty acids from fish oils using HPLC: An overview. *Proc. 12th Ann. Conf. Trop. Subtrop. Fish. Technol. Soc.,* pp. 74–77.

Langmuir, J. 1916. Evaporation, condensation and reflection of molecules, and the mechanism of adsorption. *Phys. Rev.* 8:149–176.

Lee, M. L., and Markides, K. E. 1987. Chromatography with supercritical fluids. *Science* 235:1342–1347.

Lehman, L. W., and Gauglitz, E. J., Jr. 1964. Synthesis of triglycerides from fish oil fatty acids. *J. Am. Oil Chem. Soc.* 41:533–535.

Linko, R. R., and Karinkanta, H. 1970A. Fatty acids of long chain length in Baltic herring lipids. *J. Am. Oil Chem. Soc.* 47:42–46.

Linko, R. R., and Karinkanta, H. 1970B. Fractionation of Baltic herring flesh oil fatty acids by urea adduct formation. *Suom. Kemistil. B* 43:311–314.

Markley, K. S. 1964. Techniques of separation. A. Distillation, salt solubility methods, low temperature crystallization. In *Fatty Acids*, 2nd ed., part III, ed. K. S. Markley, pp. 1983–2123. New York: Interscience Publishers.

Martin, A. J. P. 1947. The principles of chromatography. *Endeavor* 1947:21–28.

Martin, A. J. P., and Synge, R. L. M. 1941. A new form of chromatogram employing two liquid phases. *Biochem. J.* 35:1358–1368.

Matic, M. 1958. South African pilchard oil. 7. The isolation and structure of an octadecatetraenoic acid from South African pilchard oil. *Biochem. J.* 68:692–695.

Mayashita, K., and Takagi, T. 1986. Study on the oxidative rate and prooxidant activity of free fatty acids. *J. Am. Oil Chem. Soc.* 63:1380–1384.

McHugh, M. 1986. Extraction with supercritical fluids. *Recent Dev. Sep. Sci.* 9:75–106.

McHugh, M. A., and Krukonis, V. J. 1986. *Supercritical Fluid Extraction—Principles and Practice*. Boston: Butterworth.

Mehlenbacher, V. C. 1960. *The Analysis of Fats and Oils*, pp. 502–504. Champaign, Ill.: Garrard Press.

Mikes, F., Schurig, V., and Gil-Av, E. 1973. Complex-forming stationary phases in high-speed liquid chromatography. *J. Chromatogr.* 83:91–97.

Monick, J. A., Allen, H. D., and Marlies, C. J. 1946. Vapor-liquid equilibrium data for fatty acids and fatty methyl esters at low pressures. *J. Am. Oil Chem. Soc.* 23:177–182.

Moreno, J. M. M., and Roncero, A. V. 1964. The application of urea inclusion compounds in fat analysis. In *Analysis and Characterization of Oils, Fats, and Fat Products*, vol. 1, ed. H. A. Boekenoogen, pp. 95–118. New York: Interscience Publishers.

Murayama, W., Kosuge, Y., Nakaya, N., Nunogaki, Y., Nunogaki, K., Cazes, J., and Nunogaki, H. 1988. Preparative separation of unsaturated fatty acid esters by centrifugal partition chromatography (CPC). *J. Liq. Chromatogr.* 11:283–300.

Murray, K. E. 1955. Low pressure fractional distillation and its use in the investigation of lipids. *Prog. Chem. Fats Other Lipids* 3:243–273.

Nichols, P. L., Jr. 1952. Coordination of silver ion with methyl ester of oleic and elaidic acids. *J. Am. Chem. Soc.* 74:1091–1092.

Nilsson, W. B., Gauglitz, E. J., Jr., and Hudson, J. K. 1989B. Supercritical fluid extraction of fish oil esters using incremental pressure programming and a temperature gradient. *J. Am. Oil Chem. Soc.* 66:1596–1600.

Nilsson, W. B., Gauglitz, E. J., Jr., Hudson, J. K., Stout, V. F., and Spinelli, J. 1988. Fractionation of menhaden oil ethyl esters using supercritical fluid CO_2. *J. Am. Oil Chem. Soc.* 65:109–117.

Nilsson, W. B., Gauglitz, E. J., Jr., Hudson, J. K., and Teeny, F. M. 1987. Supercritical fluid CO_2 fractionation of fish oil esters. Paper read at the 194th ACS Meeting, Aug. 30–Sept. 4, 1987, at New Orleans, La.

Nilsson, W. B., Stout, V. F., Gauglitz, E. J., Jr., Teeny, F. M., and Hudson, J. K. 1989A. The use of SF-CO_2 in the synthesis of trieicosapentaenoylglycerol from fish oil. In *Supercritical Fluid Science and Technology*. ACS Sym. Ser. 406:434–448.

Patokina, E. V., Alekseev, S. M., Sarycheva, I. K., Karpova, G. V., and Evstigneeva, R. P. 1988. Adductive crystallization of fatty acids with urea. 3. Calculation of equilibrium phase-composition in multicomponent mixtures of fatty acid esters (in Russian). *Khim. Farm. Zh.* 22(9):1129–1132.

Perrut, M. 1988. Purification of polyunsaturated fatty acid (EPA and DHA) ethyl esters by preparative high performance liquid chromatography. *LC-GC* 6:914, 916, 920.

Peter, S., and Brunner, G. 1978. The separation of nonvolatile substances by means of compressed gases in countercurrent processes. *Angew. Chem. Int. Engl.* 17:746–750.

Privett, O. S., and Nickell, E. C. 1963. Preparation of highly purified fatty acids via liquid-liquid partition chromatography. *J. Am. Oil Chem. Soc.* 40:189–193.

Privett, O. S., Weber, R. P., and Nickell, E. C. 1959. Preparation and properties of methyl arachidonate from pork liver. *J. Am. Oil Chem. Soc.* 36:443–449.

Rakoff, H., and Emken, E. A. 1978. Silver resin chromatographic separation of methyl *cis*- and *trans*-mono- and dihydroxy fatty esters. *J. Am. Oil Chem. Soc.* 55:564–566.

Ratnayake, W. M. N., Olsson, B., Matthews, D., and Ackman, R. G. 1988. Preparation of omega-3 PUFA concentrates from fish oils via urea complexation. *Fat Sci. Technol.* 90:381–386.

Rizvi, S. S. H., Chao, R. R., and Liaw, Y. J. 1988. Concentration of omega-3 fatty acids from fish oil using supercritical carbon dioxide. In *Supercritical Fluid Extraction and Chromatography*. ACS Sym. Ser. 366:89–108.

Rose, A. 1936. Distillation efficiency in 3- and 6-mm fractionating columns. *Ind. Eng. Chem., Ind. Ed.* 28:1210–1212.

Saito, S. 1986. Supercritical gas extraction of food and natural products. II. Application to condensation of ethanol and to separation of polyunsaturated fatty acids (in Japanese). *Kagaku to Seibutsu* 24:201–210.

Schlenk, H. 1954. Urea inclusion compounds of fatty acids. *Progr. Chem. Fats Other Lipids*, 2:243–267.

Schlenk, H. 1961. Crystallization of fatty acids. *J. Am. Oil Chem. Soc.* 38:728–736.

Schlenk, H., and Gellerman, J. L. 1961. Column chromatography of fatty acids. *J. Am. Oil Chem. Soc.* 38:555–562.

Schlenk, H., and Holman, R. T. 1950. Separation and stabilization of fatty acids by urea complexes. *J. Am. Chem. Soc.* 72:5001–5004.

Schlenk, H., and Sand, D. M. 1962. Collection of gas liquid chromatography fractions by gradient cooling. *Anal. Chem.* 34:1676.

Schlenk, H., and Sand, D. M. 1967. Fractionation Methods. In *Fish Oils, Their Chemistry, Technology, Stability, Nutritional Properties, and Uses*, ed. M. E. Stansby, pp. 75–106. Westport, Conn.: Avi Publishing Co.

Schlenk, W., Jr. 1949. The urea addition of aliphatic compounds (in German). *Justus Liebigs. Ann. Chem.* 565:204–240.

Scholfield, C. R. 1975. High performance liquid chromatography of fatty methyl esters: Preparative separations. *Anal. Chem.* 47:1417–1420.

Scholfield, C. R. 1979. Silver nitrate-high performance liquid chromatography of fatty methyl esters. *J. Am. Oil Chem. Soc.* 56:510–511.

Sen, N., and Schlenk, H. 1964. The structure of polyenoic odd- and even-numbered fatty acids of mullet (*Mugil cephalus*). *J. Am. Oil Chem. Soc.* 41:241–247.

Silk, M. H., and Hahn, H. H. 1954A. South African pilchard oil. 3. The fatty acid composition of South African pilchard oil. *Biochem. J.* 57:577–582.

Silk, M. H., and Hahn, H. H. 1954B. South African pilchard oil. 4. The isolation and structure of a hexadecatetraenoic acid from South African pilchard oil. *Biochem. J.* 57:582–587.

Silk, M. H., Sephton, H. H., and Hahn, H. H. 1954. South African pilchard oil. 2. Concentrates of highly unsaturated fatty acids and alcohols derived from South African pilchard oil. *Biochem. J.* 57:574–577.

Singleton, W. S. 1948. Phase investigations of fats. II. Systems containing oleic and stearic acids and an organic solvent. *J. Am. Oil Chem. Soc.* 25:15–20.

Singleton, W. S. 1949. Phase investigations of fats. III. Systems containing oleic and palmitic acids and an organic solvent. *J. Am. Oil Chem. Soc.* 26:332–336.

Singleton, W. S. 1960. Solution properties. In *Fatty Acids*, 2nd ed., part I, ed. K. S. Markley, pp. 609–678. New York: Interscience Publishers.

Skau, E. L., and Boucher, R. E. 1954. An interpolative method of calculating solubilities of missing members of homologous series. *J. Phys. Chem.* 58:460–468.

Smith, A. E. 1952. Crystal structure of the urea-hydrogen complexes. *Acta Cryst.* 5:224–235.

Spinelli, J., Stout, V. F., and Nilsson, W. B. 1987. Purification of fish oils. U.S. Patent 4,692,280, Sept. 8, 6 pp.

Stout, V. F. 1963. A simple procedure for obtaining docosahexaenoic acid. *J. Am. Oil Chem. Soc.* 40:40.

Stout, V. F., and Spinelli, J. 1987. Polyunsaturated fatty acids from fish oils. U.S. Patent 4,675,132, June 23, 6 pp.

Sumerwell, W. N. 1957. Liquid-solid countercurrent distribution of fatty acids with urea. *J. Am. Chem. Soc.* 79:3411–3415.

Suzuki, Y. 1988. Fractionation of fish oil esters by using supercritical carbon dioxide (in Japanese). *Kagaku Kogaku* 52:516–518.

Swern, D. 1964. Techniques of separation. E. Urea complexes. In *Fatty Acids*, part III, ed. K. S. Markley, pp. 2309–2358. New York: Interscience Publishers.

Takahashi, K., Hirano, T., and Saito, M. 1988. Application of partition chromatographic theory for the analysis of marine triglyceride molecular species. *Nippon Suisan Gakkaishi* 54(3):523–528.

Tokiwa, S., Kanazawa, A., and Teshima, S. 1981. Preparation of eicosapentaenoic and docosahexaenoic acids by reversed phase high performance liquid chromatography. *Bull. Jap. Soc. Sci. Fish.* 47:675.

Traitler, H., Wille, H. J., and Studer, A. 1988. Fractionation of black currant seed oil. *J. Am. Oil Chem. Soc.* 65:755–760.

Treybal, R. E. 1951. *Liquid Extraction.* New York: McGraw-Hill.

Treybal, R. E. 1980. *Mass Transfer Operations.* New York: McGraw-Hill.

Utzinger, G. E. 1943. Concerning a new molecular distillation apparatus and short-path fractionation (in German). *Angew. Chem.* 56:130–131.

Utzinger, G. E. 1954. Short-path fractionation (in German). *Chem. Ing. Tech.* 26:129–131.

Weitkamp, A. W. 1947. The amplified distillation of methyl esters of fatty acids. *J. Am. Oil Chem. Soc.* 24:236–238.

Weitkamp, A. W. 1955. Distillation. *J. Am. Oil Chem. Soc.* 32:640–646.

White, H. B., Jr., and Quackenbush, F. W. 1962A. Isolation of pure linolenate as its mercuric acetate adduct. *J. Am. Oil Chem. Soc.* 39:517–519.

White, H. B., Jr., and Quackenbush, F. W. 1962B. Separation of fatty ester-mercuric acetate adducts on alumina. *J. Am. Oil Chem. Soc.* 39:511–513.

Wille, H. J., Traitler, H., and Kelly, M. 1987. Production of polyenoic fish oil fatty acids by combined urea fractionation and industrial scale preparative "HPLC." *Rev. Fr. Corps Gras* 34:69–74.

Winstein, S., and Lucas, H. J. 1938. The coordination of silver ion with unsaturated compounds. *J. Am. Chem. Soc.* 60:836–847.

Wright, S. W., Kuo, E. Y., and Corey, E. J. 1987. An effective process for the isolation of docosahexaenoic acid in quantity from cod liver oil. *J. Org. Chem.* 52:4399–4401.

Wurster, C. F., Jr., Copenhaver, J. H. Jr., and Shafer, P. R. 1963. Separation of the methyl esters of oleic, linoleic, and linolenic acids by column chromatography using cation exchange resin containing silver ion. *J. Am. Oil Chem. Soc.* 40:513–514.

Zosel, K. 1978. Separation with supercritical gases: Practical applications. *Angew. Chem. Int. Ed. Engl.* 17:702–709.

Chapter 5
DETERIORATION

Maurice E. Stansby

INTRODUCTION

Fish oils are much more subject to deterioration than are other fats or oils. Such deterioration will be discussed in this chapter. After a brief description of the mechanism of such changes and its reduced action as a result of the presence of natural or added antioxidants, the types of odors and flavors will be discussed. This will be followed by a section on methods of measurement of such changes. Not only the use of chemical measurements will be included, but also the use of organoleptic (sensory) procedures.

MECHANISM OF OXIDATION AND ACTION OF ANTIOXIDANTS

When polyunsaturates in an oil are exposed to air, there is a time interval called the induction period during which it appears that no oxidation is occurring. At the end of the induction period, rapid uptake of oxygen, called autoxidation, takes place. These changes occur in accordance with the following reactions:

Initiation step

$$
\begin{array}{ccc}
\text{H} \quad \text{H} \quad \text{H} & & \text{H} \quad \text{H} \quad \text{H} \\
\text{R—C}{=}\text{C—C—R}_1 \rightarrow & \text{R—C}{=}\text{C—C—R}_1 & \text{(hydrocarbon} \\
\text{H} & \cdot & \text{chain radical)}
\end{array} \qquad (1)
$$

Propagation steps

$$
\begin{array}{ccc}
\text{H} \quad \text{H} \quad \text{H} & & \text{H} \quad \text{H} \quad \text{H} \\
\text{R—C}{=}\text{C—C—R}_1 + \text{O}_2 \rightarrow & \text{R—C}{=}\text{C—C—R}_1 & \text{(hydroperoxy} \\
\cdot & \text{O} & \text{radical)} \\
& \cdot &
\end{array} \qquad (2)
$$

$$\underset{\substack{| \\ O \\ | \\ O \\ \cdot}}{\overset{\text{H H H}}{R-C=C-C-R_1}} + \underset{\substack{| \\ H}}{\overset{\text{H \quad H}}{R-C=C-C-R_1}} \rightarrow \qquad (3)$$

$$\underset{\substack{| \\ O \\ | \\ OH}}{\overset{\text{H H H}}{R-C=C-C-R_1}} + \underset{\substack{\\ \cdot}}{\overset{\text{H H H}}{R-C=C-C-R_1}}$$

Propagation of the chain involves both hydrocarbon and hydroperoxy free radicals yielding as an end product a nonradical hydroperoxide. As a result of further decomposition of the hydroperoxide, additional radicals are formed, which in turn initiates new chains.

$$\underset{R_1}{\overset{H}{R-C-OOH}} \rightarrow \underset{R_1}{\overset{H}{R-C-O\cdot}} + \cdot OH \qquad (4)$$

This accounts for the accelerating rate of oxidation at the end of the incubation period. The length of the induction period is determined by the temperature, the availability of oxygen, and the presence or absence of pro- or antioxidants. The length of the induction period is decreased by increases of temperature, by the amount of light, and by the presence of heavy-metal salts, peroxides, or other sources of free radicals.

Enzymatic Involvement of Lipid Oxidation

The mechanism of oxidation of fatty acids in fish oils, which in the past has been assumed to be a purely chemical change, is at least in some cases involved with enzymatic activity. Many recent papers have shown that certain enzymatic activities in some cases initiate the oxidation reaction. A paper by Josephson et al. (1984) was perhaps the earliest one to point out that most of the previous work suggested that the initiation of lipid oxidation was a purely chemical reaction. However, many indications that enzymes might possibly be involved appeared in earlier papers. They showed that oxidation of the freshwater fish, emerald shiner, was initiated through enzymatic action. A paper by Hsieh and Kinsella (1986) contains a very good summary of work up to 1986 on oxidation of oils, especially where enzymatic action is involved, and these authors describe their own experiments on the lipoxygenase-catalyzed oxidation of ω6 and ω3 fatty acids, especially with relation to the action in fish tissue. Since then many investigators have published papers along these lines.

ANTIOXIDANTS

Antioxidants are substances which interfere with the chain of reactions that occur when oils are oxidized. The antioxidant reacts with the original free radical or one forming early in the oxidation process in such a way as to form an intermediate that is unable to continue the chain. Where AH is the antioxidant, the following is a simplified version of what goes on:

$$
\begin{array}{c}
\overset{H\ \ H\ \ H}{R-C-C=C-R_1} + AH \rightarrow \overset{H\ \ H\ \ H}{R-C-C=C-R_1} + A\cdot \\
\underset{\cdot}{} \qquad\qquad \underset{H}{}
\end{array} \tag{5}
$$

$$
\begin{array}{c}
\overset{H\ \ H\ \ H}{R-C-C=C-R_1} + AH \rightarrow \overset{H\ \ H\ \ H}{R-C-C=C-R_1} + A\cdot \\
O \qquad\qquad\qquad O \\
O \qquad\qquad\qquad O \\
\cdot \qquad\qquad\qquad H
\end{array} \tag{6}
$$

$$
A\cdot + \overset{H\ \ H\ \ H}{R-C=C-C-R_1} \quad \text{(does not react)} \tag{7}
$$
$$
\underset{H}{}
$$

$$
A\cdot + A\cdot \rightarrow AA \quad \text{(terminates)} \tag{8}
$$

Various substances that have been found to have properties enabling them to enter into these oxidizing equations and act as antioxidants are used to slow down the rate of oxidation of fish oils. For use in food, an antioxidant must be one approved by governmental agencies as being safe to use. The following antioxidants are currently approved for use in foods in the United States by the U.S. Food and Drug Administration:

Butylated hydroxyanisole (BHA)
Butylated hydroxy toluene (BHT)
Dehydroacetic acid (Ethoxyquin)
Tertiary butylhydroquinone (TBHQ)
2,4,5-Trihyroxybutyrophenone (THBP)

Synergists are substances that have little or no antioxidant properties by themselves, but, when added to an antioxidant, greatly increase its activity. Some substances that may exert synergistic effects are ascorbic acid, ascorbyl palmitate, lecithin, citric acid, isopropyl citrate, and phosphoric acid.

Natural Antioxidants

The antioxidants mentioned so far are ones that do not occur in the fish oils but that are added to them to increase the length of their induction period. Most fish oils contain naturally occurring antioxidants, the most common of which is tocopherol. Table 5-1 lists the tocopherol content of the oils of several species of fish.

The fact that sablefish has the highest content of tocopherol in the oil of the muscle may account for the great stability against oxidation of this species (Dolev and Olcott 1965).

ODORS AND FLAVORS IN DETERIORATED FISH OILS

Objectionable odors of fish oils sometimes hinder their use in industry. With other factors such as price and adaptability to use being equal, the oil chosen for a given application is apt to be one having no undesirable odor or flavor characteristics. Where the application is in a strictly industrial area, this facet may not be given great weight. Where the use affects the general public, the presence of fishy odors usually excludes such uses. For example, wider use of fish oils in paint, especially for wall paints used in building interiors, has been hindered by objectionable reversion odors appearing during drying of the paint.

In rare instances, however, the reverse situation occurs, and a charac-

Table 5-1. Tocopherol Content of the Muscle of Several Species of Fish[a]

SPECIES	TOCOPHEROL CONTENT, μ/g OIL
Sardine	40
Menhaden	70
Tuna	160
Herring	140
Whale	220
Sablefish	630

[a] Einset, Olcott, and Stansby (1957).

teristic fish odor is considered desirable. Leather for shoes, for example, as a result of the use of fish oils in the tanning process, acquires a faint odor now considered characteristic of new shoes. This odor actually is a diluted "fishy" odor. When efforts made to develop a superior fish oil for leather tanning resulted in a nonfishy odor that did not impart the desirable "new shoe" odor, the new fish oil product was rejected by the tanning industry. Such instances are very rare; far more often the use of fish oils is discouraged by undesirable odors.

Undesirable flavor of extracted fish oils greatly hampers their use for any sort of human consumption. Preparation of cod-liver oils lays great stress on the use of well-preserved fish livers, with initial rendering sometimes carried out at sea to minimize undesirable flavors. Faint flavors in fish liver oils sometimes have to be masked by the addition of peppermint or other flavors. The use of fish body oils for their cholesterol depressant activity in the form of salad or cooking oils has been discouraged by their adverse flavor characteristics.

ODOR AND FLAVOR PROBLEMS IN UTILIZING EDIBLE FISHERY PRODUCTS

Odors and particularly flavor of fresh and frozen fish as well as other fishery products, especially those destined for human consumption, play a major role in determining quality. The presence of normal flavor components in the oil of fresh or frozen fish, for example, makes the major difference between a prime, highest-quality product and a run-of-the-mill one, readily marketable but lacking attributes of a first-class product. The presence of oxidized or otherwise altered fish oil in such products often marks the principal dividing line between a barely acceptable and completely unmarketable one. One of the principal aims of fishery food science, in fact, is to minimize undesirable flavor alteration in fishery products. A major cause of such alterations results from the deterioration of oils in the fish.

As with odor, sometimes an altered or deterioration flavor in the oil of fish, as a result of an acquired taste, is preferred to the natural one. The characteristic flavor of most salt fish, for example, results from the presence of some rancidity derived from partially oxidized oil in the flesh.

"FISHY" ODORS AND FLAVORS IN NONFISHERY PRODUCTS

Flavors and odors similar or identical to those occurring in fish sometimes are found in other foods. This may result from consumption of fish oil in the feed of animals or poultry later used as human food. In some cases disagreeable odors or flavors in other foods may be described as "fishy" even when their characteristics bear only a remote, if any, relationship to those occurring in fish.

Farm animals fed fish oil at moderate to high levels in the diet have the chemical makeup of their depot fat altered so that a higher proportion of fatty acids characteristic of fish oils appears in the animal fat. The same situation develops when the diet of poultry includes any considerable proportion of fish oil. Accompanying this phenomenon is the development of off-flavors in the meat (Oldfield and Anglemier 1957) or poultry (Klose et al. 1951) flesh which are sometimes described as "fishy." The off-flavors apparently do not result from post mortem oxidation of the somewhat more unsaturated fat of the meat or poultry flesh but rather appear immediately after slaughter.

When considering the relevancy of "fishy" odors and flavors in non-fishery products to our problems concerning flavors and odors in fish oil, we must be sure that the odors and flavors described are the same or at least bear some relationship to those occurring in fish oil. Mere descriptions of flavors and odors are often ambiguous since different investigators may use the same descriptive term to mean quite different things. A sample of pork described as "fishy" by a panel of tasters at a laboratory engaged in meat research was not considered "fishy" by a panel at a laboratory working exclusively with fish, but rather was described by some members of the latter panel as having odors and flavors reminiscent of mutton.

These considerations bring up the question of just what is meant by the term "fishy." Is it some one odor and flavor or type of odor and flavor, is it a term used for several types, or is it an almost meaningless word perhaps reserved for almost any obnoxious odor or flavor?

WHAT ARE "FISHY" ODORS AND FLAVORS?

It has been suggested by Stansby (1962) that there are several quite distinct odors and flavors that are described as "fishy." These several distinct and separate odors or flavors may each separately have some definite to vague relationship to fish handled or treated in some way, yet each one may be quite different from the others. Odors and flavors occurring in fish oils are, in general, the same as occur in other fishery products. Stansby and Jellinek (1965) have classified odors and flavors found in various fishery products as shown in Table 5-2. Although as indicated in this table some of the listed odors and flavors are found primarily in fish

Table 5-2. Flavors and Odors in Fishery Products

TYPE	DESCRIPTION	PRINCIPAL SOURCE	PREDOMINANCE AS FLAVORS (F) OR ODOR (O)	
			PRIMARY	SECONDARY
A	Aminelike	Slightly stale to spoiled fish	O	—
B	Burnt	Fish oils and fish meals	O	F
F	Freshwater fish	Freshly caught freshwater fish, in skin and to lesser extent in flesh	O	F
G	Green	Fish oils	F	O
I	Iodinelike	Certain species such as sole, especially after they have been feeding on some particular types of food	F	O
N	Natural species giving characteristic flavors and odors	Flesh and oil of many fish such as salmon or herring	F	O
O	Pure oxidation types, occurring at early stages of oxidation	Fish oils and meals and oily fish, especially after extended storage primarily in the frozen state	F	O
P	Putrid or spoiled; very obnoxious types of flavor and odors such as those derived from certain sulfur compounds	Spoiled fish and fishery products	O	F
R	Pure oxidation types occurring at late states of oxidation	Fish oils, fish meals, frozen and other preserved fish	F	O
S	Sweet; an intense sweet odor that at extremes may border on the putrid but at low concentration is generally quite unobjectionable	Well-iced fish kept for a relatively long time	O	F

flesh, any of these various "fishy" components may occur at least in small quantities of fish oils. Some odors and flavors occur naturally in the fish or fish oil while others result from one or another kind of deterioration. Some arise from bacterial spoilage of the fish from which the oil was manufactured, whereas others arise from changes in the oil after manufacture such as result from oxidation. These various odors and flavors associated with fish oils are combinations of these several types. Since these odors and flavors arise from a variety of different causes, a logical way of discussing them is to consider them according to manner of origin.

ODORS AND FLAVORS ASSOCIATED WITH PURE FISH OIL TRIGLYCERIDES

Natural Flavors

Oxidized Flavors and Odors.   When fish oil triglycerides oxidize, two quite distinct types of odors and flavors develop. At high levels of oxidation a rancidity occurs that is similar to that which develops in other unsaturated oils. At very early stages of rancidity a quite different flavor, sometimes vaguely described as "fishy," occurs.

Fish oils, like other natural oils, oxidize in such a way that when the degree of oxidation is plotted against storage time a more or less typical induction type of curve results with an accelerating rate of oxidation as the oxidation proceeds. The break in the induction curve for fish oils is less sharp than that obtained with most other oils. The beginning of the increase in peroxide number also occurs sooner than for most other oils such that the early lag phase, which with most oils is nearly parallel to the time axis, shows a small but definite upward slope. During this early oxidation period when peroxide numbers are still very low, a type of oxidative flavor develops that is quite characteristic of fishery products and that can best be described as similar to the flavor of a good grade of cod-liver oil.

This characteristic flavor, described in Table 5-2 as type O, is best noted as a flavor, with only a poorly defined odor counterpart. The flavor in a given sample ordinarily has only transitory duration. In a stored fish oil sample exposed to air, the original flavor characteristic of the species first usually gradually diminishes, followed by the occurrence of this type O flavor, which, however, is quite soon overshadowed by the development of stronger-flavored substances of later occurring oxidation type ordinarily referred to as rancid (type R in Table 5-2). If other types of flavors, caused by the presence of impurities, occur in the fish oil, it is unlikely that the less pronounced type O flavor will be recognized as such, but rather it will blend into the overall composite flavor.

This type O flavor forms to a more pronounced extent when the fish oil is stored with a limited access to air, for example, in a stoppered vessel containing some head space above the oil but with no possibility for additional air to enter the container. Under such conditions, the type O "fishy" flavors will develop, but with insufficient oxygen present to produce the ordinary rancidity flavors, the type O flavor will remain almost indefinitely.

Rancidity in fish oils is quite similar in characteristics to the rancid flavors and odors in many vegetable oils, yet it possesses some properties, especially in regard to flavor, that are somewhat different. The flavor differences are so subtle as to be most difficult to describe. Perhaps there is a carryover of some of the type O "fishiness" from the early oxidative change which, although effectively masked by the more pronounced characteristic rancidity, nevertheless renders a slightly different note to rancid fish oils. The overall type R flavor is certainly one that anyone familiar with extremely rancid cottonseed oil or with oxidized linseed oil would unquestionably describe as rancid. There is the sharp initial, unpleasant flavor followed by a prolonged aftertaste.

Different degrees of fish oil rancidity are readily detectable. Even untrained observers can readily recognize such degrees (Table 5-3), ranging from the barely distinguishable rancidity with no aftertaste, described as very slight, to the extremely rancid one characterized by exceedingly disagreeable flavor and aftertaste.

Relatively little research has been carried out to determine the chemical substances responsible for rancid odors and flavors in fish oils. What little work has been done along such lines has been largely concerned with substances occurring as a result of advanced stages of oxidation with compounds identified after aeration of the oil for long periods of time.

Yu et al. (1961) and Wyatt and Day (1963) isolated and identified from an oxidized salmon oil many carbonyls with carbon chain lengths of C_1 to C_{12}, alkenals (C_4 to C_{12}), several alk-2-enals, and C_6 to C_{10} alk-2, 4-dienals. Chipault (1959) found in oxidized menhaden oil alkenals of

Table 5-3. Readily Distinguishable Fish Oil Rancidity Degrees

DEGREE	FLAVOR DESCRIPTION	AFTERTASTE DESCRIPTION
Very slight	Barely distinguishable	Usually absent
Slight	Flavor weak but quite definite and somewhat objectionable to many	Slight
Moderate	Unpleasant to most	Lasting; undesirable to most
Pronounced	Undesirable to almost everyone and quite objectionable to many	Persistent, annoying
Extreme	Exceedingly disagreeable	Very disagreeable

carbon chain length up to six, C_3, C_4, and C_5 methyl ketones, and several diketones. Chipault and McMeans (1965) identified from oxidized menhaden oil formic, acetic, acrylic, propionic, crotonic, butyric, and valeric acids.

In recent years the oxidation products of linolenic acid have been studied more than the oxidation of fish oils. However, linolenic acid oxidation is important toward understanding what may happen to oxidation of fish oils. Linolenic acid occurs to a small extent in fish oils but, more importantly, it is an $\omega 3$ fatty acid that is analogous to the longer-chain $\omega 3$ fatty acids in fish oils. Neff et al. (1988) made a detailed study of oxidation of methyl linolenate, and Ulbrich and Grosch (1988) studied the oxidation of methyl linolenate carried out for 48 hours at 22–24°C. They found that the highest flavor units of the oxidized products produced came from the following four compounds: (1) *trans, cis*-2,6-nonadienal; (2) 1, *cis*-5-octadien-3-one; (3) *trans, cis*-3-5-octadien-2-one; and (4) *cis*-3-hexenal. After further oxidation to a total of 102 hours 1, *cis*-5-octadien-3-one was by far the most important odor compound, followed by *cis*-3-hexenal and *trans, cis*-2,6-nonadienal.

Another very recent report, Hsieh et al. (1989) gives great detail on volatile components from crude menhaden oil (see Table 5-4). Crude, undeodorized 1985 manufactured menhaden oil was purged in a dynamic head space sampler system with helium at 65°C for 1 hour. The components removed by this procedure were determined by gas chromatography. A total of 55 different chemical compounds (see Table 5-4) were found. While these results correlate descriptive odors with compounds contained in menhaden oil, the results still leave much that needs to be determined. What really is desired is a comparison between the components of a refined menhaden oil having little or no rancidity odor and a menhaden oil that has been oxidized to yield a product showing definite fishy or rancid flavors and odors. To a considerable extent, however, this difficulty is overcome by the results of a very recent paper by Karahadian and Lindsay (1989) in which odors and flavors were examined in oxidizing menhaden oil. They reported that their results on such flavors and odors coincided closely to those reported by the much earlier paper of Stansby and Jellinek (1965). However, by use of more recently developed capillary GC methods for the analysis of volatile products, they identified many of these (such as are listed in Table 5-2). The green flavor they found to be caused primarily by *trans, cis*-2,6-nonadienal. To some extent two other components, *trans*-2-hexenal and 1, *cis*-5-octadiene-3-one, were partially responsible for the green odor. They found that *cis*-4-heptanal was responsible for the burnt flavor.

Table 5-4.   Volatile Components in Crude Menhaden Oil as Determined by DHS/GC/MS

PEAK NO.	COMPOUND NAME	RETENTION INDEX	ODOR CHARACTERISTICS	ION M/Z	CONC. PPB
1	octane[a]	800		43	20
2	nonane[a]	900		43	2
3	pentanal[b]	979		58	360
4	decane[a]	1000		57	90
5	2-methyl-5-ethylfuran[c]	1014		110	10
6	1-penten-3-one[a]	1022		84	240
7	(E)-but-2-enal[a,e]	1040	painty	70	130
8	hexanal[a]	1085	cut grass, green	56	1380
9	undecane[a]	1100		57	130
10	(Z)-2-pentenal[b,e]	1110		84	70
11	(E)-pent-2-enal[a,e]	1130	greasy green, musty	84	930
12	heptan-3-one[a]	1162	sickly sweet, cooling	57	8530
13	heptanal[a]	1186	waxy green, grassy	70	410
14	dodecane[a]	1200		57	280
15	(E)-hex-2-enal[a,e]	1218	sharp green, oily	69	540
16	2-pentylfuran[b]	1233		138	10
17	1,3,5-trimethylbenzene[a]	1242	pesticidelike	120	20
18	1,2,4-trimethylbenzene[a]	1279	pesticidelike	120	40
19	octanal[a]	1290	citrus, fatty, orange	57	240
20	tridecane[a]	1300		57	370
21	(E)-hept-2-enal[a,e]	1323	sharp green, greasy	83	140
22	1,2,3-trimethylbezene[a]	1332	pesticidelike	120	20
23	nonan-2-one[a]	1390	musty with citrus topnote	58	620
24	nonanal[a]	1395	fatty floral	57	500
25	tetradecane[a]	1400		81	230
26	(E,E)-hexa-2,4-dienal[c,e]	1402		81	100
27	(E)-oct-2-enal[a,e]	1429	musty, waxy floral	70	280
28	acetic acid[a]	1471	irritating, vinegarlike	60	1380
29	hepta-2,4-dienal[c,d,f]	1467	vegetable green	81	1880
30	decanal[a]	1488	sweet, green fruity, fatty with citrus topnote	57	640
31	(E,E)-hepta-2,4-dienal[a,e]	1493		81	2180
32	pentadecane[a]	1500		57	520
33	(Z,Z)-octa-3,5-dien-2-one[c,e]	1520		124	130
34	benzaldehyde[a]	1521	cherry, almond, sweet fruity	105	60
35	nonenal[a]	1535	fatty, waxy, musty	70	200
36	propanoic acid[a]	1547	astringent, acidic	74	2410
37	octa-2,4-dienal[a,d,f]	1563		81	10
38	(E,E)-octa-3,5-dien-2-one[c,e]	1570		124	40
39	isobutanoic acid[c]	1579	sweaty, dirty socks	73	100
40	(E,Z)-nona-2,6-dienal[a,e]	1587		70	240

Table 5-4 (continued)

NO.	PEAK COMPOUND NAME	RETENTION INDEX	ODOR CHARACTERISTICS	ION M/Z	CONC. PPB
41	(E,E)-octa-2,4-dienal[c,e]	1590		81	40
42	hexadecane[a]	1600		57	10
43	butanoic acid[a]	1636	dirty socks	60	8110
44	decenal[c]	1645		55	410
45	heptadecane[a]	1700		85	80
46	pentanoic acid[a]	1747	Parmesan cheese, dirty socks	60	330
47	5-ethyl-2(5H)-furanone[c]	1755		112	20
48	deca-2,4-dienal[a,d]	1764	oxidized oil	81	150
49	deca-2,4-dienal[a,d]	1806	oxidized oil	81	250
50	hexanoic acid[a]	1850	sweaty, dirty socks	60	810
51	nonatrienal[c,d,f]		oxidized oil	79	60
52	nonatrienal[c,d,f]		oxidized oil	79	130
53	decatrienal[c,d,f]		oxidized fish oil	79	70
54	decatrienal[c,d,f]		oxidized fish oil	79	8
55	phenol[a]	2014	medicinal, disinfectant	94	110

Source: Hsieh et al. 1989.
[a] Identified by GC retention index and MS (standard and literature).
[b] Identified by GC retention index and MS (literature).
[c] Identified by MS (literature).
[d] Configuration of geometric isomers not determined.
[e] Prefix (E)- denotes a *trans*-isomer and prefix (Z)- denotes a *cis*-isomer.
[f] Calculation of MS response factors based on *trans, trans*-hepta-2,4,-dienal.

Fish Oil Odors and Flavors Arising from the Presence of Spoilage Impurities

Commercial fish oils are sometimes manufactured from fish brought into the oil-rendering plant without refrigeration. Sometimes the fish are stored at high temperatures for sufficient time that considerable bacterial or enzymatic spoilage has occurred. At early stages of decomposition, the spoilage products most likely to predominate are of nitrogenous origin and include ammonia and amines, particularly trimethylamine. At more advanced states of spoilage, various sulfur compounds including hydrogen sulfides and various mercaptans occur. Both the nitrogenous and sulfur compounds, if present in the fish at the time of processing, will pass over in part into the oil and occur in trace amounts sufficient to alter flavor and odor. The sulfur compounds possessing the more obnoxious odors cause more serious alterations in the quality of the oil, but in well-handled fish their presence is minimal. Ammonia and amines, almost always present to some extent, are common components of fish oils although the quantities present may be very small. Their presence undoubtedly affects the odor and flavor of fish oils.

Trimethylamine and "Fishy" Odors. There is a common opinion that trimethylamine possesses a pronounced characteristic "fishy odor." This is only partially true. As has been shown by Stansby (1962) the odor of trimethylamine that is spoken of as "fishy" occurs only at narrow ranges of dilution of this gas with air (between about 1 : 1500 and 1 : 8000). At higher concentrations the odor resembles that of ammonia gas in high concentrations. At air dilutions greater than 1 : 8000, the odor of trimethylamine is usually undetectable. Ammonia gas itself when diluted with air to about 1 : 2000 possesses an odor essentially the same as a 1 : 6000 diluted trimethylamine mixture. The odor of both trimethylamine and ammonia diluted as indicated, while resembling that of some stale fish, is not nearly as strong as that from spoiled fish. It was also shown by Stansby (1962) that the amount of trimethylamine that analysis shows to be present in spoiled fish does not, by itself, impart the characteristic "fishy" odor to fish. Furthermore, certain fishery products (e.g., canned salmon) may contain far more trimethylamine than any spoiled fish and yet have none of this odor.

Davies and Gill (1936) carried out exhaustive experiments on the fishy flavor of certain butters and ascribed this flavor to trimethylamine released from choline. These authors were the first to show that the characteristic fishy odor ascribed to trimethylamine is greatly intensified when trimethylamine occurs with unsaturated fat that is allowed to oxidize. They failed to show just what occurs during such an alleged reaction, and subsequent research still has not elucidated the mechanism. Nevertheless, it appears that the general observation of Davies and Gill (1936) is correct and that trimethylamine, present with oxidizing fish oil, produces a characteristic "fishy" odor similar to that of diluted trimethylamine (or ammonia) but much more intense.

Advanced Spoilage Odors. When fish oils are manufactured from fish held for long periods of time or for shorter periods without refrigeration, extensive bacteriological spoilage leads to production of obnoxious substances, particularly sulfur compounds some of which end up in the oil. When present to any appreciable extent in fish oils these types of substances (sulfides, mercaptans, etc.) will furnish the predominant odor or flavor noted, or if present at exceedingly low levels may still alter the pattern and, being with other odors or flavors components, give an altered odor type. Such flavors and odors can be eliminated completely by using only relatively fresh raw material. Clay bleaching removes some of these components, but it is better to avoid their presence in the first place by controlling the quality of fish employed for the manufacture of the oil.

Odors and Flavors from Nontriglyceride Components of Oil

Pure fish oils contain, in addition to triglycerides, usually smaller quantities of other components such as phospholipids and various unsaponifiables. Most of the nontriglyceride components of fish oil, if concerned with odor or flavor at all, act in an analogous way to the triglycerides. Phospholipids when present in or associated with fish oils may undergo very slow hydrolysis to yield odiferous compounds or, more likely, precursors to such compounds. Often much of the most highly polyunsaturated fatty acids, the ones having the greatest susceptibility to oxidation, are tied up as phospholipids. During storage, these phospholipids may slowly release the highly unsaturated fatty acids, which may then have greater instability. Furthermore, choline is a component of phospholipids, and it may release trimethylamine, which, as discussed in a preceding section, may contribute either directly or indirectly to the development of undesirable odors in fish oils.

In the preparation of such products as fish protein concentrate, removal not only of triglycerides but also of phospholipids is necessary to avoid stability against oxidative deterioration of lipids and the resulting flavor reversion. Fat solvents that readily remove triglycerides may fail to extract all of the phospholipids that are a potential source of odor problems.

MEASURING CHANGES IN LEVELS OF ODORS AND FLAVORS

Handling and Sampling Commercial Fish Oils

Handling.   Fish oils, because of their content of highly polyunsaturated fatty acids, are far more unstable, or subject to very rapid oxidation, than are most other oils. This instability necessitates very careful attention by the analyst to storage methods suitable to prevent oxidation or other changes from occurring either during storage prior to analysis or even during the analysis itself. Oxidation can occur not only from very small traces of oxygen or air present in any headspace above the oil but even from air dissolved in the oil itself. Fish oil that is to be stored before analysis should, therefore, be provided with an inert atmosphere. Most commonly used for this purpose is nitrogen, which is best applied by bubbling through the oil in the container in which it is to be stored. In order to displace air dissolved in the oil, bubbling should be at such a rate that some circulation of the oil in the container takes place. For prolonged storage of the oil, bubbling should continue for at least one hour.

It is, of course, important that the nitrogen used for this purpose be as free as possible of any small traces of oxygen. While it is possible to purchase specially purified nitrogen containing only about 0.01% oxygen, it is usually better to use a regular commercial grade of nitrogen and to pass it over heated copper (Wiberg 1960) before use. In laboratories doing considerable work with fish oils it is desirable to pipe nitrogen, passed first over heated copper, to outlets at workbenches.

Since exceedingly minute traces of oxygen are sufficient to cause alteration in fish oils, in providing an inert atmosphere not only must oxygen-free inert gas be used and bubbled through the oil to displace dissolved oxygen, but also great care must be taken in sealing or stoppering of the container to be sure that minute amounts of air are not admitted at the point where the container is sealed or stoppered. Carbon dioxide offers some advantage over nitrogen at this stage because with a density greater than air it is less likely that air will diffuse into the container at the moment of closing.

Sampling. Fish oil manufacturers require that homogeneous samples be taken of oil from very large lots such as in storage tanks usually ranging from 50,000 to 750,000 gallons or in barge shipments of 200,000 gallons or more. In order for the sample to be representative of such large lots, considerable care is needed to get uniformity. Samples are most frequently taken using a Bacon bomb sampler thief that is attached to a drop cord and lowered down through the tank at a uniform rate. This type of thief consists of a cylindrical body of about 12 in. (305 mm) long and $2\frac{3}{4}$ in. (66 mm) outside diameter. An opening at the bottom admits the oil through an attached center tube as the bomb sinks to the bottom of the tank. An adjustable needle valve at the top controls the filling speed by throttling the escape of air. The thief has a 16-oz capacity. It gives a sample representative of a cross section from top to bottom of the tank.

It is important that in passing down to the bottom of the tank, the bomb should not quite be filled with oil; otherwise it might become completely filled before reaching the bottom and thereby not give a true cross-section sample.

A problem in sampling fish oil, especially at low temperatures, is caused by the presence of stearine, which exists as a solid or semisolid under such conditions. Under severe sampling conditions this problem is overcome by stirring the oil for several hours by means of a side-entry agitator or, rarely, by heating the oil.

A sample of one pint is generally taken as being representative from tanks or lots up to 10,000 gallons. For larger lots, the sample size is increased, and for a 200,000-gallon barge load of fish oil, four quarts is considered adequate.

For cross-section sampling the "average"-type Bacon bomb thief is employed. Where samples representative of the oil at different levels in the tank are desired, a special type of thief is used.

Analytical Extraction of Oil from Fish Flesh

A sample is prepared for oil extraction by comminution in some sort of cutting-type grinder. Although it is possible to use equipment similar to the common kitchen meat grinder in which the material, fed by a spiral shaft, is forced through a plate with holes, better grinding leading to a more homogeneous sample results from use of a sausage-type grinder in which the flesh is cut by a rotating, circular knife. Ordinarily fish samples for oil content determinations consist of bone-free material such as fillets. If bone is present, the above-mentioned types of grinders are unsuitable unless the fish can be cooked under pressure, which will soften the bones. If raw fish containing bone must be ground, more powerful mills such as of the hammer type may be necessary.

Moisture is rapidly lost by evaporation from fish, especially after the flesh has been minced. In any quantitative work, therefore, it is important to keep the minced sample in tightly closed containers until the sample has been weighed for analysis.

In some cases, especially when dealing with fish that has been frozen, the flesh releases moisture slowly after mincing, and fluid collects gradually. It is, therefore, important to stir the flesh thoroughly immediately before sampling in order to incorporate any separated fluid uniformly throughout the flesh.

For quantitative determination of the oil content of fish flesh the method of the AOAC (1984), involving acid hydrolysis followed by extraction in the cold with ethyl and petroleum ethers and using Mojonnier equipment, is quite generally employed.

Where the extracted oil is to be used for some subsequent analysis, a more gentle extraction procedure is usually indicated. In order to obtain the fish oil with a minimum of change during extraction, the minced flesh can be dried in a vacuum desiccator over concentrated sulfuric acid after mixing with sand, as is done in the AOAC (1984) method for moisture in grain and stock feeds, followed by extraction in the cold by an appropriate fat solvent.

Alternately the Bligh and Dyer (1959) method involves extraction of the undried, minced fish flesh with a blended mixture of chloroform and methanol.

Extraction of Oil from Fish Meal

The AOAC (1984) acetone extraction method should be used for determination of the oil content of fish meal. This is a two-step procedure involving initial extraction with acetone, then an acid hydrolysis with $4N$ hydrochloric acid followed by a second acetone extraction. This type of procedure is needed because as most fish meals are stored after manufacture, their lipid gradually reacts with the protein to form compounds that cannot be extracted until after an acid hydrolysis is performed. In such cases a fish meal with an initial lipid content of 12% may, after prolonged storage and using a single extraction, appear to have a lipid content of 2% or less.

Evaluation of Flavors and Odors Using Chemical Tests

Chemical Tets for Oxidative (Rancidity) Odors and Flavors. There are no chemical tests at present for which a given value will invariably correspond to a definite degree of rancidity. Nevertheless, there are several tests that are used and, when their limitations are kept in mind, can be of value. The three most frequently used such tests are peroxide number, thiobarbituric acid (TBA) value, and the measurement of gain in weight of the oil sample during the course of oxidation. Of these methods the measurement of the peroxide value is the most usually used. Of the several procedures for this determination, the method of Wheeler (1932) is perhaps the most convenient. It must always be remembered, however, that a given peroxide value may correspond under different conditions to quite different degrees of rancidity. For example, when fish are stored at different temperatures (e.g., held frozen vs. stored unfrozen in ice), a given peroxide number for a slight degree of rancidity will be quite different between fish stored at the different temperatures.

Consequently, it is necessary to use sensory examination at frequent intervals when peroxide number or other chemical tests are used.

Chemical Tests for Nonrancidity Flavors and Odors

Our knowledge of the causes of "fishy" flavors in fish oils, other than those that arise from oxidative deterioration, is so very meager that there are few tests that can be considered. A measurement of trimethylamine or tertiary nitrogen would probably be helpful, but unfortunately, the quantity present in fish oils is usually so exceedingly small that its quantitative measurement is most difficult. Usually it is sufficient to measure the total nitrogen content of the oil. Even this, with the quantity of nitrogen present being very small, is not easy to do. A micro-Kjeldahl nitrogen digestion folowed by a colorimetric determination of liberated ammonia has been used by Chipault (1960) for determining traces of nitrogen in fish oils. The quantity present is sometimes considerably smaller than the amount of nitrogen present as impurities in the Kjeldahl reagent chemicals, which may result in larger blanks than in the sample. Use of a Dumas nitrogen determination method avoids this difficulty and often gives better results.

SENSORY EXAMINATION METHODS

Importance

A number of chemical methods are available for evaluating the flavor of fish oils, especially where flavor results from oxidative rancidity. Such objective methods, however, are of practical value only when they are standardized and frequently checked against the actual flavor of the fish oil. As has been pointed out by Stansby (1963), values obtained for rancidity tests in fish oils at identical flavor stages vary depending on such conditions as storage temperature and the presence or absence of antioxidants. Thus, unless sensory tests are used in conjunction with scientific tests, the latter alone may give meaningless results.

Sensory Panels

As with sensory judgment of flavor in other food products, appraisal made by a single observer of the flavor or odor of fish oil is not sufficiently consistent to give reproducible results. It is necessary, therefore, to use a panel of several individuals. Panel members for evaluations of this kind should be experienced and familiar with the different types of odors and flavors normally encountered in fish oils. Thus, a consumer preference type of panel is not applicable to such work. Flavors and odors of fish oil are generally made up of a blending of a number of different components. Unless panel members are fully familiar with these individual flavor or odor components, no adequate evaluation is possible.

Judging Flavor of Fish Oils

A panel of at least four persons (preferably more), experienced in flavors of fish oils, is necessary in order to get a satisfactory evaluation. It is important to limit the number of oil samples compared at one time in order to reduce fatigue. As a rule, reproducibility of results falls off rapidly if more than about six samples are compared at one time. Since it is sometimes difficult to completely remove previously examined oil from glassware, it is convenient to present fish oil samples to the panel members in 9-cm disposable plastic petri dishes as suggested by Stansby and Jellinek (1965). These dishes give a large area for preliminary odor examination and can be discarded after use. Using plastic spoons, samples of oil can be conveniently tasted, a small portion of the oil being taken on the tip of the spoon. This procedure prevents excess oil from adhering to the lips, which might interfere with successive tasting of several oil samples. Since fish oil often has a persistent aftertaste, it is helpful to remove flavor between oil samples in some suitable manner. For this purpose apple juice is useful. It is just tart enough to readily remove the fish oil flavor without excess acidity, such as is present in citrus juices, which interferes with subsequent sample tasting.

Judging Flavor of Oil in Fishery Products

When comparing flavor or samples of fish oil contained in such products as cooked fish, many of the same considerations pointed out in the preceding section on fish oil flavor evaluation apply. In addition, it is important to remember that the oil in fish is not uniformly distributed throughout the flesh and, furthermore, that oxidative rancidity occurs to a far greater extent in oil in areas of dark flesh than in the light tissue; with some species virtually all the oxidation takes place in the oil in the dark muscle (Brown et al. 1957). In tasting samples of such fish it is important that these facts be well recognized. Otherwise, one panel member may be judging exclusively the dark flesh. It is possible to present to the panel a homogenized sample in which light and dark meat are blended together so that each panel member receives essentially identical samples. This procedure, while eliminating much discrepancy in judgments among panel members, also decreases sensitivity in picking up off-flavors. The dark tissue ordinarily occurs in fish in much smaller quantities than the light tissue. Hence the oxidized dark sample containing most of the flavor component is diluted with the light flesh containing largely unaltered oil. It is usually much better to have panel members each separately evaluate the flavor of some of the dark as well as of the light flesh. This same principle applies to chemical rancidity tests where it is advisable to run peroxide numbers, TBA, etc., on oil samples extracted from light and dark flesh separately rather than on a composited sample. Often minimal or zero values are obtained on oil from the light flesh whereas the corresponding oil from the dark flesh gives high rancidity values.

Induction Period Measurements

Often fish oils may, at the time they are analyzed, all have good flavor but, upon oxidation, some oils will develop rancid or other flavors more rapidly than others. A measure of the induction period will give an estimation of stability of the oil, and sometimes sensory tests offer the best means of judging when the end of the induction period has been reached.

Ordinarily the oil is stored under some reproducible, accelerated condition to hasten oxidation. This is usually accomplished by aeration, heating to some elevated temperature at which the oil is stored, or a combination of both. The use of elevated storage temperatures usually alters the pattern of oxidation. Thus, if two oils have an induction period ratio of 1 : 3 at the elevated temperatures, this ratio may be quite different at some lower temperature, at which the oil is apt to be stored. Another method sometimes more suitable for accelerating oxidation rate in induction period measurement is by increasing the surface of oil exposed to air. For example, fish oil spread on filter paper may oxidize 100 times as fast as when stored in a beaker. Samples stored on filter paper can be tasted at intervals of storage at room or lower temperature until flavor changes have occurred to give a measure of the induction period, or chemical tests can be applied.

REFERENCES

AOAC. 1984. *Official Methods of Analysis of the Association of Official Analytical Chemists*, 14th ed., Sidney Williams. Washington, D.C.: Association of Official Analytical Chemists.

Bligh, E. G., and Dyer, W. S. 1959. A rapid method of total lipid extraction and purification. *Can. J. Biochem. Physiol.* 37:911–917.

Brown, W.D., Venolia, A. W., Tappel, A. L., Olcott, H. S., and Stansby, M. E. 1957. Oxidative deterioration in fish and fishery products. II. Progress on studies concerning mechanism of oxidation of oil in fish tissues. *Commercial Fisheries Rev.* 19(5A):27–31.

Chipault, J. R. 1959. The odors of oxidized fish oils. *Annual Report*, The Hormel Institute 1958–1959:7–8.

Chipault, J. 1960. The odors of oxidized fish oils. *Annual Report*, The Hormel Institute, University of Minnesota, for 1959–1960:7–8.

Chipault, J. R., and McMeans, E. 1965. Volatile acids from menhaden oil. *J. Agric. Food Chem.* 13:15–17.

Davies, W. L., and Gill, E. 1936. Investigations on "fishy" flavors. *Chem. and Ind.* (*London*) 55:141T–146T.

Dolev, A., and Olcott, H. S. 1965. The triglycerides of sablefish (*Anaploma fimbria*). I. Quantitative fractionation by column chromatography on silica gel impregnated with silver nitrate. *J. Am. Oil Chemists' Soc.* 42:624–627.

Einset, E., Olcott, H. S., and Stansby, M. E. 1957. Progress on studies concerning oxidation of extracted oils. *Commercial Fisheries Rev.*, 19(5):35–37.

Hsieh, R. J., and Kinsella, J. E. 1986. Lipoxgenase-catalyzed oxidation of N-6 and N-3 polyunsaturated fatty acids; relevance to and activity in fish tissue. *J. Food Sci.* 51:940–945, 996.

Hsieh, Thomas C. Y., Williams, Stephen S., Vejaphan, Warinda, and Meyers, Samuel P. 1989. Characterization of volatile components of menhaden fish (*Brevoortia tyrannus*) oil. *J. Am. Oil Chemists' Soc.* 66:114–117.

Josephson, D. B., Lindsay, R. C., and Stuiber, D. A. 1984. Biogenesis of lipid-derived, volatile aroma compounds in emerald shiner (*Nolropis atherinopides*). *J. Agric. Food Chem.* 32:1347–1352.

Karahadian, C., and Lindsay, R. C. 1989. Evaluation of compounds contributing characterizing fish flavors in fish oils. *J. Am. Oil Chemists' Soc.* 66:953–960.

Klose, A. A., Mecchi, E. P., Hanson, H. L., and Lineweaver, H. 1951. The role of dietary fat in the quality of fresh and frozen storage turkeys. *J. Am. Oil Chemists' Soc.* 28:162–164.

Neff, W. E., Frankel, E. N., and Fujimoto, K. 1988. Autoxidative dimerization of methyl linoleate and its monohydroperoxyepidioxides and dihydroperoxides. *J. Am. Oil Chemists' Soc.* 65:616–623.

Oldfield, J. E., and Anglemier, A. F. 1957. Feeding of crude and modified menhaden oils in rations for swine. *J. Animal Sci.* 16:917–921.

Stansby, M. E. 1962. Speculations on "fishy" odors. *Food Technol.* 16(4):28–32.

Stansby, M. E. 1963. Results of some organoleptic tests on pork from pigs fed experimental diets containing menhaden oil. Unpublished report. U.S. Bureau Commercial Fisheries Technological Laboratory, Seattle, Wash.

Stansby, M. E., and Jellinek, G. 1965. Flavor and odor characteristics of fishery products with particular reference to early oxidation changes in menhaden oil. In *The Technology of Fishery Products*, ed. Rudolph Kreuzer. London: The Fishing News (Books) Ltd.

Ulbrich, F., and Grosch, W. 1988. Identification of the most intense compounds found during autoxidation of methyl linolenate at room temperature. *J. Am. Oil Chemists' Soc.* 65:1313–1317.

Wheeler, D. H. 1932. Peroxide formation as a measure of auto-oxidative deterioration. *Oil and Soap* 9:89–97.

Wiberg, K. B. 1960. *Laboratory Techniques in Organic Chemistry*. New York: McGraw-Hill.

Yu, T. C., Day, E. A., and Sinnhuber, R. O. 1961. Autoxidation of fish oils. I. Identification of volatile monocarbonyl compounds from auto-oxidizing salmon oil. *J. Food Sci.* 26:192–197.

Chapter 6
PRODUCTION OF FISH OIL

Anthony P. Bimbo

INTRODUCTION

This chapter will deal primarily with U.S. production of fish oil; however, since the world production of fish oil is relatively small, the domestic and international industries are so intimately related that one cannot talk about one without references to the other. Since liver oils and marine mammal oils have a historical place in the U.S. industry, they will be covered briefly.

HISTORICAL BACKGROUND

Fishing is probably America's first industry and can be traced back to the early colonies. Lee (1953) mentions that the Indians used fish for fertilizer long before the colonists arrived. In fact, references to such use can be found in colonial writings of 1621. Frye (1978) describes a legend of how the early Plymouth settlers learned of the use of fish as fertilizer from an Indian sometimes called Squanto or Tisquantum. This use supposedly saved the colony from disaster during those early years.

According to Stansby (1978), whale oil was the first marine oil produced in the United States, with initial production in a small way originating as early as 1640. However, whale oil is not a fish oil, it is a marine mammal oil. The American fish oil industry actually began around 1811 in Rhode Island. According to early literature, the fish were unloaded from nets cast from the shore or from small boats by pitchfork into tanks or kettles on the shore and boiled. The boiled fish were then transferred to casks, and the oil and water were pressed out by placing stones on top of boards on the fish. The oil was then skimmed off the top and placed into barrels.

Later, as production increased and operations began to take on a small factory appearance, the fish were unloaded directly into small wooden tram cars holding about 20 barrels each. These cars were hauled to the upper floor of the plant, where the fish were dumped into large holding bins. From there, the fish flowed into the cooking tanks, which were constructed of wooden staves, sometimes with a false bottom, and had perforated pipes in the bottom for the introduction of steam. Improvements in the boiling step came in 1842 when steam cooking was first used, and in 1855 the first fully mechanical screw press was introduced at a plant on Long Island.

Lee (1953) mentions that with the development of the screw press, the production of fish oil moved from a farm sideline to a small factory operation. Frye (1978) says that by mid-century disposal of the residue after the oil was removed became a problem. Thus the term "guano," or fertilizer, was born. The residue was removed and given to farmers to manure the fields, and this replaced the use of whole fish.

In 1860 a modern plant at Narragansett Bay, Rhode Island, was utilizing steam cookers and mechanical screw presses. Fishing was done primarily from the shore prior to 1860. Sailboats were used up until 1873, but steam was beginning to catch on. By 1912 the Atlantic coast industry consisted of 48 factories extending from Rhode Island to Florida. During the period 1873–1911 the U.S. production of fish oil remained stable at about 2 million gallons per year produced from between 110,000 and 115,000 metric tons (mt) of fish. In 1912 it increased to 6.6 million gallons from 323,000 mt of fish and remained at that level until the mid 1940s, when it began to increase rapidly (Fitzgibbon 1969). By 1917, because of animal feed shortages, the fish scrap began to find use in animal feeds, and by 1935, virtually all of it was used in this way.

Smith (1940) describes the rapid changes that were beginning to take place in the industry along the Atlantic coast. Prior to 1940 the process consisted of cooking the fish in large vats, pressing the cooked fish, and catching the pressed liquor in a series of settling tanks. By a series of skimmings, the oil was separated from the water phase and an emulsion layer was recooked to recover oil. The remaining "gurry" was then allowed to decompose to form dark, low-grade oil that was removed by hand dippers. In 1940, the industry began to use centrifuges to separate oil from water and thus eliminate this emulsion phase. The oil was the most valuable product recovered from the fish and was used in soap, paints, and linoleum. It was this introduction of the centrifuge that started the rapid increase in production of menhaden oil in the United States, the "Industrial Revolution" of the menhaden industry.

Vaughan et al. (1988) described the menhaden fishery from the post-World War II period as follows. The 1950s were years of stock expansion, the age structure widened, and several dominant year classes entered the Atlantic fishery. Landings surpassed 500,000 mt in 1953, producing over 17 million gallons of oil, and peaked at 712,000 mt in 1956 with 22.5 million gallons of oil produced. By 1962 dominant year classes disappeared and the stock's age structure began to contract, and by 1969 only 162,000 mt of fish were landed on the Atlantic. Before World War II purse seine landings in the Gulf of Mexico were few and sporadic, ranging from 2,000 to 12,000 mt between 1918 and 1944. During the late 1940s new plants were built in Mississippi, Louisiana, and Texas, and landings increased to 103,000 mt by 1948 and 481,000 mt by 1962. In 1963 Gulf landings surpassed Atlantic landings. Today Gulf landings represent about 70% of the total menhaden landings and almost 90% of the oil production.

Parallel with the development of the menhaden fishery on the east coast of the United States, there was a rapid rise in landings of the Pacific sardine. Prior to 1915, landings of this species were not even recorded; however, by the late 1920s there were sizable landings which peaked from the mid-1930s to the mid-1940s. The fish was used for canning, but offal and rejected fish were converted to fish meal and oil. In 1936 oil from the Pacific sardine accounted for 60% of the U.S. fish oil production. The landings rapidly declined after 1945, and by the early 1950s, the production of oil from this species was insignificant (U.S. Bureau of Commercial Fisheries 1967). Much of the early edible fish oil research was done with the oil from this species. In 1925, 45 metric tons (mt) were processed into margarine. By 1928 usage had risen to about 7,300 mt, and in 1936 it peaked at 18,200 mt. Use in shortening involved the preparation of hydrogenated mono- and diglycerides. These were added to the shortening at a level of 2.5–3% in the preparation of a superglycerinated shortening. This type of shortening was in great demand in the baking industry, especially for use in cakes, since it permitted a higher sugar-flour ratio without harming the final texture of the product. It was produced during the 1930s and 1940s and reached a peak level of 45,000 mt per year (Stansby 1978). The total U.S. consumption of marine oil for all edible purposes during this peak period was approximately 75,000 mt. In 1951, because of the declining availability due to the disappearance of the Pacific sardine, the large processing plants on the west coast of the United States ceased operations. With this decreased availability, fish oil was no longer used as an edible oil (Bimbo 1983).

Pressures on the industry from the major European markets and a need to expand markets for menhaden oil led to a decision by the menhaden industry to seek reaffirmation of edible status for menhaden oil in the United States. At a meeting of the U.S. menhaden industry and representatives of the U.S. National Marine Fisheries Service (NMFS) in June 1977, a task force was formed to develop the strategy necessary to obtain approval of menhaden oil as an edible product. During the early meetings of the task force, avenues of approach to a food additive or GRAS petition were explored. Preliminary meetings were held with the U.S. Food and Drug Administration (FDA) during the 1977–1979 planning stages to discuss information requirements, types of studies necessary, and the FDA's position on fish oils in general.

Although marine oils had been consumed in the United States over a 20-year period and in Europe for the last 60 years, FDA still felt that fish oils were totally new ingredients and a comprehensive and time-consuming series of toxicological tests would be required to be certain that adding such products to the food supply would not present an unacceptable risk to the public. Based on these discussions, and the then current FDA philosophy, a series of long-term studies were planned to affirm the safety of menhaden oil (Bimbo and Bauersfeld 1982). The studies were completed in 1985.

On June 13, 1986, the National Fish Meal and Oil Association (NF-MOA) filed a petition with FDA to affirm that menhaden oil is generally recognized as safe (GRAS) as a direct human food ingredient (U.S. FDA 1986). The petition defined two product areas for consideration: partially hydrogenated menhaden oil (PHMO) which covers the family of products currently in use worldwide as ingredients in margarines, shortenings, soft spreads, cooking fats, salad oils, emulsifiers and waxes; and refined menhaden oil (RMO) where the fatty acids remain intact (NFMOA 1986). In essence menhaden oil would be used wherever edible fats and oils are currently being used (Bimbo 1987b).

On September 15, 1989, the U.S. FDA affirmed the GRAS status of partially hydrogenated and hydrogenated menhaden oils as direct human food ingredients (U.S. FDA 1989). Citing the current Code of Federal Regulations, the agency stated that general recognition of safety may be based only on the views of experts qualified by scientific training and experience to evaluate the safety of substances directly or indirectly added to food. The basis for such views may be either (1) scientific procedures or (2) in the case of a substance used in food prior to January 1, 1958, experience based on common use of the substance in food. General recognition of safety based on scientific procedures requires the same quantity and quality of scientific evidence that is required to obtain approval of a food additive. It must ordinarily be based on published studies, which may be corroborated by unpublished studies and other data and information. General recognition of safety through experience based on common use in food prior to January 1, 1958, may be established without the quantity or quality of scientific evidence required for approval of a food additive regulation but must be based on generally available data and information. The FDA revised its procedures for establishing general recognition of safety of the use of a substance that was commonly used for that purpose in food before 1958 to include consumption outside the United States on May 10, 1988. As a result, the long history of safe food use in Europe was accepted, thus indicating a "prior sanction" for the oil. This historical use coupled with the four toxicological studies conducted in the United States and Europe were sufficient to demonstrate the safety of menhaden oil. The FDA went on to say that the final rule responds only to the portion of the petition requesting GRAS affirmation of the use of partially hydrogenated menhaden oil as an edible fat or oil and not to the portion pertaining to refined menhaden oil. Issues relevant to the GRAS status of refined menhaden oil will be dealt with in a future Federal Register document.

This initial approval of PHMO by the U.S. FDA represents a milestone for the world fats and oils industry because, for the first time, the leading regulatory agency in the world has placed its approval on fish oil (menhaden) in modern times and reopened the U.S. market to a product that has been consumed for a long period of time in many parts of the world. With current pressures on various fats and oils for a number of reasons both real and imaginary, this approval becomes a unique milestone in the history of fats and oils.

FISH OILS IN PERSPECTIVE

Over 90 million metric tons (mmt) of fish and shellfish are landed annually worldwide. Table 6-1 gives a breakdown of the 1986 landings by geographical area. Herring-type fish make up 26% of the total world landings, whereas menhaden, the largest-volume species landed in the United

Table 6-1. World Landings
of Fish and Shellfish by
Geographical Area, 1986,
in 1000 Metric Tons

AREA	LANDINGS
Latin America	15,572
United States	4,945
Western Europe[a]	6,511
Scandinavia	6,072
Eastern Europe[b]	12,494
Africa	3,264
Far East	31,464
Middle East	722
Others	11,924
Totals	92,968

Source: IAFMM 1988.
[a]Excluding Scandinavia.
[b]Including the USSR.

Table 6-2. Disposition of World and U.S. Catch of Fish and Shellfish, % of Use, 1985

DISPOSITION	WORLD	U.S.
Marketed fresh and frozen	41.6	32.2
Canned	13.4	18.3
Cured	15.2	1.1
Whole fish reduced to fish meal and oil[a]	28.6	43.4
Other	1.2	4

Source: U.S. Dept. of Commerce 1987A.
[a]Whole fish only, does not include fish waste.

States, is probably tenth in volume worldwide (USDC 1988A). On average, about 29% of the world catch is converted into fish meal and oil. In the United States, this figure is higher, 43%, because of the large catch of menhaden. Table 6-2 gives the U.S. and world disposition of fish by end use for 1985, the latest year for which this data is available (USDC 1988B).

Commercial fish and shellfish landings by U.S. fishermen at ports in the 50 states were 3.1 mmt in 1987. This total was composed of 1.8 mmt of edible fish and shellfish and 1.3 mmt of fish for reduction to meal and oil of which 92%, or 1.2 mmt, were menhaden (USDC 1988A). An eight-year breakdown of the U.S. catch versus Atlantic and Gulf menhaden landings is shown in Table 6-3.

The world produces around 75 mmt of fats and oils annually. Soybean oil and animal fats make up almost 50% of the total while marine oils, consisting of marine mammal oils, fish liver oils, and fish body oils, account for a little over 2% of the world supply of fats and oils, with fish

Table 6-3. Availability of Fish, Shellfish, and Menhaden, 1980–1987, in 1000 Metric Tons

YEAR	FISH AND SHELLFISH	ATLANTIC MENHADEN	GULF MENHADEN	TOTAL MENHADEN
1980	2940	430	702	1132
1981	2711	402	553	955
1982	2888	400	854	1255
1983	2921	420	924	1344
1984	2920	329	983	1311
1985	2839	359	884	1243
1986	2736	256	829	1085
1987	3128	323	907	1230

Source: U.S. Dept. of Commerce 1988A.

body oils making up 97% of the total marine oil supply. Fish oils usually rank twelfth out of the 17 major fats and oils, just ahead of corn oil and behind olive oil in volume (Bimbo 1989A). Table 6-4 gives the 1988–1989 season forecast for the 17 major fats and oils of commerce.

According to preliminary data, the U.S. production of edible fats and oils was about 7.6 mmt in 1988, with soybean oil accounting for about 67% of the total production of all fats and oils. The U.S. production of marine oils totaled 135 thousand metric tons in 1987 and was composed of 134 thousand metric tons of menhaden oil (99%) and 1.5 thousand metric tons of oil from miscellaneous fish (USDC 1988A). Table 6-5 shows the U.S. fish oil production data for an eight-year period.

While marine oils make up only about 2% of the world supply of fats and oils, nonetheless they represent a major source of fat in many countries and a valuable export commodity to others. Table 6-6 gives the major fish oil producing, exporting, and importing countries for 1987 (IAFMM 1988).

Marine oils are usually competitive with other fats and oils available on the world market (IAFMM 1988) and have a wide range of functionality,

Table 6-4. World Forecast of Production of Oils and Fat for the 1988–1989 Crop Year in 1000 Metric Tons

OIL OR FAT	PRODUCTION
Soybean	15,171
Cottonseed	3,730
Groundnut	3,588
Sunflower	7,905
Rapeseed	7,659
Sesame	587
Corn	1,321
Olive	1,647
Coconut	2,889
Palm kernel	1,133
Palm	9,148
Butter as fat	6,157
Lard	5,291
Fish	1,479
Linseed	744
Castor	381
Tallow and grease	6,514
Totals	75,344

Source: Oil World Weekly Statistics Update 1988.

Table 6-5. U.S. Production of Fish Oils and Menhaden Oil, 1980–1987, in 1000 Metric Tons

YEAR	PRODUCTION	
	FISH OIL	MENHADEN OIL
1980	141	132
1981	83	77
1982	157	153
1983	181	174
1984	169	165
1985	129	126
1986	153	151
1987	135	134

Source: U.S. Dept. of Commerce 1988A.

Table 6-6. Major Fish Oil Producing, Exporting, and Importing Countries, in 1000 Metric Tons, 1988 Estimated

COUNTRY	PRODUCTION	EXPORTS	IMPORTS
Belgium	0	1	36
Denmark	80	42	16
Fed. Rep. Germany	12	12	156
Other EEC	22	20	38
Iceland	120	114	0
Netherlands	0	19	172
USSR	92	1	0
Canada	7	6	0
Mexico	6	0	1
Ecuador	26	4	0
Japan	398	172	7
United Kingdom	9	4	197
Norway	83	85	65
Rep. South Africa	48	34	0
U.S.	148	120	11
Colombia	0	0	18
Chile	205	100	0
Peru	138	52	36
Panama	16	9	0
Faeroe Is.	9	9	0
Sweden	4	3	7
Morocco	7	5	0
Argentina	4	0	0
Turkey	12	8	0
East Europe	2	0	29
Others	46	19	44
Totals	1494	839	833

Source: Oil World Annual 1988, April 88 Commodities 133.

Table 6-7. Prices of Selected Fats and Oils in U.S. $/Metric Ton, CIF Rotterdam

YEAR	FISH	PALM	SOYA	COCONUT	RAPESEED	LARD
1976	370	415	460	450	415	482
1977	488	545	593	627	584	618
1978	453	550	580	733	593	626
1979	445	650	660	1020	636	716
1980	445	595	605	749	571	648
1981	415	560	525	581	483	610
1982	340	450	460	482	417	574
1983	385	545	573	743	500	503
1984	370	773	775	1120	687	575
1985	303	520	573	655	540	553
1986	275	318	417	358	340	465
1987	237	343	334	NA	305	NA
1988	373	445	489	NA	432	NA

Source: International Association of Fish Meal Manufacturers 1975–1988.

especially in the partially hydrogenated form for the baking industry (Bimbo 1987B, 1989A). Table 6-7 gives a price comparison for six oils on the world market for the years 1976–1988.

THE PRODUCTION OF FISH MEAL AND OIL

Raw Material

According to the Food and Agriculture Organization of the United Nations (FAO 1986), raw material used for reduction to meal and oil falls into several categories:

1. Fish caught specifically for reduction to meal and oil such as menhaden, anchovy, and sardines.
2. Incidental or by-catch from another fishery, for example shrimp by-catch which could range from 5 to 15 mmt annually (James 1989, personal communication).
3. Fish offal or waste from the edible fisheries such as cuttings from filleting operations, fish cannery waste, roe fishery waste, and more recently surimi processing.

The three categories all have several things in common: The fish are of little edible use or the raw material is a waste and of no edible value, and in fact may present a potential disposal problem, and the raw material contains a high percentage of oil and or bones (FAO 1986). The latter two categories, by-catch and offal, produce small volumes of oil compared to the volume produced from whole fish because the traditionally edible species are primarily nonfatty and generally classified as "white fish."

Menhaden is the primary U.S. species converted to fish meal and oil and represents almost 50% of the total fish and shellfish landings. They are small, oily, herringlike fish similar in appearance to the alewife and shad. They are dark blue to brown in color with silver along the sides, and are distinguished from other fish of the herring family by the presence of a dark shoulder spot on both sides of the body. A typical menhaden appears in Fig. 6-1. Menhaden are migratory fish and appear in dense schools in the open waters of large bays and along the shores of the Atlantic and Gulf coasts of the United States. They feed primarily on plankton and efficiently convert this food into energy, which is then stored as fat (Bimbo 1986).

The menhaden resource is relatively stable when compared with the other pelagics that are used to produce fish meal and oil (Vaughan et al. 1988). Records on menhaden go back to the mid-1800s, and there has been a steady increase in landings since that time. The menhaden industry has not experienced the precipitous rise and fall in landings that has been experienced with the South American anchovy or even the Pacific sardine. Table 6-8 shows a comparison of historical menhaden, Peruvian anchovy, and Pacific sardine landings for the period 1875–1985.

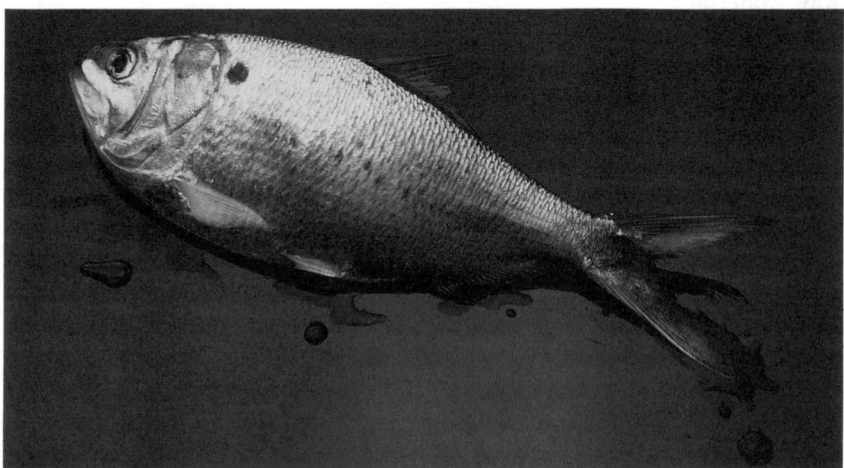

Fig. 6-1. Menhaden, *Brevoortia* sp. (*Source:* Zapata Haynie Corporation, Hammond, Louisiana.)

Table 6-8. Menhaden, Peruvian Anchovy,
and Pacific Sardine Landings, 1875–1985,
in 1000 Metric Tons

YEAR	MENHADEN[a]	SARDINE[b]	ANCHOVY[c]
1875	171	—	—
1880	236	—	—
1890	162	—	—
1900	277	—	—
1910	307	—	—
1915	323	2	—
1920	314	54	—
1925	241	143	—
1930	186	224	—
1935	197	530	—
1940	288	415	—
1945	344	386	—
1950	454	281	—
1955	838	66	100
1960	907	26	3,500
1965	749	1	7,700
1970	805	0	13,100
1975	793	0	3,300
1980	1,103	0	700
1985	1,188	0	1,000

[a]Fitzgibbon 1969.
[b]U.S. Bureau of Commercial Fisheries 1967.
[c]U.S. Dept. of Commerce 1988A.

Harvesting

Industrial fish used for reduction to meal and oil are often caught by vessels working fairly close to the processing plant, but usually not more than three days away. Purse seining is the principal catch method used. Since menhaden feed and live near the surface (pelagic) they are easily visible from the vessel or from the air. Airplanes are used to spot the schools and direct the fishing vessels to them. When a school is located, the vessel releases two purse boats that have a net stretched between them. The purse boats encircle the school, and then close the net to form a purse or bag. This can be seen in Fig. 6-2. The net is then retrieved to concentrate the catch, after which the mother ship comes alongside and pumps the fish and seawater aboard, as shown in Fig. 6-3. The water is separated and discharged back overboard, and the fish are dropped into refrigerated holds. The nets can vary from 10 to 60 tons each, and the

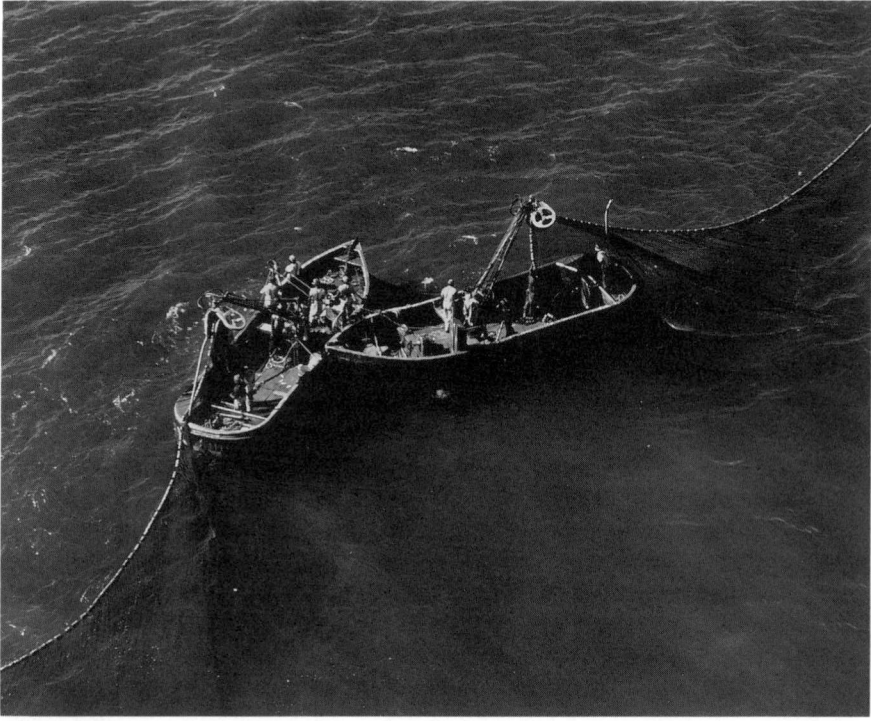

Fig. 6-2. Purse seining using two purse boats. (*Source:* Zapata Haynie Corporation, Hammond, Louisiana.)

fishing vessel can carry 400–600 tons of refrigerated fish. A typical modern menhaden vessel appears in Fig. 6-4. This vessel is the latest generation of fishing vessel that has evolved from sailing ships and steamboats in the post-Civil War era to today's modern diesel-powered vessels.

Other catch methods involve trawls that can be hauled at various depths depending on the location of the fish or single-vessel purse seines shown in Fig. 6-5. In every case, the fishing method will depend on the species of fish being sought, its location and depth, and the size of the schools.

Unloading Methods

Once the fish are delivered to the factory, they are unloaded from the vessel by one of several methods. These can be divided into wet and dry methods.

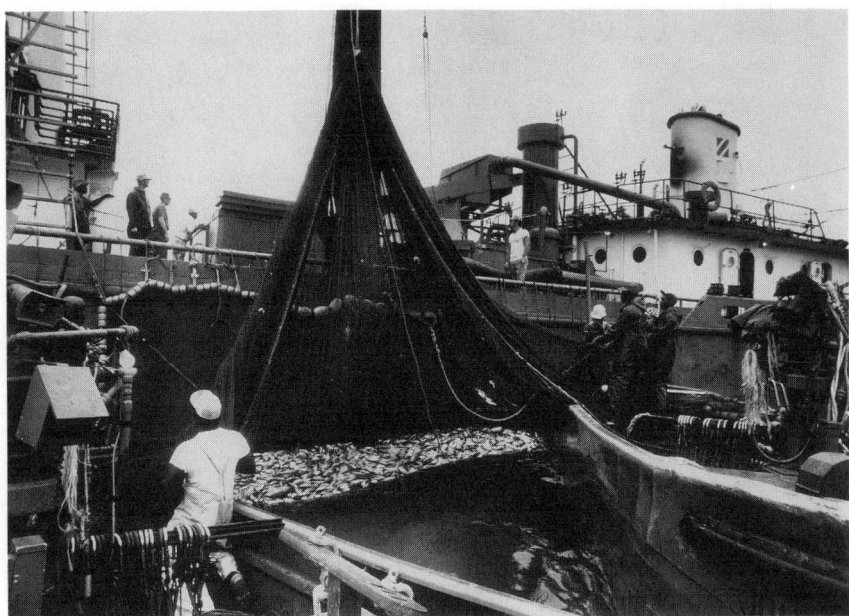

Fig. 6-3. Pumping fish from the net aboard the steamer. (*Source:* Zapata Haynie Corporation, Hammond, Louisiana.)

Dry Unloading.   There are a number of dry unloading methods available today. The grab method involves use of a crane and "grab" to remove fish directly from the hold of the vessel. The elevator method employs a bucket elevator and conveyor to remove fish directly from the vessel. The air suction and vacuum method of unloading are somewhat similar; both employ suction to remove the fish from the vessel and a cyclone to separate air from fish. The air suction method employs a suction nozzle and vacuum pump to move the fish in a current of air. The vacuum method employs a vacuum pump and rotating valve to maintain the seal and works well with fish that move easily. Direct pumping without water employs a pump either on the vessel or on shore. The pump is specially constructed to convey the fish in a sealed pipeline so that there is little crushing of the fish and no need for transport water (Sola 1978).

Wet Unloading.   In the water-pumping method, sea or fresh water is added to the vessel's hold to create a seal so that a vacuum pump can suck the fish and water from the hold of the vessel. The water is used as a transporting medium to convey the fish into the plant, then is separated

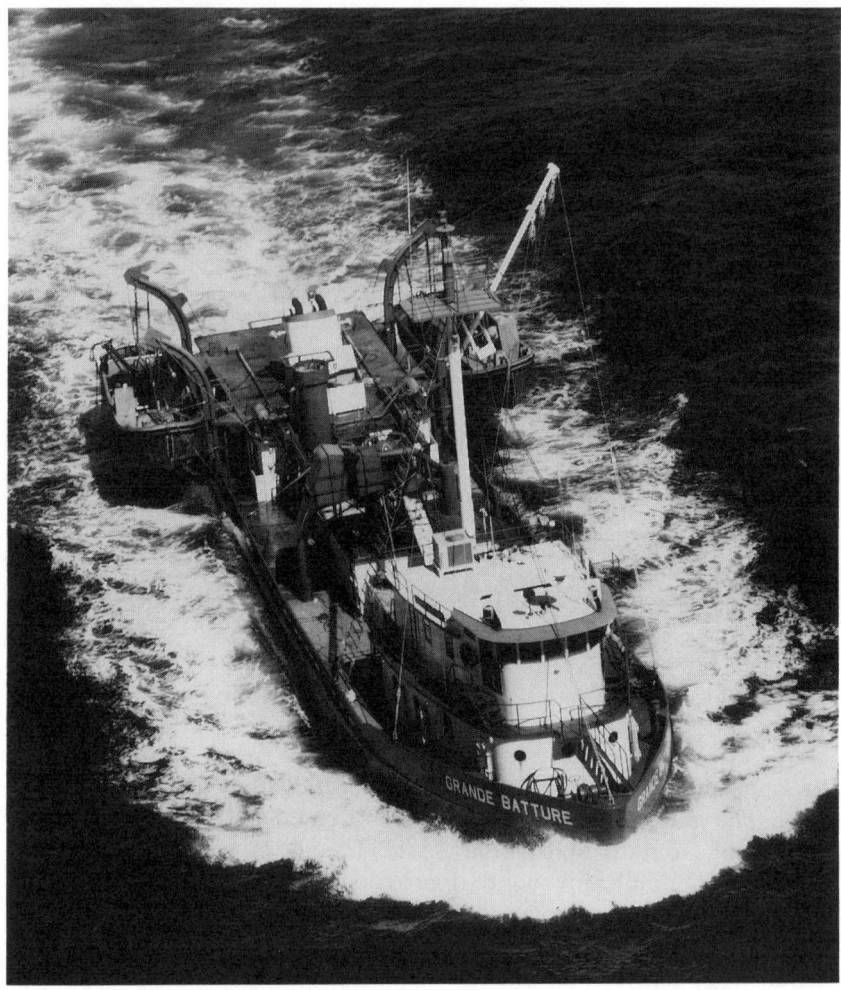

Fig. 6-4. Modern menhaden vessel with purse boats. (*Source:* Zapata Haynie Corporation, Hammond, Louisiana.)

from the fish by screening, and recycled back to the vessel and reused. In areas where salt from the water will not present a problem in the fish meal, the water is eventually added to the process and converted into product. In areas where salt from ocean water presents a problem, the unloading water is pumped on board the vessels and returned to the sea, where it enters back into the food chain. A relatively new wet-pumping system was used for unloading menhaden at the Zapata Haynie surimi demonstration plant in Reedville, Virginia. The pump operated on a

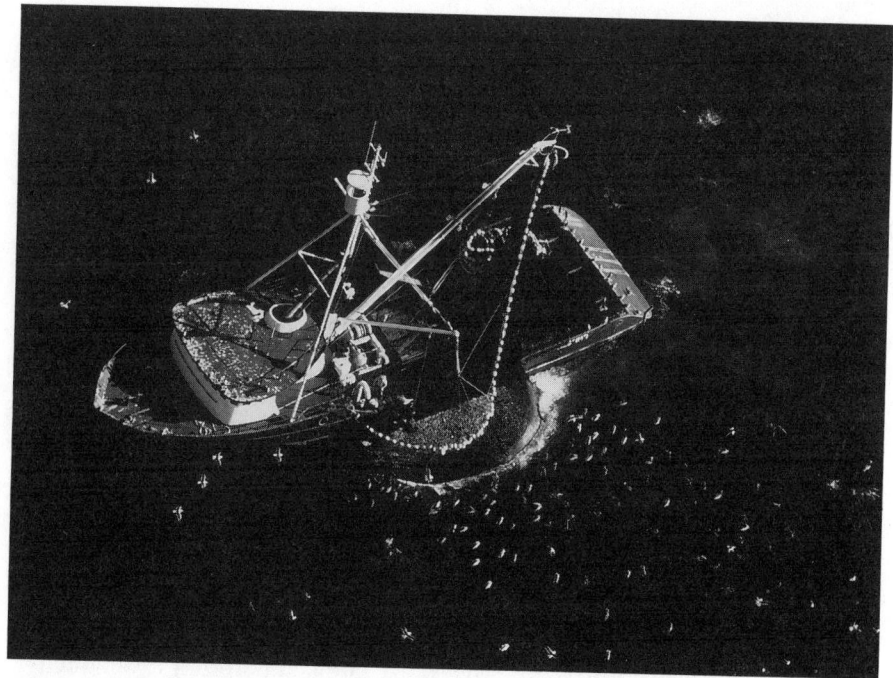

Fig. 6-5. Purse seining with a single purse boat. (*Source:* Pesquera Zapata SA de CV, Ensenada BC, Mexico.)

pulsed cycle, vacuum unloading the fish in a mass of water to a sealed tank and then pumping the fish and water under pressure to the dewatering screens and finally storage, with no damage to the fish (Bimbo 1988B).

The Wet Reduction Process

The processing techniques involved in the commercial production of edible fats and oils vary according to the type of raw material. The simplest, butter production, involves only churning of the matured cream from cow's milk. Tallow and lard can involve lengthy high-temperature rendering of waste carcass parts. Extraction of oil from oil seeds entails precooking of the crushed seed at temperatures reaching 120°C, followed by pressing to remove about half the oil. Further treatment of the pressed cake with a solvent, such as hexane, removes the remaining oil. This process requires oil recovery from the hexane solution, usually in several stages. The crude oil is then refined by degumming, alkali treatment, bleaching, and deodorizing to produce refined vegetable oil.

Fish reduction to produce oil and fish meal, except for solvent extraction, generally employs the same principles, techniques, and equipment common to the production of the other edible fats and oils. In general, fish are processed by the wet reduction method, in which the principal operations are cooking, pressing, separation of the oil and water emulsion with recovery of oil, and drying of the residual protein material. Continuous processing from the time the fish are landed optimizes efficiency and maximizes product quality (FAO 1986).

There are a number of processes that can be used to convert raw fish and cuttings into fish meal and oil. These fall into several categories defined as wet rendering, hydrolysis, silage production, dry rendering, and solvent extraction. The wet-rendering process is used in the majority of the factories that produce fish oil worldwide. This process is universal; factories all over the world both on land and on ships employ it with slight differences in equipment type, but the major steps of cooking, pressing, separating, and drying are always present. We will look at the process in two phases, solids flow and liquid flow.

Solids Flow

Cooking.   Raw fish enter the process by conveyor from a raw holding area to the cookers. The purpose of the cooking step is to coagulate the protein of the fish, so that liquids and solids can be mechanically separated. Fat cells are also ruptured, releasing the oil into the liquid phase. A typical continuous indirect cooker is shown in Fig. 6-6. The cooker is a cylinder having a steam-heated jacket enclosing a steam-heated auger, with hollow flights. The cooker is equipped with covers for inspection and cleaning and a nozzle system for blowing direct steam into the fish. The liquid drained from the cooked fish is screened and pumped with the water from the presses (Fosbol 1980, 1988).

Pressing.   The cooked fish are usually conveyed to the press by an inclined screw conveyor with perforations for dewatering the cooked mass. The purpose of pressing is to separate, as completely as possible, the liquid phase from the remaining solids contained in the cooked fish. Both continuous single- and twin-screw presses are used in the fish meal industry today. The screw in the single-screw press is designed with a taper and exerts an increasing pressure on the fish pulp by reducing the volume as it progresses through the press. Some problems are experienced when the fish are soft and slip through the press without being squeezed.

The twin-screw press consists of a press chamber with two hollow interlocked cylinders. The cylinder wall contains heavily supported strainer plates, and the two screws have tapered shafts that are pitched

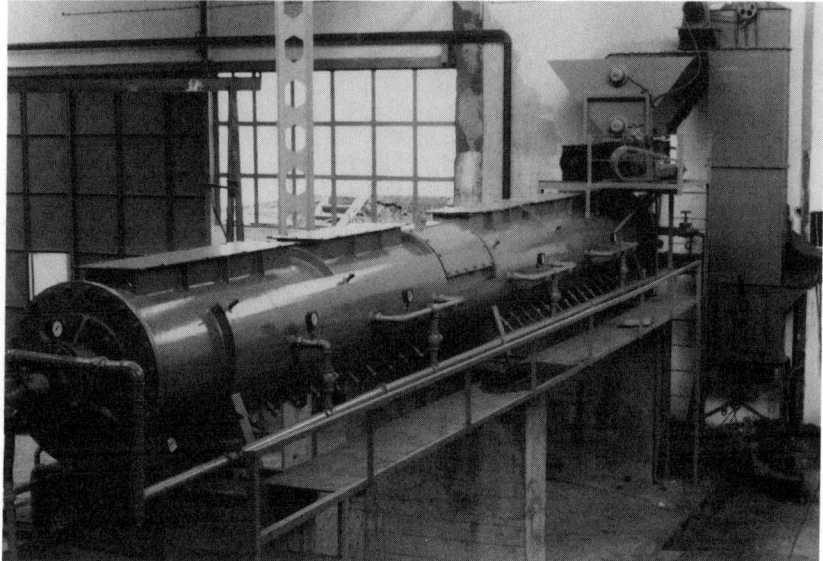

Fig. 6-6. Indirect heated cooker. (*Source:* Zapata Haynie Corporation, Hammond, Louisiana.)

opposite to the shaft taper. The screws operate in opposite directions and appear more capable of handling soft fish (Onarheim and Utvik 1979). Figure 6-7 shows a typical twin-screw press.

Drying. The pressed fish are then dried to produce fish meal. Drying reduces the moisture content so that the fish meal is stable to microbiological decomposition. There are two main types of dryers in commercial use: direct and indirect (Jason 1980). The direct or flame dryer utilizes a current of flue gases from the furnace to evaporate water from the pressed cake. A typical flame dryer can be seen in Fig. 6-8. Indirect dryers rely on an intermediate material to convey the heat from the furnace to the dryer. Initially this was done with steam, but major improvements in drying technology have taken place during the last five years and today, low-temperature, gentle drying seems to be getting more popular in the industry. These improvements have led to increased utilization of indirect hot-air, vacuum, and fluid bed dryers (Sand and Burt 1987). Figure 6-9 gives a schematic of a new-generation indirect hot-air dryer equipped with waste heat recovery and incineration of fumes in the furnace (Wiedswang 1988).

Modern fish meal plants may utilize both types of dryers. The direct-fired flame dryer is used to reduce the moisture in the presscake to 20–25%. Stickwater concentrate is then added to the partially dried cake,

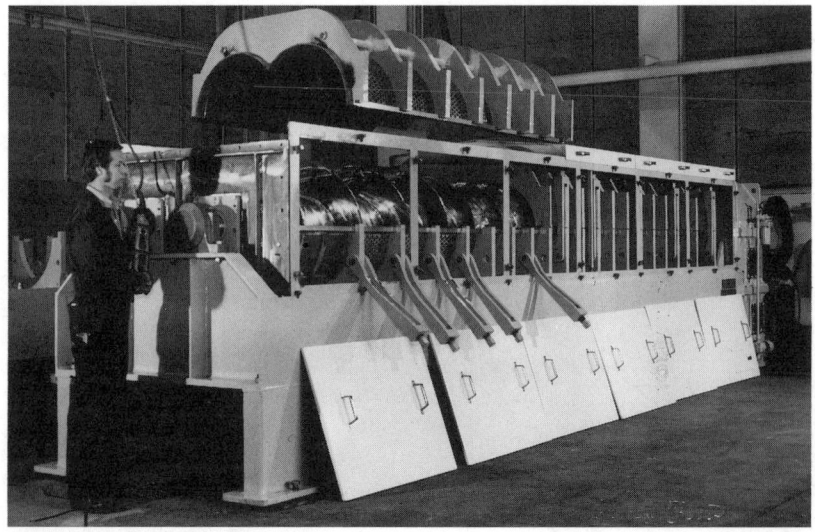

Fig. 6-7. Twin-screw press with inspection covers off. (*Source:* Stord Bartz A.s, Bergen, Norway.)

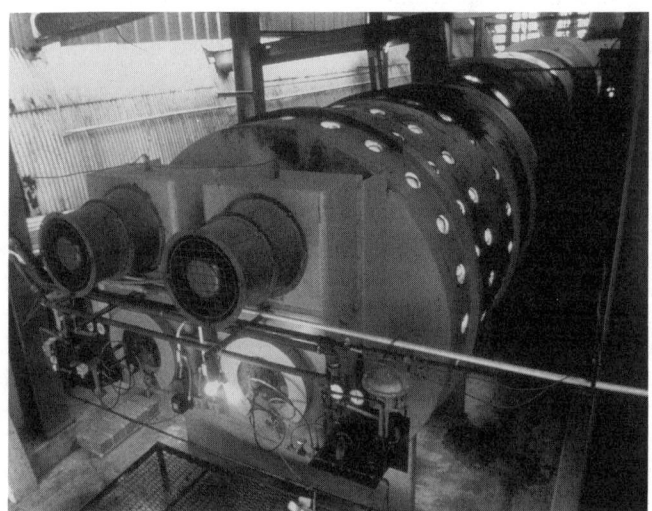

Fig. 6-8. Typical hot-air dryer. (*Source:* Zapata Haynie Corporation, Hammond, Louisiana.)

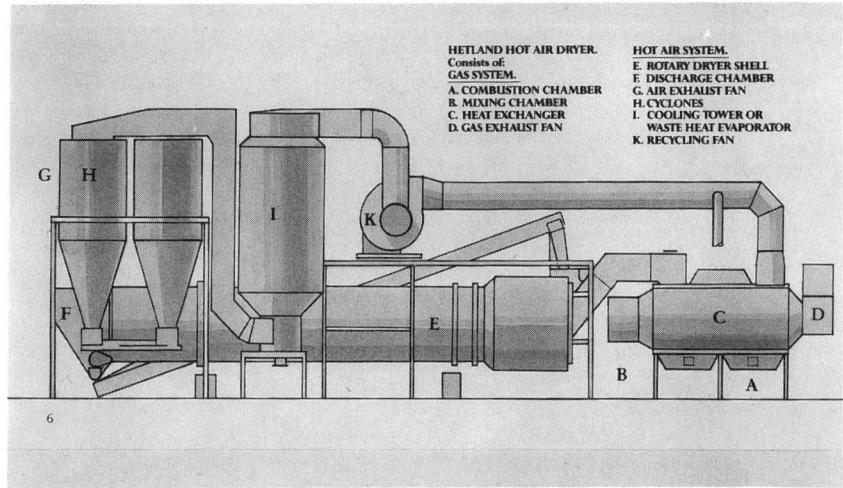

HETLAND HOT AIR DRYER.
Consists of:
GAS SYSTEM.
A. COMBUSTION CHAMBER
B. MIXING CHAMBER
C. HEAT EXCHANGER
D. GAS EXHAUST FAN

HOT AIR SYSTEM.
E. ROTARY DRYER SHELL
F. DISCHARGE CHAMBER
G. AIR EXHAUST FAN
H. CYCLONES
I. COOLING TOWER OR
WASTE HEAT EVAPORATOR
K. RECYCLING FAN

Fig. 6-9. Schematic of an indirect hot-air dryer with waste heat evaporator and discharge gas return. (*Source:* Kvaerner Eureka A/S, Hetland Process Division, Bryne, Norway.)

which is then further dried in an indirect dryer. In this way, one or two direct-fired dryers can be used to feed a battery of indirect dryers (Hetland 1980). Other plants may use one or the other type of dryer or reverse the flow so that the indirect dryer is used first followed by the direct-fired dryer. Figures 6-10 to 6-12 illustrate several types of dryers in use today.

Antioxidant Addition. The meal is cooled when it leaves the dryer and an antioxidant is added to prevent oxidation of the residual fat. The amount of antioxidant required to avoid spontaneous heating depends on the degree of unsaturation of the residual fat in the meal and the species of fish processed. Northern species of fish with relatively low unsaturation in the fat, such as herring or capelin, require low concentrations of antioxidant, while southern species such as anchovy, sardine, and menhaden require higher dosages of the antioxidant (FAO 1986).

The proper treatment of fish meal is very important in obtaining the maximum protective value. This involves applying the correct quantity of antioxidant to the meal and thoroughly mixing. The proper point of addition to fish meal in the processing system will vary, but in general the antioxidant is added after the meal has passed through the dryer to minimize the effects of steam distillation and prevent loss of the antioxidant by volatilization. Some plants use coolers after the dryer to help with this. It

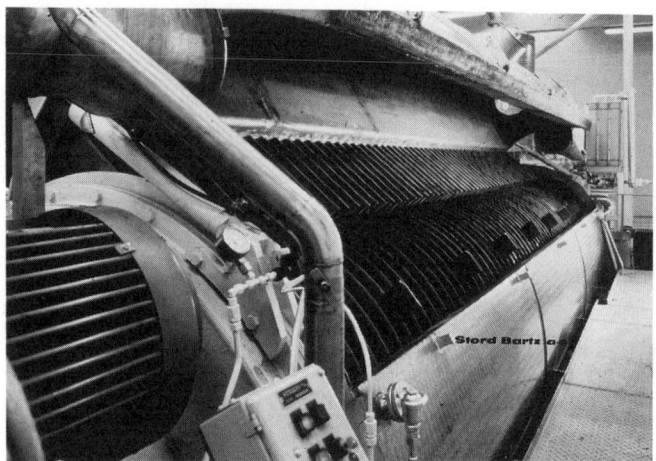

Fig. 6-10. Rotadisc dryer with inspection doors off. (*Source:* Stord Bartz A.s, Bergen, Norway.)

has been suggested that some antioxidant should be added prior to the dryer so that any oxidation within the dryer can be avoided, but so far the results are inconclusive. Liquid antioxidants are added to the meal through a metering and spraying system so that the antioxidant is reduced to a fine mist for easy mixing in the product. Dry antioxidants can be

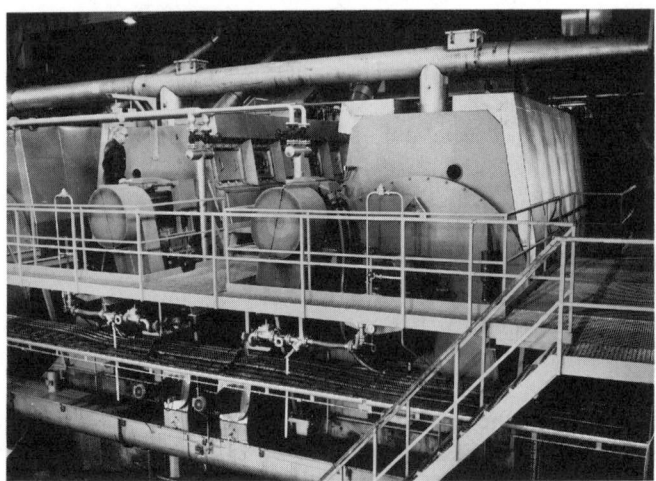

Fig. 6-11. Rotaplate dryers. (*Source:* Stord Bartz A.s, Bergen, Norway.)

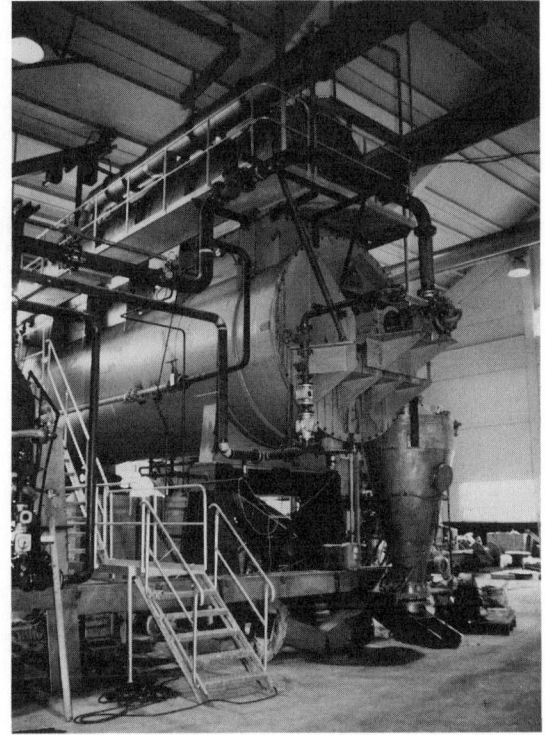

Fig. 6-12. Rota-vacuum dryer. (*Source:* Stord Bartz A.s, Bergen, Norway.)

metered in by any number of proportioning systems that feed trace amounts of chemicals into mixtures.

Ethoxyquin (6-ethoxy-2,2,4-trimethyl-1,2-dihydroquinoline) is the major antioxidant used in the fish meal industry. Ethoxyquin is approved for use as an additive in the feeds of animals in the United States up to 150 ppm (Code of Federal Regulations 1982). Other antioxidant systems consisting of synergistic blends of several antioxidants, emulsifiers, and metal chelating agents are currently being evaluated in several areas of the world (Vargas 1988).

Storage and Shipping. Storage methods for fish meal vary, depending on climate, production capacity, and transportation facilities to the marketplace. Fish meal must be stored in weatherproof, well-ventilated areas. About half of the world's fish meal is stored in bulk in sheds and silos.

Storage sheds may be of single- or multiunit construction with concrete outer walls and floors. Silo storage is also used. The fish meal is kept in continuous motion by extracting it from the bottom of the silo and returning it to the top by means of automatic conveyors. Because of the poor flow properties of fish meal, silos must be constructed in special ways so that the product will flow (FAO 1986). Although used in different parts of the world, silos are not currently used in the United States. Fish meal is also stored in multiwall paper, burlap, and woven plastic bags containing 50–100 pounds each on pallets. A newer concept is the bulk bag, which can hold about one ton of product. A typical flow diagram of the solids portion of the wet reduction plant can be seen in Fig. 6-13.

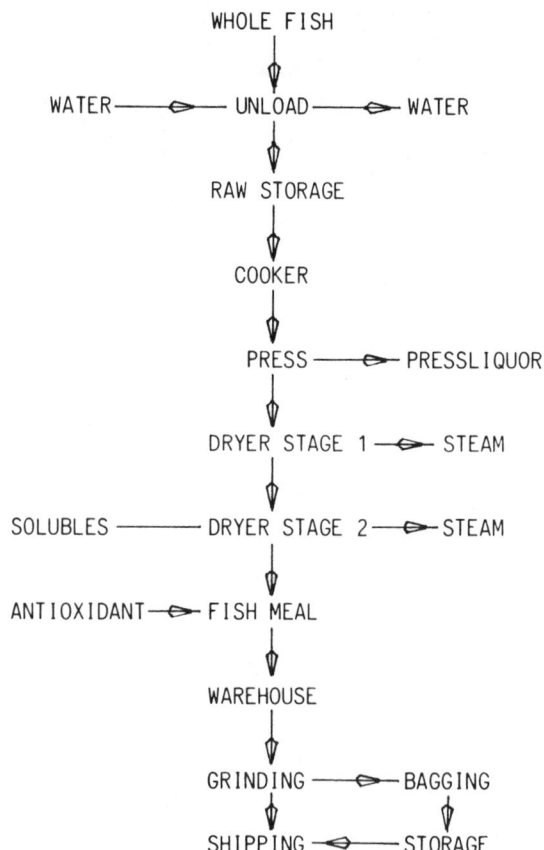

Fig. 6-13. Solids flow diagram in the wet reduction process.

Liquid Flow

During the pressing operation, two intermediate products are produced: presscake and pressliquor. As shown previously, the presscake is dried to produce fish meal. The pressliquor that is squeezed from the cooked fish contains coarse particles of fish and bone which must be removed before the liquor can be centrifuged. These solids are removed by passing the liquor over a vibrating screen with 5–6-mm perforations. The recovered solids go back on the presscake and are dried.

Separation of the screened presswater is then carried out in three steps involving:

1. Decanters, which are used to remove fine suspended solids including sand from the pressliquor in order to obtain a liquor suitable for the separation step.
2. Separators, which are used to remove as much oil as possible from the pressliquor and thus produce a stickwater with the least amount of fat.
3. Polishers or purifiers, which are used to remove the final traces of moisture and impurities from the oil prior to its pumping to storage.

In some plants there is also a fourth step, the subsequent separation of oil (deoiling) from the solubles after partial evaporation (Bimbo 1987A).

Solids Removal. Decanters are cylindrical bowls with a cylindrical conveyor turning inside. Figure 6-14 shows a typical decanter. The pressliquor is pumped into the bowl, and the solids are forced to the outer

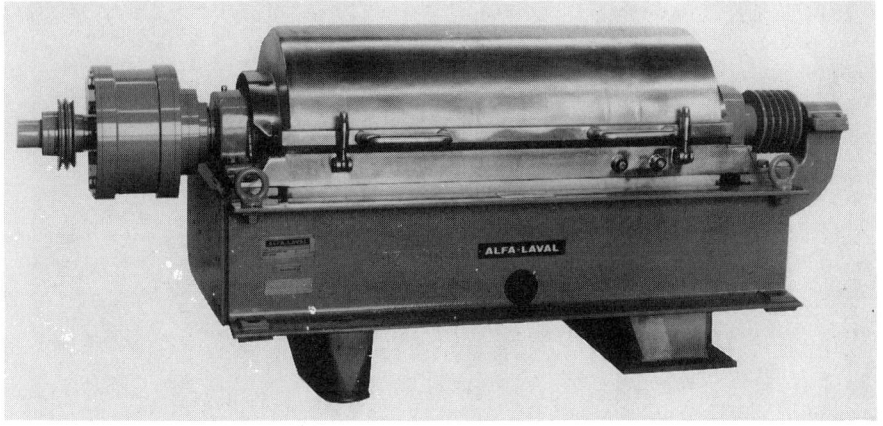

Fig. 6-14. Decanter. (*Source:* Alfa- Laval AB, Tumba, Sweden.)

periphery and conveyed out of the system by the conveyor. The conveyor turns at a slower speed than the bowl, and through a combination of conveyor speed and liquid depth, the desired clarifications can be achieved. Solids removed from the decanters are mixed with the press-cake and dried (Bimbo 1987A).

Separation.   Pressliquor discharged from the decanters is pumped into a holding tank, heated if necessary, and then fed either by gravity or by pump to the separators. Today, the separator is a modern, high-capacity machine capable of handling many times more gallons of feed per hour than the machines described by Smith in the 1940s. These machines are self-cleaning; that is, either they have a sensor in the bowl capable of interrupting the separation cycle long enough to discharge the solids accumulated in the bowl, or they discharge the contents of the bowl on a timed cycle. The machines make a three-phase separation of the pressliquor into an oil phase, water phase, and sludge phase. The sludge phase is pumped away either to the cooker or to the presscake, where it is dried back on the fish meal (Bimbo 1987A). Figure 6-15 shows a typical oil room with self-cleaning separators in a modern fish meal factory.

Evaporation.   The water phase, which is rich in soluble proteins and vitamins, is stored in large holding tanks and then pumped to continuous vacuum evaporators that concentrate the solids content to 50%. This concentrate is called fish solubles. Today both high-speed multieffect and

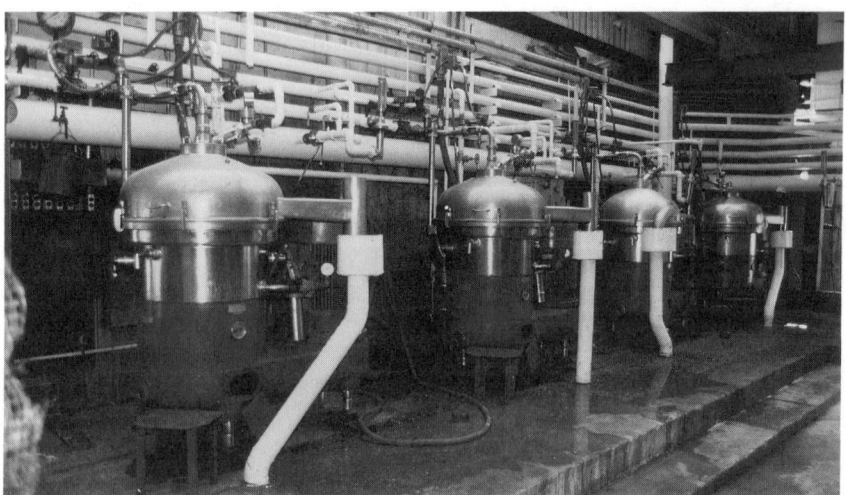

Fig. 6-15. Centrifuges used to separate pressliquor into fish oil and stickwater.

falling-film evaporators are capable of producing product as fast as the water is produced, thus ensuring that fresh product is added back on the fish meal. A typical falling-film evaporator can be seen in Fig. 6-16 and a schematic diagram of its operation in Fig. 6-17. A multieffect high-speed evaporator can be seen in Fig. 6-18.

The stickwater concentrate may then be added back on the presscake and dried to produce whole or full meal, or it can be centrifugally deoiled to further reduce the fat content, concentrated back to 50% solids, acidulated to pH 4.2, and sold as condensed fish solubles. Today, most of the solubles are added back on the presscake to produce whole meal (Christensen 1978).

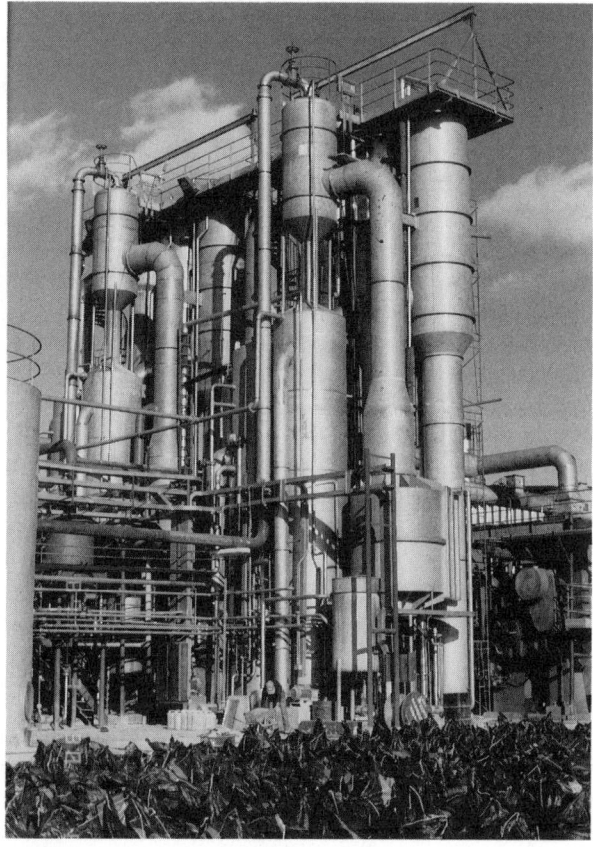

Fig. 6-16. Falling-film waste heat evaporator plant. (*Source:* Kvaerner Eureka A/S, Hetland Process Division, Bryne, Norway.)

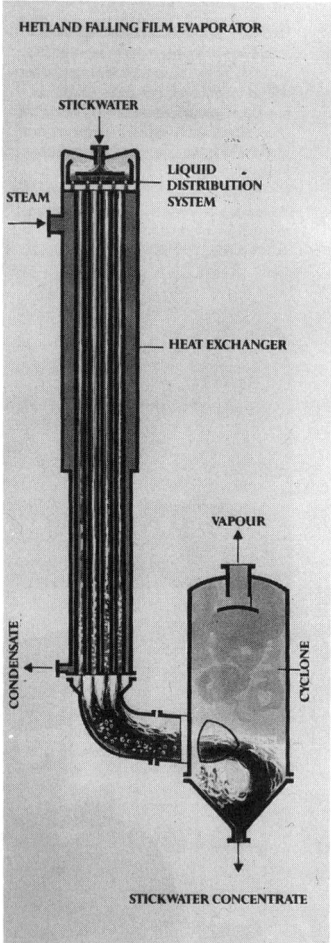

HETLAND FALLING FILM EVAPORATOR

STICKWATER

STEAM

LIQUID
DISTRIBUTION
SYSTEM

HEAT EXCHANGER

VAPOUR

CONDENSATE

CYCLONE

STICKWATER CONCENTRATE

Fig. 6-17. Schematic diagram of falling-film evaporator. (*Source:* Kvaerner Eureka A/S, Hetland Process Division, Bryne, Norway.)

Polishing or Purifying. The oil phase recovered from the separators is continuously washed and separated into two phases, water and crude fish oil. The water phase is mixed with the stickwater and evaporated. The fish oil is pumped into storage tanks, where it is tested and sold for a variety of uses. The crude oil can also be further refined and processed

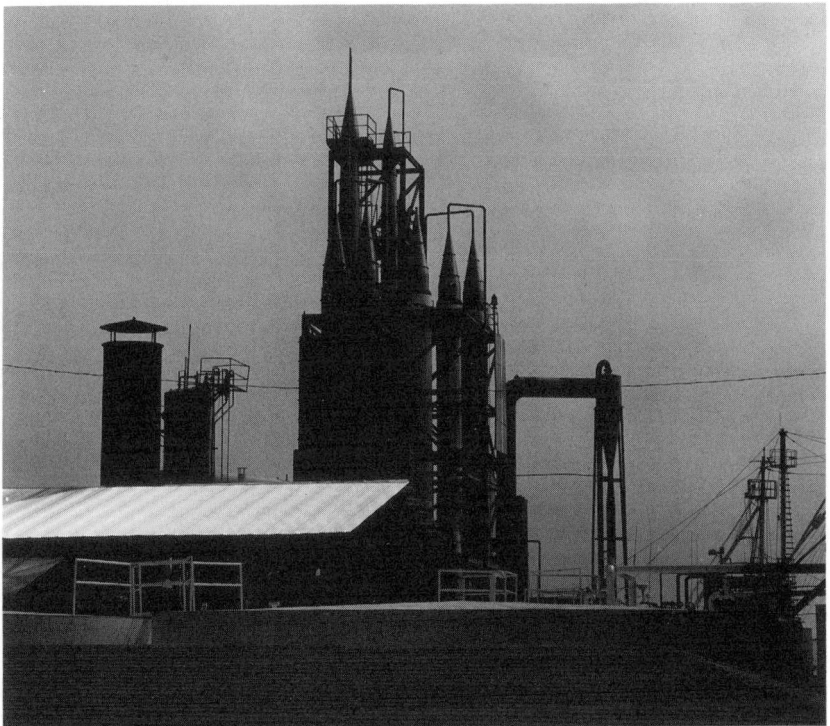

Fig. 6-18. Conventional multieffect high-speed evaporator. (*Source:* Zapata Haynie Corporation, Hammond, Louisiana.)

into a number of other food and industrial raw materials (Bimbo 1988A, 1989B). A typical flow diagram of the liquid phase of fish reduction is shown in Fig. 6-19.

We have now reviewed the wet-rendering process in some detail. The major steps are cooking, pressing, separation, and drying. A typical flow diagram of such a plant is seen in Fig. 6-20.

OTHER PRODUCTION METHODS

There are several alternative production methods primarily designed to produce fish meal or its equivalent with the oil phase as a minor by-product. They are mentioned here because they have some general use for the recovery of protein and oil from fish and fish waste, and historically these uses come up for review now and then.

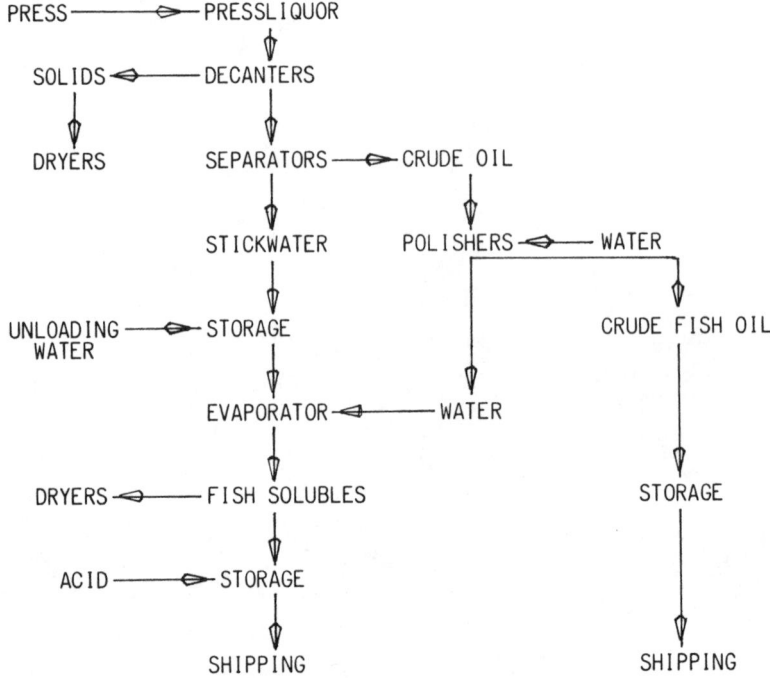

Fig. 6-19. Liquid flow diagram in the wet reduction process.

Hydrolysis

Hydrolyzed fish proteins are produced by employing proteolytic enzymes either from the fish themselves (autolysis) or from other sources (hydrolysis), either animal, vegetable, or microbial, to accelerate the breakdown of the proteins into smaller units. Hydrolysis can also be accomplished chemically under acidic or alkaline conditions. According to Windsor and Barlow (1981), the process is generally slow and uncontrolled. By use of some of the newer enzymes available on the market, a process can be developed to recover proteins in varying degrees of breakdown of the fish. Although the process could be used with any fish, it is primarily used for white fish or offal low in oil. In cases where oily fish are hydrolyzed, the processor faces a dilemma. He must recover the oil phase without denaturing the proteins or face supplying a high-fat hydrolyzed protein product or a protein product with reduced functionality. It has been difficult to achieve a commercially viable product from fatty fish that is both functional and low in fat. Perhaps the newer processing technol-

THE PRODUCTION AND REFINING OF MENHADEN OIL

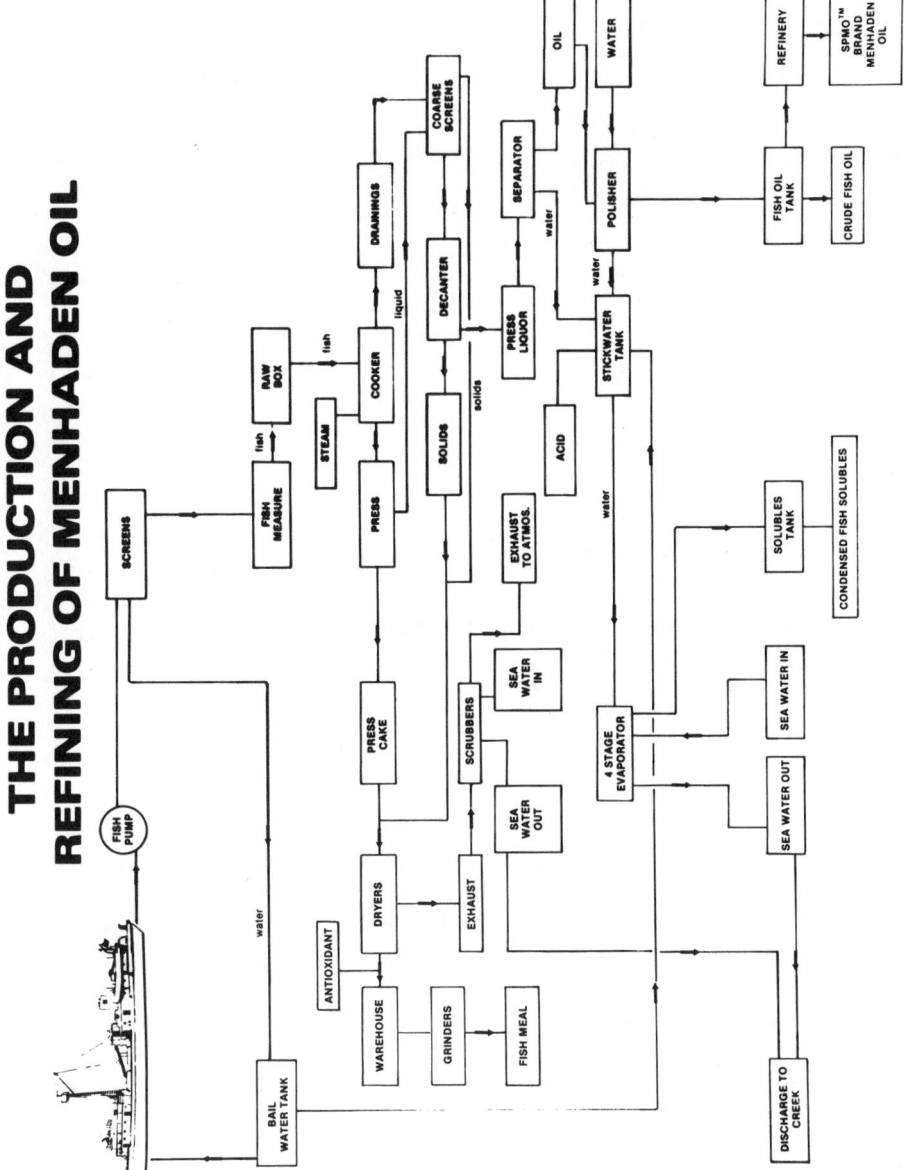

Fig. 6-20. Flow diagram of a typical menhaden reduction plant.

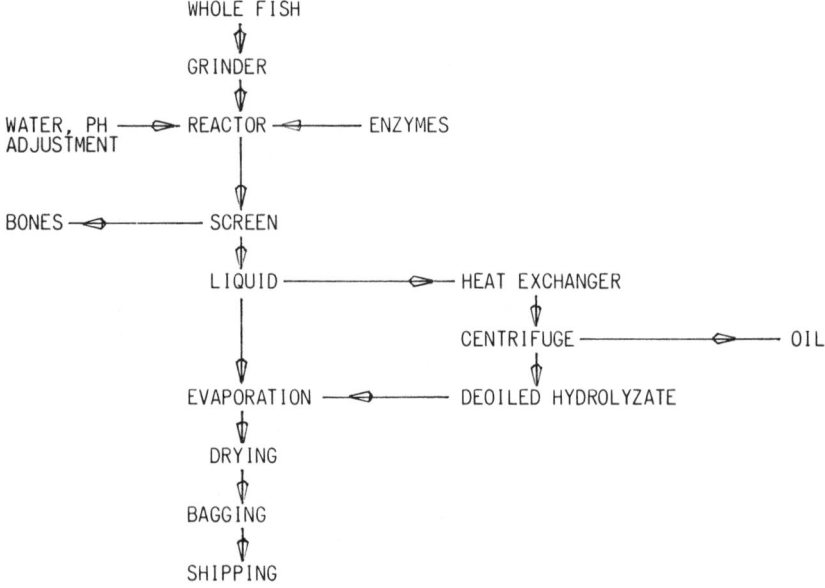

Fig. 6-21. Flow diagram of hydrolyzate production.

ogy designed for producing surimi or minced fish could be used to pretreat fish before the hydrolysis step. Figure 6-21 gives a typical flow diagram for the hydrolysis process.

Silage Production

Fish silage is liquified fish stabilized against bacterial decomposition by an acid. The process involves mincing of the fish followed by the addition of an acid for preservation. The enzymes in the fish break down the fish proteins into smaller soluble units, and acid helps to speed up their activity while preventing bacterial spoilage. Formic, propionic, sulfuric, and phosphoric acids have been used. Normally, about 3–4% of acid is added so that the pH remains near 4.0. Strong mineral acids require neutralization before feeding the final product. The process is outlined in Fig. 6-22. Silage might be defined as a crude form of hydrolyzate.

Silage made from white fish offal does not contain much oil, but when made from fatty fish such as herring it is necessary to remove the oil. The composition of the silage will be very similar to the material from which it is made. Fish silage of the correct acidity is stable at room temperature for at least two years without decomposition. The protein becomes more

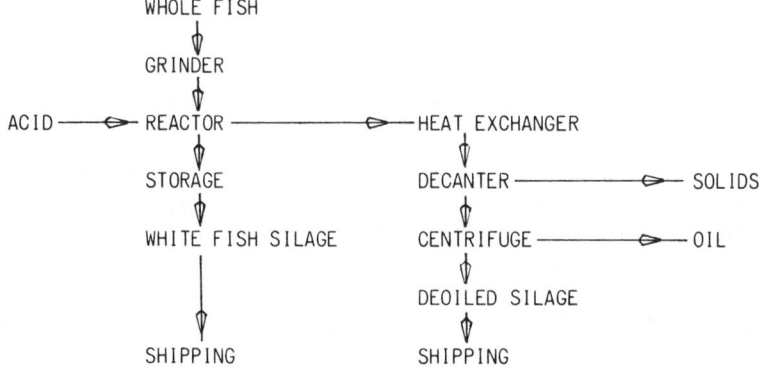

Fig. 6-22. Flow diagram of silage production.

soluble, and the amount of free fatty acids increases in any fish oil present during storage (Tatterson and Windsor 1974). Silage production offers a solution to the handling of fish waste when the logistics of delivering to a fish reduction plant are not economical. Silage can be produced in large or small containers both on the vessel and on shore.

Dry Rendering

The dry-rendering process that is commonly used to prepare meat and bone meal is not normally used in the manufacture of fish meal and oil. If used at all, it would find some limited use when the raw material is extremely low in oil. The process is usually batch type, involving a combined cooking and drying step. The cooker is usually a steam-jacketed, paddle-stirred rotary-operated device, sometimes operated under vacuum. The cooked and dried product is then conveyed to a hydraulic press, where the oil is removed. The recovered oil is generally dark in color and must be further refined before it can be used (Pigott 1967).

A commercial improvement in the dry-rendering process is the patented Carver-Greenfield process, which produced a low-temperature, dehydrated, semideoiled meat and bone meal (Anonymous 1962). The process was used commercially at two fish reduction plants in the United States during the 1960s and 1970s. Whole fish were unloaded from the vessel and stored in raw holding bins. The fish then passed through a prebreaker, which chopped the fish into pieces. The chopped fish were then slurried with fish oil and pumped into a disintegrator where the size was further reduced to $\frac{1}{8}$ inch or less. This slurry of ground fish and fish oil was then heated and pumped via a level control tank to a two-stage falling-film evaporator, where the moisture in the fish was reduced from 70% to 1%. Fish oil was used as the heat transfer medium. The slurry of dried fish solids and fish oil was then pumped to a centrifuge feed tank and then a decanter, where it was partially deoiled. The decanter separated the free oil from the solids, the oil returned to the recycle tank and then back to the disintegrator to slurry more fish, and the solids were conveyed to expeller presses, where the remaining oil was removed. This expressed oil, rich in solids, was also pumped back to the disintegrator to slurry more fish. Excess recycle oil was pumped to a series of hydration tanks and finally to polishers before storage. The hydration step removed phospholipids along with fines. Solids discharged from the polisher returned to the disintegrator with the expeller oil.

The expelled meal, in the form of cracklings or chunks, was conveyed to a warehouse, where antioxidant was added prior to bulk storage. After a short curing time, the product was ground and either bagged or shipped in bulk. The oil product required further refining before it could be sold; this was a major drawback to the process.

The beauty of the process was its simplicity and versatility; where the wet reduction plants are spread out horizontally, this plant was built vertically. All operations were carried out in one processing building. The entire plant was run from an air-conditioned control room that contained a panel of temperature recorders, tank level sensors, and communications with all other parts of the plant. Essentially, it was a pushbutton operation. Its versatility lay in its intermediate product, the centrifuge cake, which could be processed to fish meal or solvent extracted to produce FPC (Bimbo 1970). It was probably the original "low-temperature" fish meal process many years ahead of its time. Unfortunately, environmental pressures in the areas where the plants were situated and high maintenance costs associated with the expeller presses forced the closing of both plants. A flow diagram of the process can be seen in Fig. 6-23.

Solvent Extraction

Solvent extraction to produce fish protein concentrate (FPC) is another process that could yield fish oil. FPC can be defined as any stable fish preparation intended for human consumption in which the protein is more concentrated than in the original fish. Water and fat together constitute about 80% of the whole fish, with the fat itself in some species being as high as 20%. The manufacture of FPC involves the removal of most of the water and some or all of the fat. Methods developed so far are based mainly on the use of chemical solvents to remove water, fat, and fishy-tasting components either from the raw fish or from fish meal. The sol-

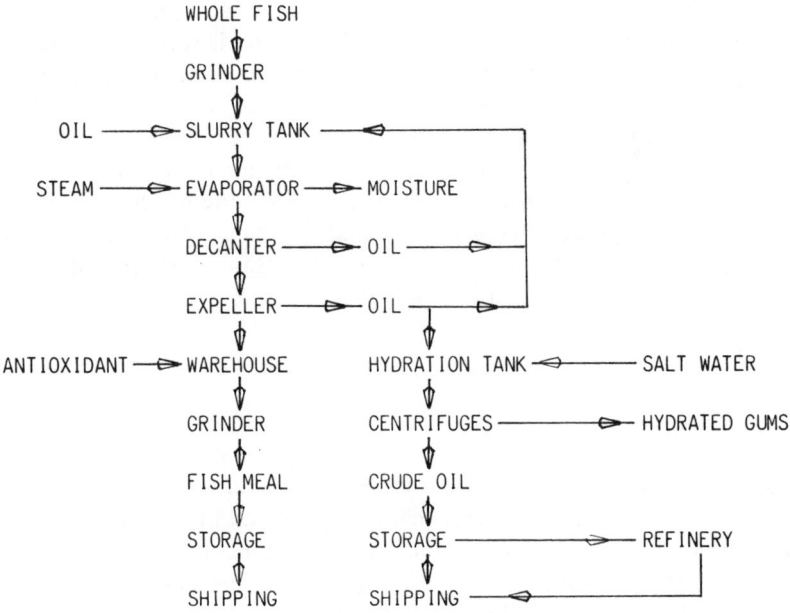

Fig. 6-23. Flow diagram of the Carver-Greenfield dry-rendering process.

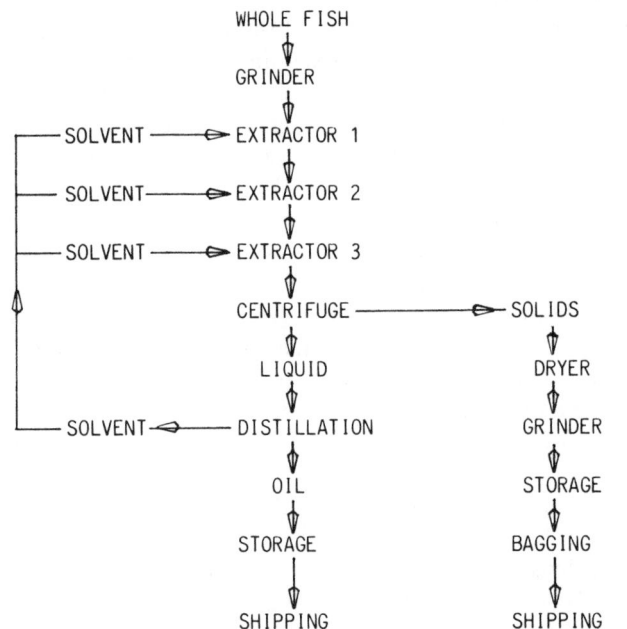

Fig. 6-24. Flow diagram of a solvent extraction process.

vents most successfully used to make FPC are ethanol, hexane, iso-propanol, or ethylene dichloride. Normally the solvent is recovered and used over again. The recovered fat is usually mixed in an azeotropic mixture with water, solvent, and water-soluble components. Separation of this azeotrope to recover the fat sometimes presents problems (Windsor 1969). Unfortunately, although FPC was nutritional, it had very poor functionality and most processes used to produce the product have been abandoned or replaced by processes that produce a functional protein concentrate, such as fish protein isolates, and surimi. A simplified solvent extraction plant can be seen in Fig. 6-24.

OTHER MARINE OILS

Fish Liver Oils

Fish liver oils were used in the treatment of rickets in the Middle Ages. As early as 1657 certain fish liver oils were believed to contain something that could cure night blindness. With the development of vitamin chemistry early in the twentieth century, it was shown that night blindness and rickets are largely caused by a dietary deficiency in vitamins A and D, respectively. Both vitamins A and D are found in certain fish liver oils at varying levels (Bimbo 1988C).

The oil is contained in the protein of the livers and is sometimes easily removed by extraction; at other times the oil is removed from the livers after digestion of the liver protein and a more complicated process of extraction is needed. Special processing is required for the extraction and separation of the vitamin-bearing material from low-fat proteinaceous liver tissue (Brody 1965).

The most important raw material for the production of liver oils comes from the fisheries for cod, coalfish, and haddock. The livers of ling, tusk, several species of shark such as dogfish, Greenland shark, and basking shark, and halibut, whale, and tuna have been used in the production of liver oils. In order to obtain high-quality, light-colored oils with good flavor and odor containing a minimum of free fatty acids, it is important to eviscerate the fish and recover the livers so that they can be processed as quickly as possible (Windsor and Barlow 1981; Brocklesby and Patrick 1958).

In the early history of the industry, the livers were allowed to stand in wooden vats or barrels and the oil was removed as it floated to the surface after being released by autolysis. The first two batches removed in this fashion were used as medicinal oil, and the remainder as industrial oil.

The residue was heated in underfired iron kettles, giving dark oil that contained large amounts of free fatty acids.

The method of heating the fish livers with steam, applied either directly in contact with the liver mass or indirectly, was introduced about 1950. This method gave lighter oils of good quality, and the many methods developed later are actually based on the sample principle (Aure 1967).

The most generally accepted way of extracting oil from cod livers is by means of a steam cooker. The method of applying the steam has been changed from time to time to meet the demand for a higher grade of oil. Low-pressure steam is piped into a tank containing the livers. The heat of the steam cooks the livers, the steam condenses, and a layer of hot water is produced upon which the oil floats. Then either the oil is dipped off or the tank is fitted with an overflow into an oil storage tank. Some liver oils are extracted at sea on board trawlers and schooners when they remain at sea for long periods of time.

The following description of Icelandic cod-liver oil production was kindly provided by Mr. Baldur Hjaltason of Lysi, HF, Reykjavik, Iceland.

Iceland first developed a process that treated the liver residue with caustic soda. After the usual treatment of the liver with steam, the oil is floated off the top and recovered as medicinal-grade oil. The residue is then treated with caustic soda. The soda destroys the protein, which becomes very dark, and oil floats to the surface and is recovered as veterinary-grade cod-liver oil. This grade is darker in color and contains a higher level of vitamins than the medicinal grade.

Lysi was the first company to utilize centrifuges in the processing of cod-liver oil. The livers are ground and pumped over magnets to remove tramp metal, especially hooks that come from the freezing plants. The livers are heated and allowed to stand for a period of time to break down the proteins. The livers are then run through decanters to remove solids, and the liquor is collected in kettles, heated to 95°C, and then separated. Modern three-way separators are used, and the crude cod-liver oil is collected and pumped to the refinery. In the refinery the oil is alkali refined to remove free fatty acids, washed and dried in a vacuum tower, and then winterized to remove stearines. The result is medicinal-grade cod-liver oil. A diagram of the Icelandic process for producing cod-liver oil is shown in Fig. 6-25.

Today the annual world production of liver oils is around 20,000 mt. Table 6-9 shows the volume of liver oils produced over several different periods both in the United States and worldwide. The peak U.S. production years were 1940–1950.

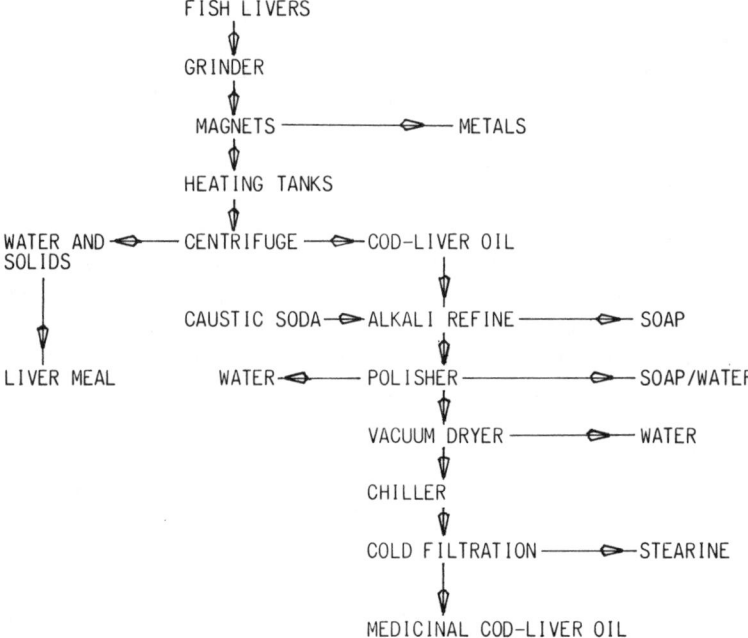

Fig. 6-25. Flow diagram of cod-liver oil production. (*Source:* Lysi HF, Reykjavik, Iceland.)

Table 6-9. World and U.S. Production of Liver Oils in 1000 Metric Tons, Historical Data

YEAR	WORLD[a,b]	U.S.[c]
1938	76	1.7
1948	65	2.5
1951	83	1.1
1952	78	0.9
1953	71	0.7
1954	70	0.8
1955	73	0.7
1975	52	—
1980	24	—
1985	16	—

[a]FAO 1954–1955.
[b]FAO 1980.
[c]Fitzgibbon 1969.

Marine Mammal Oils

According to Gilmore (1960), the first great whaling nation of the world was England, followed closely by Holland. In the seventeenth and eighteen centuries the English and Dutch caught right and bowhead whales worldwide. The early American industry initially caught right and bowhead whales but soon began searching for the sperm whale. In 1846 there was as many as 746 whaling ships registered in America and fishing out of New England ports. The Norwegians began to use the powder harpoon-cannon and winch on steamships in the 1860s, and this made whaling both profitable and efficient.

Once accounting for as much as 75% of the total marine oil production, today the oil from marine mammals accounts for less than 2% of the total aquatic animal oil production. Table 6-10 gives a breakdown of marine mammal oil production for several periods both in the United States and worldwide. This reduction in production is primarily due to conservation and a worldwide moratorium on whaling. The U.S. production of whale oil was at its peak between 1936 and 1940. Abegglen et al. (1963), Brocklesby and Patrick (1958), and Bimbo (1989B) have described the production and uses of marine mammal oils in great detail.

Table 6-10. World and
U.S. Production of
Marine Mammal Oils, in
1000 Metric Tons,
Historical Data

YEAR	WORLD[a,b]	U.S.[c]
1938	624	26
1948	624	0.5
1951	624	0.2
1955	502	—
1965	352	1
1966	261	0.6
1967	253	1
1968	213	1
1970	210	0
1975	133	0
1980	12	0
1985	6	0

[a]FAO 1954–1955.
[b]FAO 1980.
[c]Fitzgibbon 1969.

REFERENCES

Abegglen, C., Roppel, A. Y., and Rice, D. W. 1963. Marine mammals. In *Industrial Fishery Technology*, ed. M. E. Stansby, pp. 209–216. New York: Van Nostrand Reinhold.

Anonymous. 1962. Inedible low-temp rendering is odor-free; product is upgraded. *The National Provisioner*, June 30.

Aure, Lars. 1967. Manufacture of fish-liver oil. In *Fish Oils*, ed. M. E. Stansby, pp. 193–205. Westport, Conn.: Avi Publishing Co.

Bimbo, Anthony P. 1970. The menhaden industry: Yesterday, today and tomorrow. Paper read at the School of Chemical Engineering, 8 October, 1970, University of Rhode Island, Kingston, R.I.

Bimbo, Anthony P. 1983. Fish oils, then and now. Paper read at the National Fish Meal and Oil Association Congressional Breakfast, 28 September, 1983, Washington, D.C.

Bimbo, A. P. 1986. Use of fish oils: Task for new technology. *N-3 News Unsaturated Fatty Acids and Health* 1(3):1–4.

Bimbo, A. 1987A. Fish meal and oil. In *The Seafood Industry: A Self-Study Guide*, pp. 1–45. Sea Grant Extension Division, Virginia Tech Univ., Blacksburg, Va.

Bimbo, A. P. 1987B. The emerging marine oil industry. *J. Am. Oil Chemists' Soc.* 64:706–715.

Bimbo, A. P. 1987C. Marine oils—Perspectives on the U.S. industry. Paper read at the American Institute of Baking Technical Seminar Fish Oil (Omega-3 Fatty Acids) and Other Unconventional Oils, 11–12 May 1987, Manhattan, Kan.

Bimbo, A. 1988A. Fish oils: Future challenges and opportunities. In *Seafood Technology—Preparing for Future Opportunities*, ed. Marvin Kragt and Donn Ward, pp. 167–203. Chicago: Institute of Food Technologists.

Bimbo, A. P. 1988B. U.S. menhaden surimi production: Third interim report. Paper read at the 29th Annual Conference of the International Association of Fish Meal Manufacturers, 11 November 1988, Lima, Peru.

Bimbo, A. P. 1988C. Historical perspectives on the development of fish oil in the USA. Paper read at the 29th Annual Conference of the International Association of Fish Meal Manufacturers, 10 November 1988, Lima, Peru.

Bimbo, A. 1989A. Fish oils as foods: Challenges and opportunities. In *Fats and Oils in Bakery Products*, ed. Okkyung Kim Chung, pp. 282–308. St. Paul: American Association of Cereal Chemists.

Bimbo, A. P. 1989B. Technology of production and industrial utilization of marine oils. In *Marine Biogenic Lipids, Fats and Oils*, vol. II, ed. R. G. Ackman, pp. 401–433. Boca Raton, Fla.: CRC Press.

Bimbo, A. P., and Bauersfeld, P. E. 1982. Rat multi-generation and life span studies with partially hydrogenated menhaden fish oil (U.S.A. first interim report). Paper read at 22nd Annual Conference of the International Association of Fish Meal Manufacturers, 9–16 September 1982, Cannes, France.

Brocklesby, H. N., and Patrick, J. R. 1958. The production of marine oils. In *Progress in the Chemistry of Fats and Other Lipids*, vol. 5, ed. R. I. Holman, W. O. Lundberg, and T. Malkin, pp. 139–148. New York: Pergamon Press.

Brody, J. 1965. Fish liver oils. In *Fishery By-Products Technology*, pp. 47–68. Westport, Conn.: Avi Publishing Co.

Christensen, Sven. 1978. Control of decanters and separators. *IAFMM News Summary* 44:104–119.

Code of Federal Regulations, Food and Drugs. 1982. Chapter 21, Part 573, Subpart B., Section 573.380, p. 581.

FAO. 1955. *Yearbook of Fishery Statistics* 5:(f4, f46).

FAO. 1980. *Yearbook of Fishery Statistics* 51:148–152.

FAO. 1986. The production of fish meal and oil. Fisheries Technical Paper 142, Revision 1.

Fitzgibbon, D. S. 1969. *Historical Statistics—Fish Meal, Oil and Solubles.* U.S. Fish and Wildlife Service, Bureau of Commercial Fisheries. Current Fisheries Statistics No. 5105, 30 pp.

Fosbol, P. 1980. Coagulation of fish protein for fish meal production. *IAFMM News Summary* 48:24–50.

Fosbol, P. 1988. Production of fish meal and fish oil. *Infofish International* 5/88:26–32.

Frye, John. 1978. *The Men All Singing.* Virginia Beach: The Donning Company.

Gilmore, Raymond M. 1960. The whaling industry—Whales, dolphins and porpoises. In *Marine Products of Commerce,* ed. D. K. Tressler and J. McW. Lemon, pp. 680–715. New York: Van Nostrand Reinhold.

Hetland, Jens. 1980. Techniques and economics of direct (flame) and indirect drying. *IAFMM News Summary* 49:35–41.

IAFMM. 1988. *Digest of Selected Statistics.* Compiled for the 28th Annual Conference, Lima, Peru.

International Association of Fish Meal Manufacturers. 1975–1985. *Digest of Selected Statistics.*

Jason, A. C. 1980. General theory of drying of fish. *IAFMM News Summary* 49:5–25.

Lee, Charles F. 1953. Menhaden industry—Past and present. Fishery Leaflet No. 412. U.S. Department of Interior, Washington, D.C.

National Fish Meal and Oil Association. 1986. Petition to the Food and Drug Administration Requesting Affirmation of Menhaden Oil and Partially Hydrogenated Menhaden Oil as Generally Recognized as Safe for Use in Foods.

Oil World Weekly Statistics Update, 1988. ISTA Mielke GmbH, Hamburg, West Germany, December 19, 1988.

Onarheim, R., and Utvik, A. O. 1979. The design and operation of screens and presses. *IAFMM News Summary* 46:105–131.

Pigott, G. M. 1967. Production of fish oil. In *Fish Oils,* ed. M. E. Stansby, pp. 183–192. Westport, Conn.: AVI Publishing Co.

Sand, G., and Burt, J. 1987. *Which Kind of Dryer Is Best.* IAFMM, Processing Bulletin 2, 11 pp.

Smith, J. Howard. 1940. Advances in menhaden reduction. *Chemical and Metallurgical Engineering* 47:99–100.

Sola, Einar. 1978. Discharge of fish for meal and oil production. *IAFMM News Summary* 42:117–136.

Stansby, M. E. 1978. Development of fish oil industry in the United States. *J. Am. Oil Chemists' Soc.* 55:238–243.

Tatterson, I. N., and Windsor, M. L. 1974. *Fish Silage.* Torry Advisory Note No. 64. Torry Research Station, Aberdeen, UK.

U.S. Bureau of Commercial Fisheries. 1967. *Summary of Pacific Sardine Fishery, 1915–1965.* U.S. Fish and Wildlife Service, Bureau of Commercial Fisheries, Statistical Digest No. 59. Fishery Statistics of the United States, 1965 pp. 694–696.

U.S. Dept. of Commerce. 1988A. *Fisheries of the United States, 1987.* Current Fishery Statistics No. 8700.

U.S. Dept. of Commerce. 1988B. *Fisheries of the United States, 1987.* Supplemental, April 1988.

U.S. Food and Drug Administration. 1986. The National Fish Meal and Oil Association; filing of petition for affirmation of GRAS status. Notice. Federal Register, 51(147):27461–27462.

U.S. Food and Drug Administration. 1989. Substances affirmed as generally recognized as safe: Hydrogenated and partially hydrogenated menhaden oils. Notice. *Federal Register* 54(178):38219–38223.

Vargas, Gaston. 1988. Oxyquin super—New synergistic antioxidant for fishmeal. *Pesca* July/August 1988:14–15.

Vaughan, D. S., Merriner, J. V., and Smith, J. W. 1988. The U.S. menhaden fishery: Current status and utilization. In *Fatty Fish Utilization: Upgrading from Feed to Food,* ed. Nancy Davis, pp. 15–35. Raleigh: University of North Carolina Sea Grant.

Wiedswang, Harald. 1988. Low temperature dryers. Paper read at the 29th Annual Conference of the International Association of Fish Meal Manufacturers, 10 November 1988, Lima, Peru.

Windsor, M. 1969. *Fish Protein Concentrate.* Torry Advisory Note No. 39. Torry Research Station, Aberdeen, UK.

Windsor, M., and Barlow, S. 1981. *Introduction to Fishery By-Products.* Surrey, England: Fishing New Books Ltd.

Chapter 7
PROCESSING OF FISH OILS

Anthony P. Bimbo

INTRODUCTION

Around 1.5 million metric tons (mmt) of fish oils is produced annually worldwide. These oils come from a variety of species from many different parts of the world. Barlow (1988) outlined the major species caught for fish meal and oil production and their location, and this can be seen in Table 7-1. Young (1985A) mentions that fish oils are normally traded under either the generic name, such as menhaden and capelin, or the name of the country where the oil is produced, for example, Peruvian or Danish. Because many of the European species migrate, variations in the composition of the catch result in oils that are mixtures of several species, for example: Icelandic (capelin and herring), Norwegian (capelin, herring, mackerel, and Norway pout), and Danish (sandeel, sprat, and Norway pout). A comparison of the fatty acid composition of some of these oils can be seen in Table 7-2.

The predominant part of the world's marine oil production is used in Europe, South America, and Japan. It is used for the production of salad oils, frying fats, table margarines, low-calorie spreads, and industrial margarines and shortenings used to make bread, pastries, cakes, cookies, biscuits, imitation creams, and emulsifiers (Bimbo 1987B, 1988, 1989A). Table 7-3 shows production, imports, and exports of marine oils for major geographical areas of the world. Other uses include feed for livestock, pets, and aquaculture species (Bimbo 1989C) as well as numerous industrial products (Bimbo 1989B). A partial list of these industrial uses is shown in Table 7-4.

In the early stages of their preparation for food use, oils and fats generally contain minor amounts of nontriglyceride substances. While some of these are considered beneficial to the stability of the oil, such as tocopherols which protect the oil from oxidation, other impurities are objectionable because they render the oil dark-colored, cause it to foam or smoke, or are precipitated when the oil is heated in subsequent processing operations (Norris 1982). Other impurities reduce acceptability because of the flavors and odors they produce in the fat or because they reduce the stability and shelf life of the foods to which the fats are added.

181

Table 7-1. Species and Quantity of Fish Used to Produce Fish Oil in 1985

COUNTRY	SPECIES OF FISH	1000 MT FISH LANDED
Japan	Pilchard	1040
	Other	3030
Peru	Anchovy	1070
	Pilchard	2520
Chile	Horse mackerel	1670
	Pilchard	3640
	Anchovy	160
Norway	Capelin	630
	Herring	160
	Norway pout	110
	Others	100
U.S.	Menhaden	1760
	Tuna	160

Source: Barlow 1988.

Hilditch (1949) suggests that some impurities are common to all fats, regardless of the source or end use, and classifies them as follows:

1. Relatively coarse suspended matter.
2. Exceedingly fine suspensions of colloidally dispersed materials.
3. Natural coloring matter.
4. Free fatty acids.
5. Semivolatile compounds dissolved in the fat or oil.

Young (1985A) classifies these nontriglyceride substances according to their effect:

1. Hydrolytic—moisture, insoluble impurities, free fatty acids, mono- and diglycerides, enzymes, and soap.
2. Oxidative—trace metals, oxidation products, pigments, to-copherols, and phospholipids.
3. Catalyst poisons—substances that inhibit the hydrogenation reaction, for example, phosphatides, oxidation products, and compounds containing nitrogen, sulfur, and halogens.
4. Miscellaneous—hydrocarbons, terpenes, resins, sterols, waxes, trace metals, and sugars whose effect is less well known but can be classified as contaminants and also may have an effect on the final flavor of the oil.

Chang (1967) says that the general objective of processing fats and oils is the removal of impurities that cause the original product to have an

Table 7-2. Principal Fatty Acids of the Major Marine Oils of Commerce (in Grams/100 Grams Oil)

RATIO	MENHADEN	SARDINE/ PILCHARD	CAPELIN	HERRING	ANCHOVY	COD LIVER[a]	MACKEREL	HORSE MACKEREL	NORWAY POUT	SPRAT	SANDEEL
14:0	9	8	7	7	9	3	8	8	6	1	7
16:0	20	18	10	16	19	13	14	18	13	16	15
16:1	12	10	10	6	9	10	7	8	5	7	8
18:1	11	13	14	13	13	23	13	11	14	16	9
20:1	1	4	17	13	5	0	12	5	11	10	15
22:1	T	3	14	20	2	6	15	8	12	14	16
20:5	14	18	8	5	17	11	7	13	8	6	9
22:6	8	9	6	6	9	12	8	10	13	9	9

Source: Bimbo 1987A.
[a]NFMOA 1986.

Table 7-3. Five-Year Average World Fish Oil
Production, Imports and Exports by Geographical
Area (1983–1987), in 1000 Metric Tons

AREA	PRODUCTION	IMPORTS	EXPORTS
Latin America	337	47	134
U.S.	154	10	138
Western Europe[a]	30	690	48
Eastern Europe[b]	89	33	0
Africa	46	48	11
Far East	417	22	239
Scandinavia	328	61	241
Others	28	10	16
Totals	1429	921	827

Source: IAFMM 1988.
[a]Excluding Scandinavia.
[b]Including the USSR.

unattractive color or taste or that causes harmful metabolic effects. Fats and oils intended for edible purposes are therefore further processed to remove these substances while retaining their desirable features. With the new emphasis on "natural" products, certain compounds in fish oils and other oils that were once undesirable are now considered desirable and often command a premium price. For example, the dark red color that appears in some fish oils at different times of the year is now considered necessary as a source of pink pigment for farmed salmon. This compound is the carotenoid asthaxanthin. Recent emphasis on the $\omega 3$ fatty acid composition of fish oils and the pending refined menhaden oil (RMO) portion of the GRAS petition (U.S. FDA 1989) has led to a number of new processes for treating fish oils. Such processes are designed to preserve the $\omega 3$ fatty acids while reducing flavor, cholesterol, and other impurities.

Table 7-4. Some Industrial Uses of Menhaden Fish Oil

Fatty acids	Fatty chemicals	Refractory compounds
Soaps	Leather tanning	Cutting oils
Protective coatings	Lubricants and greases	Plasticizers
Rubber compounds	Ore floatation	Printing inks
Caulking compounds	Insecticidal cds.	Linoleum
Glazing compounds	Fermentation substrates	Presswood fiber boards
Automotive gaskets	Illuminating oils	Oiled fabrics
Core oils	Fuel oils	Ceramic deflocculants
Tin-plating oils	Mushroom culture	Attractants
Rust proofing	Fire retardants	Polyurethane foams

Source: Bimbo 1989A.

In some cases these new processes are very expensive and for the present can only produce oils suitable for premium markets such as cosmetics, health food supplements, and laboratory analytical standards.

Young (1978) defines the processing steps used to purify fats and oils and the impurities reduced or removed as follows:

1. Oil storage—insoluble impurities.
2. Degumming—phospholipids, sugars, resins, proteinaceous compounds, trace metals, and others.
3. Alkali refining—free fatty acids, pigments, phospholipids, oil insolubles, water solubles, and trace metals.
4. Washing—soaps.
5. Drying—moisture.
6. Bleaching—pigments, oxidation products, trace metals, sulfur compounds, and trace soaps.
7. Deodorization—free fatty acids, mono- and diglycerides, aldehydes and ketones, chlorinated hydrocarbons, and pigment decomposition products.

The food and Agriculture Organization (FAO) of the United Nations (1977) adds:

8. Fractionation for removing higher-melting triglycerides and enhancing the unsaturated triglycerides.
9. Hydrogenation for reducing the level of polyunsaturates so that the resultant product has a stable flavor.
10. Interesterification for rearrangement of the triglycerides to a more random distribution.

Recent interest in the cholesterol content of foods and possible environmental contamination of fats and oils including fish oils has focused attention on processing steps that might be used to remove these compounds from fish oils and other fats and oils. These steps include vacuum stripping, steam deodorization, low-temperature crystallization, and supercritical fluid (SCF) extraction.

PREREFINING

Hilditch (1949) states that the refining of each individual oil or fat must be considered separately and that the procedure used will vary with the type of fat and should be determined by experimental trial in each particular case to attain the best results. In Chapter 6 we described the production of crude fish oil. When it leaves the production facility, crude fish oil is stored in large bulk storage tanks that can vary in capacity from 100,000 to 2,000,000 gallons. From these tanks the oil is either shipped as crude oil or delivered to the refinery for further processing.

Young (1985A) defines the refining of the oil as starting in these crude oil storage tanks because both quality and yields are affected by storage conditions. Particular areas of concern are free fatty acid (ffa) increases, oxidation, color setting, and contamination by insoluble impurities. He mentions that oxidation can be reduced by extending intake pipelines to the bottom of the storage tanks, and eliminating contact with iron, copper, and copper alloys which are pro-oxidants. The tank should be equipped with a sump at its lowest point so that moisture and other insoluble impurities can be drained off, thus preventing ffa increases. Since some fish oils contain large quantities of high-melting triglycerides (stearines), the tanks should be equipped with side-mounted agitators and hot-water heating coils so that a homogeneous product is obtained. His suggestion for specifications for crude fish oils appears in Table 7-5.

Fish oil is similar to other oils with regard to the effects of the various impurities on processing and on the quality of the final product. Fish oils contain the same types of fatty acids as other fats and oils, differing only in the content of the longer-chain polyunsaturated fatty acids; this can be seen in Table 7-6. Fish oils are therefore processed in much the same way as the other edible fats and oils. A typical flow diagram for the processing of fish oils appears in Fig. 7-1.

Table 7-5. Typical Crude Fish Oil Guideline Specifications

Free fatty acids, %	2–5
Moisture and impurities, %	0.5–1.0
Peroxide value, Meq/kg	3–20
Anisidine number	4–60
Iodine value, WIJS	
Capelin	95–160
Herring	115–160
Menhaden	150–200
Sardine	160–200
Anchovy	180–200
Color, Gardner scale	12–14
Iron, ppm	0.5–7.0
Copper, ppm	0.3 maximum
Phosphorous, ppm	5–100
Sulfur, ppm	30 maximum

Source: Young 1985A.

Table 7-6. Principal Fatty Acids of Some Edible Fats and Oils in Grams/100 Grams

	MEN-HADEN	SOYA	CORN	CANOLA	PALM	COTTON-SEED	SUN-FLOWER	OLIVE	LARD
C14	9				3				1
C16	19	11	11	5	39	22	6	1	24
C16:1	13			1	2	1		2	3
C18	4	4	2	2	5	2	4	2	13
C18:1	16	23	25	53	43	18	22	72	41
C18:2	2	51	57	22	8	50	66	8	10
C18:3	1	7	1	11				1	1
C20:5	13								
C22:6	8								

Source: Bimbo 1987A.

DEGUMMING

Carr (1988) defines degumming as the treatment of crude oils with water, salt solutions, or dilute acids such as phosphoric to remove phosphatides, waxes, and other impurities. Degumming exploits the affinity of the phosphatides for water by converting them to hydrated gums that are insoluble in oil and readily separated by a centrifuge. These impurities are soluble in the oil in the anhydrous form and can be precipitated and removed if they are hydrated. Hydration is accomplished by steaming the oil or mixing it with water or a weak acid solution. It can also occur in the

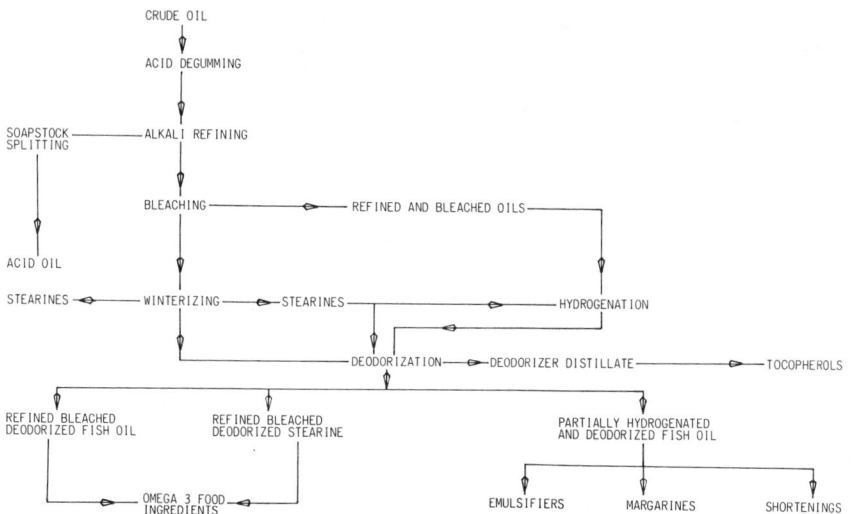

Fig. 7-1. Flow diagram of the processing of fish oil.

crude oil storage tank if sufficient atmospheric moisture is present. This results in foots settling out in the bottom of the storage tank.

Degumming is a prerefining treatment designed to remove phosphatides and other "slimes" from the oil so that a more efficient refining can be done. In some cases—for example, soybean oil—the degumming step produces crude lecithin, which is then further refined and processed to yield commercial lecithin. If these gums are left in the oil, they tend to produce high refining losses and occasionally trouble from settling out in storage tanks. Norris (1982) suggests that the degumming step should be carried out before the oil goes to storage to prevent the formation of foots in the tank.

Degumming is not ordinarily carried out with animal fats and fish oils, because they are low in phosphatides. In some refineries, however, an acid pretreatment designed to hydrate gums and remove phosphorous and other trace metals is applied to the oil as it enters the alkali-refining plant. The subsequent alkali treatment neutralizes the acid and mixes the gums with the soapstock. The pretreatment of fish oils with phosphoric acid ahead of caustic refining is a standard practice in Europe. The pretreatment precipitates natural calcium, magnesium, and other trace elements as insoluble phosphates and involves adding from 0.02% up to 1% of concentrated 85% phosphoric acid at a temperature of 158°–195°F. The reaction time can be very short, about one minute if the acid and oil are thoroughly mixed. Or the acid can be added to the refinery feed oil tank with agitation four hours before the start-up of the refining process. The mixture is then pumped to the refining process without removal of the precipitated solids, using enough caustic soda to neutralize the phosphoric acid as well as the free fatty acids. When used this way, the phosphoric acid pretreatment alters iron and other compounds so that they are more completely removed in the refining and bleaching steps and improves the quality of the final product (Brekke 1980A). A flow diagram of this acid pretreatment step appears in Fig. 7-2.

Dijkstra and van Opstal (1989) describe a novel degumming process that can be used with undegummed as well as water-degummed oils. The process lowers the iron and phosphorous content so that the oil can be physically refined and bleached to produce a stable oil similar to alkali-refined oils. In the process, phosphoric or citric acid is dispersed into the oil, and after sufficient contact time, caustic soda is added and the mixture pumped to a centrifuge where the gums are removed with little oil loss. The oil stream is then pumped to a second centrifuge, where the remaining gums are removed, and after normal washing and drying, the oil is either alkali or physically refined. Based on their data, approximately a 0.5% improvement in yield is obtained.

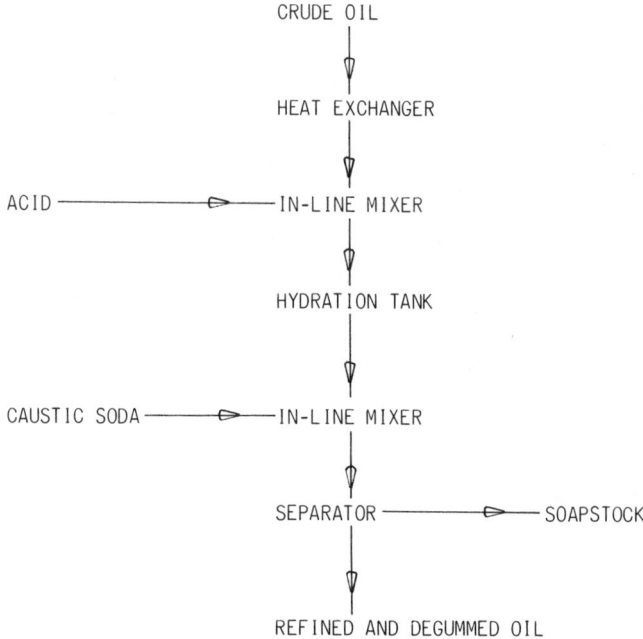

CRUDE OIL

HEAT EXCHANGER

ACID ──────────▷── IN-LINE MIXER

HYDRATION TANK

CAUSTIC SODA ─────▷── IN-LINE MIXER

SEPARATOR ────────▷── SOAPSTOCK

REFINED AND DEGUMMED OIL

Fig. 7-2. Flow diagram of the acid pretreatment (degumming) process and refining process.

Since dry rendering of fish removes water in the initial step of the process, the phosphatides are not hydrated. They remain in the oil phase, whereas in the wet-rendering process they are hydrated and go with the stickwater phase. It is therefore necessary to put dry-rendered oils through a degumming step prior to alkali refining.

Nilsson et al. (1989) state that a good degumming step is necessary before an oil can be physically refined. They mention that both citric and phosphoric acid solutions are suitable for degumming because they are powerful complexing agents that are hydratable and dissolve in the water phase during washing. They describe a water hydration process where the oil is heated to 70°C and 1–3% water is mixed into the oil. The mixture is agitated slowly for about 30 min in a tank and then centrifuged to remove the gums. In acid degumming, the oil is heated to 70°–85°C and about 0.1% of 85% phosphoric acid or 0.3% citric acid is added and intensively mixed with the oil. Water is then added followed by centrifugal separation.

Elson, and Ackman (1978) and Elson et al. (1981) evaluated the changes in trace metals that take place with the processing of herring and menhaden oils, respectively. In the case of menhaden oil, they found that the degumming step effectively reduced lead, copper, arsenic, and zinc but had very little effect on the low levels of cadmium. In the case of herring oil, the degumming step was not used and the effects on trace metals did not show up until the alkali-refining step.

THE REFINING PROCESS

Alkali Refining (Neutralization)

The addition of an alkali solution to crude oils results in both chemical reactions and physical changes:

1. The alkali combines with the free fatty acids present in the oil to form soaps.
2. The gums absorb the alkali and are coagulated by hydration.
3. Much of the coloring matter is degraded, absorbed on the gums, or made water soluble by the alkali.
4. The insoluble matter is entrained with the other coagulated material.

When the oil is heated in subsequent operations, these impurities could cause the oil to darken, foam, or smoke or to become cloudy because of precipitated solids. They must be removed to prevent problems later on. The alkali most commonly employed for refining oils is caustic soda, which is much more effective in its decolorizing action than weaker alkalis. Caustic soda, however, saponifies some of the neutral triglycerides, causing a higher refining loss. Norris (1982) says that the amount of neutral oil lost in alkali refining depends primarily on the amount and kind of impurities that are present. It is relatively low in the refining of tropical oils and fish oils that are low in phospholipids and similar-type products, amounting to 1.5–2.0 times the free fatty acid content, and high in vegetable oils such as cottonseed and soybean oils, because of the presence of phosphatides, and could amount to as much as 5–10 times the free fatty acid content.

Fish oil can be alkali refined by either a batch or continuous process. Essentially all the oil is refined by the continuous process, with the batch process used for oils high in free fatty acids. A typical batch kettle used for both alkali refining and bleaching can be seen in Fig. 7-3. The crude oil is supplied to the refinery either from storage or from the phosphoric acid pretreatment tank. The oil is pumped through a heat exchanger to adjust the temperature to about 120°F. Depending upon the ffa in the oil, the

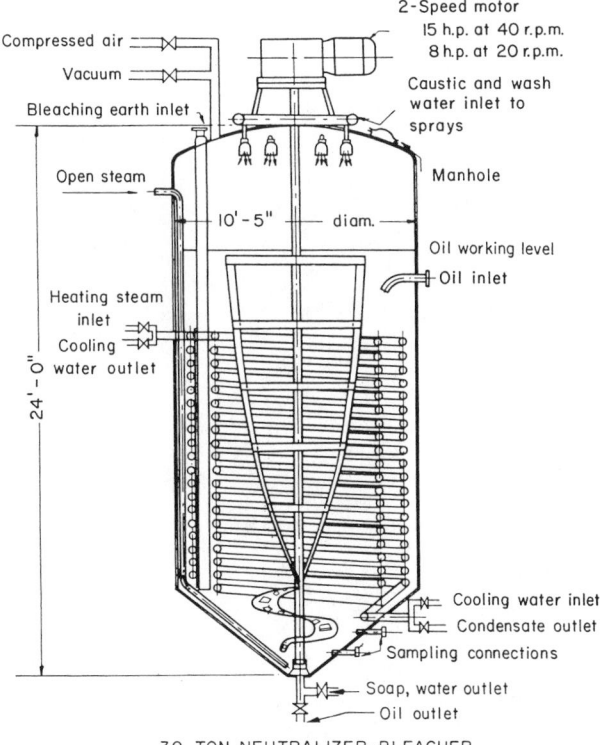

Fig. 7-3. Kettle for refining and bleaching. (*Source:* Devine and Williams, *Chemistry and Technology of Edible Fats and Oils,* 1961. Courtesy of Pergamon Press Ltd.)

correct strength and volume of caustic soda is metered into the oil stream so that the right proportion of alkali to oil is maintained. The mixture is pumped through a high-shear in-line mixer so that intimate contact between oil and alkali is maintained. The soap/oil mixture is heated to 180°F and pumped to the primary separator, which separates oil from soapstock. The refined oil discharged from the primary separator is heated to 190°F and mixed with 10–20% by weight of soft water that has been heated to 200°F. This mixture passes through a second high-speed shear mixer to obtain intimate contact of soap and water. The water/oil mixture is then pumped to a secondary separator, which clarifies the oil. At this point about 90% of the soap has been removed from the oil phase. In some plants a second water washing is used before the oil is sprayed into a vacuum dryer to reduce the moisture below 0.1%. The dryer operates at

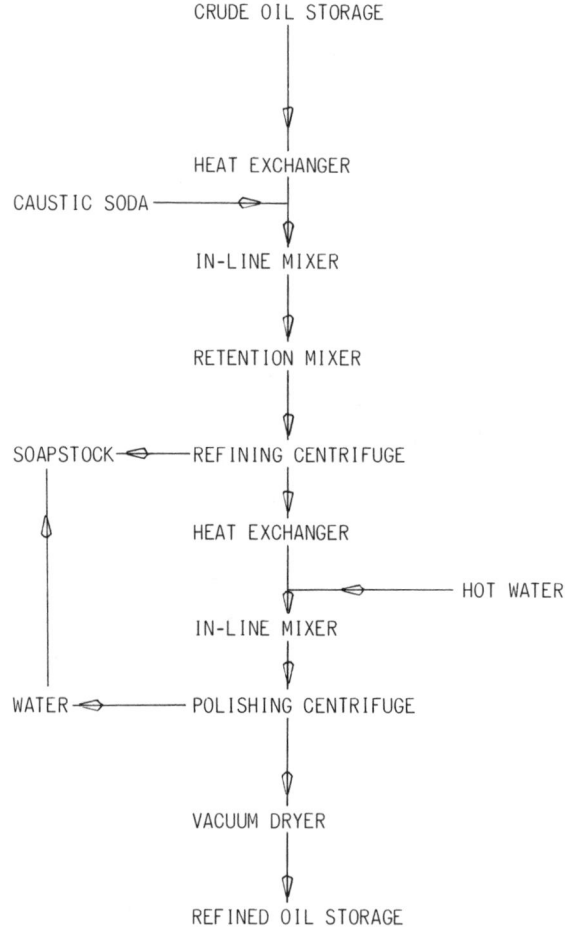

Fig. 7-4. Flow diagram of the alkali-refining process.

28 in. vacuum. The refined and dried oil is then transferred to the bleaching tank (Mounts 1980). A flow diagram of the alkali-refining process is shown in Fig. 7-4.

The major by-product of any refining operation is the fatty acids removed by the process. After the free fatty acids have been saponified with caustic soda, the soapstock is separated from the neutral oil in a centrifuge or by gravity. Water is used to thin the soapstock either in a batch or continuous process, acid is added to split the soap, and the resultant fatty acids are separated from the aqueous phase by either gravity or centrifuge, then dried and sold to fatty acid producers, soap makers, or feed

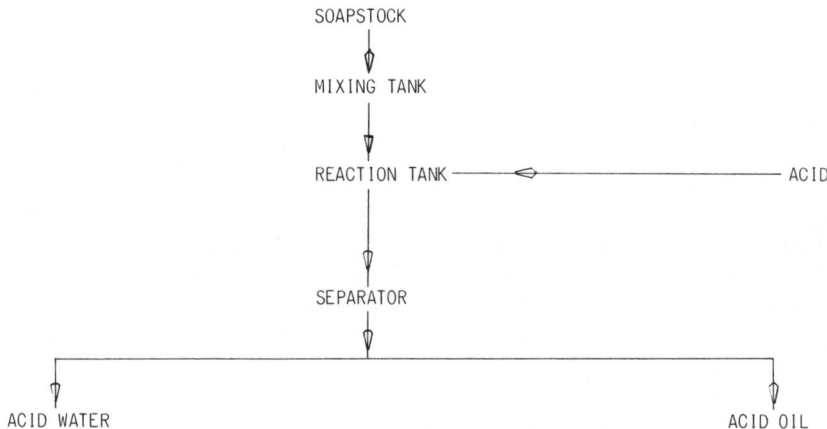

Fig. 7-5. Flow diagram of the soapstock-splitting process.

manufacturers. This product is called acid oil or acidulated soapstock. A flow diagram of the process can be seen in Fig. 7-5.

There are several other methods of refining fish and other fats and oils which although not used routinely in large scale commercial operations do offer some possibilities in special cases.

Supercritical Fluids Extraction

Spinelli et al. (1987) described an alternative process for the "purification" of fish oils using supercritical carbon dioxide as the processing medium. According to these researchers, current processes for purifying fish oils are inappropriate, cumbersome, and detrimental to the relatively labile polyunsaturated fatty acids unique to fish oils.

Supercritical carbon dioxide, which is carbon dioxide under high pressure above its critical temperature of 31°C, that is, carbon dioxide gas nonliquefiable under pressure, is known to have selective solvent properties for the preparation of human food-grade products. Commercially it is used to extract caffeine from coffee and in the extraction of the essence of hops for use in the brewing of beer. It is also used to prepare essential oils for the cosmetic industry (Eckert et al. 1986).

Spinelli et al. (1987) say that supercritical carbon dioxide is a superior substance for purifying fish oils because it is selective for the removal of odor bodies, pigments, and products of autoxidation that contribute to off-flavors. In the first step of their process, supercritical extraction removes the volatile and odor-causing constituents of fish oil while the second step selectively extracts fatty acid glycerides from oxidized and colored materials. Repetition of the extractions yields a relatively high quality triglyceride. The patent utilizes color data, odor, and fatty acid composition as the criteria for measuring the improved quality of the oil. There is no mention of removal of trace metals, pesticides, cholesterol, or other nontriglyceride components. Krukonis (1989) says that fish oils can be made "too pure" by carbon dioxide extraction because natural antioxidants such as tocopherols and phospholipids are separated from the oil during processing. The tocopherols have a similar distribution coefficient and selectivity to that of PCB and are thus extracted from the fish oil by the carbon dioxide. If the fish oil is subjected to complete solution in carbon dioxide, the phospholipids will be separated since they are not soluble. The extraction of tocopherols and the simultaneous separation of phospholipids results in a highly purified fish oil fraction that exhibits very low stability to autoxidation.

Bimbo (1988) mentions that very little economic data is available about this system as a replacement for conventional oil technology. It is difficult to determine where the supercritical fluid process would fit into the refining of fats and oils. Questions that continue to come up are: Could this process replace all of the refining steps, or is it an add-on or finisher step? Has the starting oil and finished oil been tested for normal components such as cholesterol, pesticides, heavy metals, peroxides, anisidine number, and stability? What is the economics? Once these areas have been evaluated, we will have a more realistic picture of the process. Supercritical fluid processing is covered in more detail in Chapter 4.

Physical Refining

When oils or fats have been degummed, alkali refined, and bleached by conventional methods, they still contain certain components responsible for their color, odor, and taste. These residual compounds, mostly volatile aldehydes and ketones, could only be removed by the deodorization process, which consists of applying vacuum steam distillation to the oil and entraining these volatiles in the steam. Since free fatty acids are more volatile than glycerides, it is also possible to remove them from the oil by high-temperature steam distillation. This process is called "physical refining."

Lee-Poy (1987) described a process of physical refining of fish oils for the removal of free fatty acids, volatile odor compounds, hydroperoxides, pesticides, PCBs, and other volatile compounds without damaging the long-chain $\omega 3$ fatty acids. The oil is pretreated by vacuum drying to remove residual moisture and precipitate water-soluble material. This is followed by filtration to remove fines, precipitated gums, and other solids.

The oil is then vacuum bleached to remove residual gums, trace metals, and pigments. This is followed by physical refining. According to Lee-Poy, economics and environmental concerns play key roles in his choice for physical refining. No soapstock is produced, thus no further processing of the waste is needed. Losses amount only to the level of free fatty acids, no neutral oil is lost, and pesticides and PCBs are directly removed without another step.

Deffense (1987) suggests that the breakeven point for using physical refining over alkali refining is 0.4–0.7% ffa. Above 0.7% ffa physical refining becomes more attractive. However, he also points out that fish oils are not normally physically refined because they are too unstable. The highly unsaturated triglycerides would tend to polymerize during the distillation and produce a rapid flavor reversion after refining. A typical physical refining plant can be seen in Fig. 7-6.

Other Refining Methods

Takao (1985) described a complete process for producing a relatively odorless, refined fish oil containing a high level of ω3 polyunsaturated

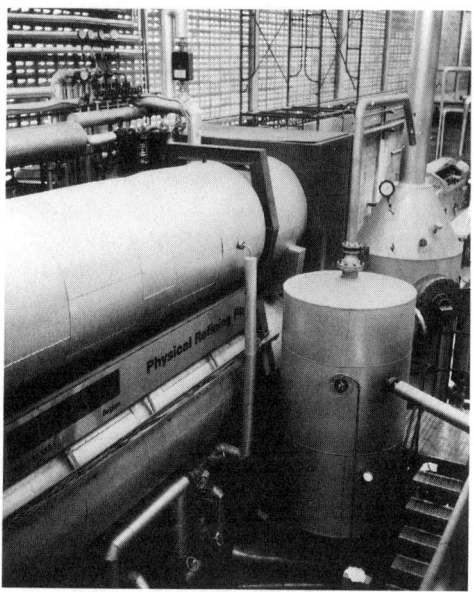

Fig. 7-6. Continuous physical refining (deodorizing) plant. (*Source:* S. A. Fractionment, Fleurus, Belgium.)

fatty acids. According to the patent, any fish oil can be used. In the process, the oil is first winterized in two steps, with the first step taking place at a temperature of 5°C down to −2°C and the second step at −2°C down to −10°C for further dewaxing. He also employed an ester interchange reaction in which the refined fish oil is reacted with a catalyst, typically sodium alcoholate 0.02–0.5%, and stirred under inert gas at 5°C down to −30°C for 3 to 36 hours. The catalyst is then neutralized with phosphoric acid. The patent then mentions the addition of a polyhydric alcohol such as glycerol and a distilled monoglyceride to the interesterified oil. The purpose of the glycerol is to attract the odor- and flavor-forming compounds so that they can be distilled out in the deodorization step.

Ward (1989 personal communication) describes a process that was developed to produce superrefined oils. The process called flash chromatography has processed 26 oils used in pharmaceutical and cosmetic products worldwide. The oils are passed through a complex adsorption column of closely controlled activity. Any polar components of the oils are retained on the column and the eluate obtained is thus neutral nonpolar lipid. According to the author, the oils exhibit behavior superior to their conventional counterparts in many areas, including oxidative stability. The process leaves a neutral oil with all the desirable properties of the crude oil but with no color or odor. The process has been used with fish oils in both the United States and Europe. There is no economic data available on the process, and the processing technique is not defined.

Fernandez (1986) described a cation strong-acid microporous resin process for the refining of fish oil for human consumption. She mentions that conventional refining processes require high temperatures which could damage the ω3 fatty acids in fish oil. Resins, on the other hand, do not require high temperature, are of consistent quality, and can be regenerated. She reports that cation strong-acid macroporous resins in columns produced superior fish oil to anything currently available to the food industry.

BLEACHING

Bleaching is used to improve the color, flavor, and oxidative stability of the oil, and to remove impurities, such as traces of soap, that interfere with the hydrogenation process. Bleaching involves the adsorption of color bodies in the oil by an activated clay. While alkali refining removes many color bodies and impurities, some still remain and the bleaching step removes them plus residual soap. Young (1985A) mentions that during bleaching the totox value (2 × peroxide value + anisidine number) can be reduced as much as 50% when 2% activated earth is used. There are two methods of bleaching, batch and continuous, and batch bleaching can be further broken down into atmospheric and vacuum bleaching.

Batch Atmospheric Bleaching

Batch atmospheric bleaching is the oldest method of bleaching still in use today. The operation is conducted in open, cylindrical, cone-bottomed kettles, holding up to 60,000 lb of oil, and equipped with an agitator and heating coils. The required amount of bleach (usually 1–4%) is added at an oil temperature of about 160°F. In some plants clay is slurried with oil and pumped into the kettle. Agitation is continued for about 30 min and then filtration is started. Filtered oil is returned to the kettle until sufficient cake has built up in the press and a clear, brilliant oil is discharged. The oil is then cooled and pumped to storage or the next processing step. Plate and frame filter presses have been used for many years and are still in use today, even though the labor requirement is very high. Other types of completely enclosed, semiautomatic or automatic self-cleaning filter units are also used because they require less labor and are easier to clean (Brekke 1980B).

Batch Vacuum Bleaching

Brekke (1980B) states that batch vacuum bleaching has a number of advantages over open-kettle bleaching:

1. Better protection of the oil against oxidation.
2. The contact or bleach time can be shortened, reducing oxidation.
3. Since oxidation is reduced, less bleaching earth is used and less oil is lost in the spent clay.
4. Under similar conditions, vacuum bleaching gives better colors than atmospheric bleaching.
5. When acid-activated earths are used, the bleached oil has less soap, and less hydrogenation catalyst will be needed.

Batch vacuum bleaching is conducted in closed, cylindrical vessels of 30,000–40,000 lb capacity, that have dished ends, a good agitator, and heating/cooling coils. The agitator is designed to roll the oil so that fresh material is constantly being brought to the surface for deaerating (Norris 1982). The vessel operates at about 26–28 in. vacuum. Incoming oil is splashed or sprayed into the vessel for immediate deaeration. Clay is added from a hopper utilizing vacuum to suck the clay into the kettle. After 15–20 min of bleaching, the oil is cooled to 160°F filtered and further cooled to 100°–150°F before exposure to air. Figure 7-7 shows the bleaching operation. The dashed line is the alternative steps for vacuum bleaching that distinguish it from atmospheric bleaching.

Continuous Vacuum Bleaching

Continuous vacuum bleaching protects the oil from oxidation even more effectively than batch vacuum bleaching since better deaeration occurs when the oil is sprayed into the vacuum chamber. The oil and bleach earth are more completely deaerated and the contact time between oil and earth is reduced. This reduces the soap content of the bleached oil, minimizes free fatty acid formation when acid earths are used, and produces an oil with improved stability.

Properly controlled streams of oil at 130°F and bleaching earth are mixed in an open slurry tank and then sprayed into the deaerating and dehydrating section of the bleaching tower, which is maintained at about 15 in. vacuum. After a retention time of about 7 min the slurry is pumped through an external heat exchanger, heated to about 200°–220°F, and then sprayed into the bleaching section of the tower. A small amount of stripping steam in each section agitates the slurry and helps remove air and moisture. After about 10 min the hot slurry is filtered and the oil is cooled and pumped to storage (Brekke 1980B).

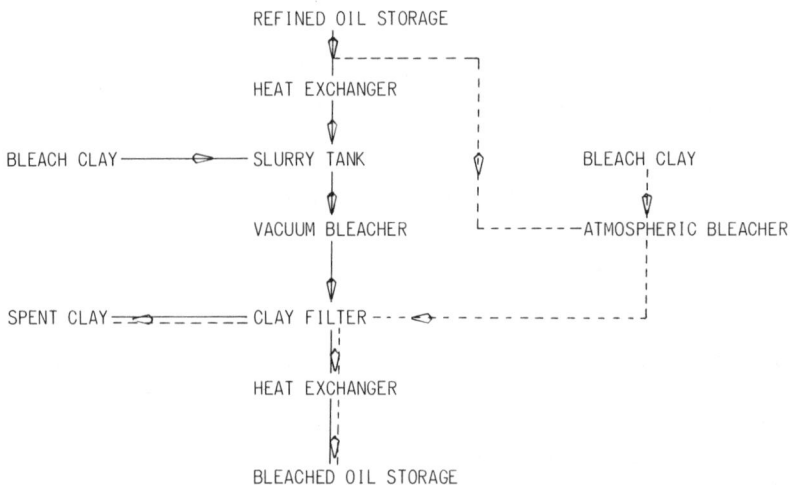

Fig. 7-7. Flow diagram of the bleaching process, vacuum and atmospheric.

FRACTIONATION OR WINTERIZATION

The process that removes the higher-melting glycerides from oils is called "winterization." Winterization is an old practice that evolved from the observation that the storage of oils in outdoor tanks during cold weather caused settling of high-melting triglycerides on the bottom, referred to as "racking" or "cold clearing." The clear oil was decanted and used as a light pressed oil. Today triglyceride oils are winterized for a number of reasons:

1. To remove waxes and other nontriglyceride constituents.
2. To remove naturally occurring high-melting triglycerides.
3. To remove high-melting triglycerides formed during partial hydrogenation or interesterification.

Letan and Koslowsky (1975) state that edible oils are usually separated into fractions of different melting characteristics either by winterization (dry fractionation), solvent fractionation with acetone or hexane, or by using aqueous solutions of surface-active agents (detergents). They say that all these methods have certain disadvantages. Winterization is a relatively low-yield process that requires a large amount of space and takes a great deal of time. The crystals entrain a large amount of free oil, are difficult to filter, and must be handled with care. Detergent fractionation requires efficient centrifugation, and the product is left with some residual detergent. Solvent fractionation with acetone and/or hexane can be continuous, will give higher yields, and produces better-quality crystals. However, very low temperatures must be used, the crystals must be filtered out, and the solvent must be recovered.

Dry Fractionation

Winterization is a specialized form of the process called fractional crystallization, which was originally developed to produce salad oil from cottonseed oil. For this reason, winterization has become economically the most important of all fractional crystallization procedures (Weiss 1983). In the case of fish oils, winterization removes the stearine fraction, which for menhaden oil could amount to anywhere from 15% to 50% of the oil. A comparison of the fatty acid composition of a starting menhaden oil and two fractions from the winterization process appears in Table 7-7. It should be noted that even though the stearine fraction is a solid at room temperature, melting around 100–110°F, it still contains a relatively large amount of the ω3 fatty acids, essentially combining the chemical proper-

Table 7-7. Simplified Fatty Acid Composition of
Menhaden Oil Fractions During the
Winterization Process

	CRUDE OIL	WINTERIZED OIL	STEARINE
C14	9	8	11
C16	21	18	31
C18	3	3	5
C16:1	11	12	9
C18:1	12	12	10
C20:1	2	2	2
C20:5	14	15	11
C22:1	1	1	1
C22:5	2	2	1
C22:6	10	11	7

Source: Zapata Haynie Corporation unpublished data 1979.

ties of a liquid oil with the physical characteristics of a partially hydrogenated fat. Menhaden stearine has an SFI and melting point similar to other
natural fats and could be a unique source of $\omega 3$ fatty acids in a variety of
products. A comparison of menhaden stearine and other naturally occurring fats can be seen in Table 7-8.

The major problem with winterized oil production is the formation of
suitable crystals for separation from the liquid oil. The process is conducted in refrigerated rooms or well-insulated refrigerated tanks in rooms
at ambient temperature. The tanks are equipped with cooling coils containing refrigerant and good temperature controls. In order to prevent
shock chilling of the oil near the coils, the temperature difference between

Table 7-8. Solid Fat Index and Melting Points of Naturally
Occurring Fats

	MELTING PT., °F	SOLID FAT INDEX				
		50	70	80	92	100
Butter	97	32	12	9	3	0
Cocoa butter	85	62	48	8	0	0
Coconut oil	79	55	27	0	0	0
Lard	110	25	20	12	4	2
Palm oil	103	34	12	9	6	4
Palm kernel oil	84	49	33	13	0	0
Tallow	118	39	30	28	23	18
Menhaden stearine[a]	102	26	17	15	8	1

Source: Weiss 1983.
[a]Zapata Haynie Corp. unpublished data.

the refrigerant and oil ranges from 10°–25°F. The coils are spaced closely since mechanical agitation of the oil is not permitted once the crystals form. It is essential that the rate of cooling be slow.

Oil is pumped into the chillers at ambient temperature. It is then cooled to 55°F in 6–12 hours, and it is at this point that crystals begin to form. The cooling rate is then reduced, and an additional 12–18 hours is allowed for the temperature to drop to 45°F. The rate of crystal formation is then rapid enough to generate heat, and a 2°–4°F rise can occur. The temperature then drops to a point below 45°F, at which time the refrigeration is turned off and the oil allowed to sit undisturbed.

Filtration of the winterized oil is usually carried out in ordinary plate and frame filter presses. In order to prevent damage to the crystals, the oil is dropped by gravity into pressure tanks and then forced to the presses using air pressure. In some of the older plants, the oil is pumped directly from the chilled tanks to the presses. Filtration is slow, and the entire winterization process from start to finish can take up to six days. After filtration is complete, the filter cake is removed from the presses and the cycle repeated (Stirton 1964). Figure 7-8 shows a typical plate and frame filter press in the process of being cleaned. The solid cake is menhaden stearine.

In the Tirtiaux winterization process, the temperature of the oil actually controls the rate of cooling. An accurate crystallization control device ensures the formation of suitable crystal seeds and their growth by regulating the heat transferred from the oil to the coolant. Unlike other pro-

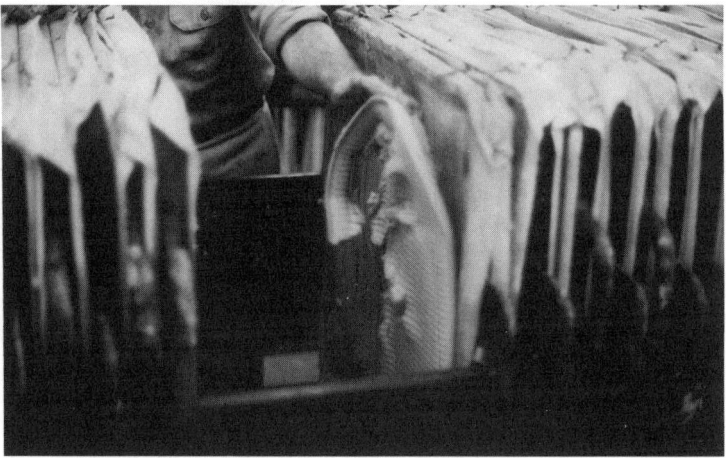

Fig. 7-8. Menhaden stearine being removed from a plate and frame filter press in the dry winterization process. (*Source:* Zapata Haynie Corporation, Reedville, Virginia.)

cesses, the oil is crystallized relatively slowly to control the latent heat of crystallization and to avoid supercooling.

The oil is fed into an agitated crystallizer tank fitted with a coil and jacket in which crystals are melted and then allowed to form and grow according to a programmed cooling procedure. The filtration takes place horizontally and continuously on an endless rotating stainless steel belt under slight vacuum. This filter, called a Florentine filter, can be seen in Fig. 7-9. The filter is self-cleaning and the filtration area is enclosed and air-conditioned. The oil mixture is maintained at the temperature of fractionation until the liquid is separated from the solid crystals. A recycling device enables the filtrate from the first filter belt section to be recycled. This results in filtration through a precoated stearine layer and improves the quality of the filtrate. The coarse mesh of the belt together with the large size of the crystals obtained allow an easy filtration under slight vacuum, even when the viscosity of the oil is high (Deffense 1985). A flow diagram of the process can be seen in Fig. 7-10.

Solvent Crystallization

Solvent winterization of triglycerides is a relatively recent development. In this process, the oil viscosity is reduced by dissolving it in a solvent such as hexane. The stearine crystals form in a few minutes and can be readily separated from the low-viscosity liquid phase.

Kokubu et al. (1984) patented a process in which fish oil can be purified by a solvent crystallization and extraction process. Crude fish oil high in

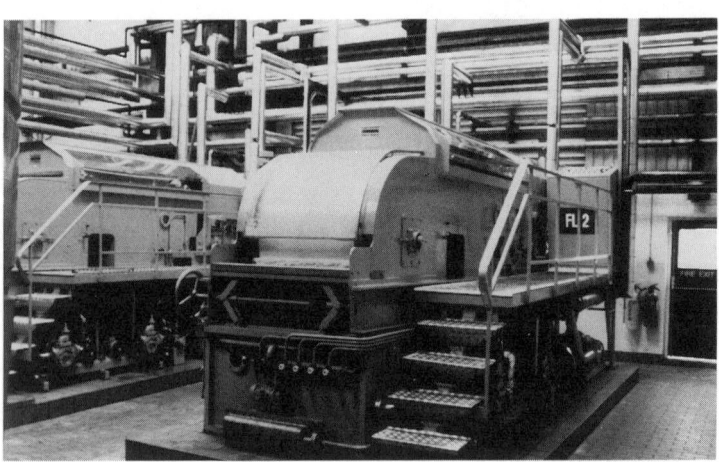

Fig. 7-9. Florentine continuous filter. (*Source:* S. A. Fractionment, Fleurus, Belgium.)

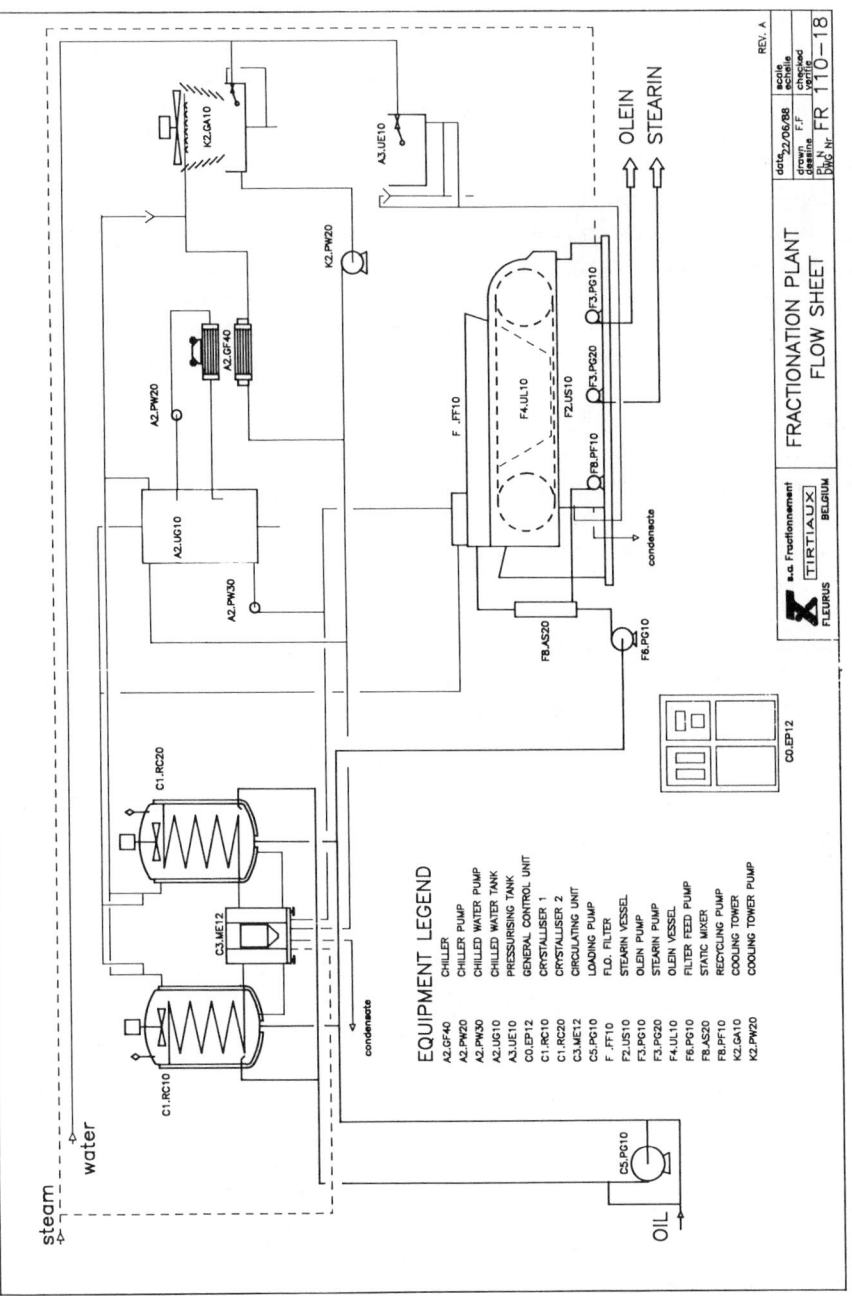

Fig. 7-10. Schematic of a continuous winterization plant. (*Source:* S. A. Fractionment, Fleurus, Belgium.)

cholesterol, vitamin A, and free fatty acids was crystallized at −60°C for 5 hr in acetone. After removal of the solid crystallized fraction, the solvent was distilled to yield a high concentrate of ω3 fatty acids, cholesterol, and vitamin A. This concentrated oil was then solvent extracted with ethanol containing about 3% water. The undissolved fraction had a reduced cholesterol and vitamin A content after about 45 min of extraction.

Noguchi and Hibino (1982) described a similar process in another patent. Fish oils are cooled in the presence of a solvent yielding high-melting crystals which are separated by filtration. In this process, acetone or some other ketone or hydrocarbon solvent is used. The solvent is added at a ratio of 2–10 times the weight of the oil and cooled to −20°C to −90°C. The crystals are filtered out at this temperature and the solvent recovered. According to the patent, levels of C20:5 and C22:6 in the winterized fraction were almost double those in the starting oil.

Sano (1984) mixed the refined and bleached triglycerides of sardine oil with hexane and chilled to 0°C overnight. The crystallized stearine fraction was removed by filtration and the filtrate held at −10°C for 24 hr. The crystallized stearine fraction was filtered out and the filtrate mixed with silicic acid in a packed bed. After removal of the hexane, a 70% yield of purified sardine oil was obtained with increased C20:5 and C22:6. Sano (1984) then treated the purified sardine oil by dissolving it in chilled hexane and mixing it with silicic acid. After filtration and washing with hexane containing 2% ethanol, the triglycerides were recovered from the silicic acid with hexane containing 20% ethanol. The concentrated triglycerides contained 25% C20:5 and 13% C22:6.

Letan and Koslowsky (1975) described a method using isopropyl alcohol in a ratio of 1:1 with the oil at 65°C. At that temperature the oil is completely soluble in the isopropanol. At lower temperatures, two phases separate, with fat crystals suspended in the alcohol in the upper phase and isopropanol dissolved in oil in the lower phase. The fractionation takes place in two stages in a short period of time, and the upper phase with the crystals can be separated by decanters. The process has worked well with palm, cottonseed, partially hydrogenated soybean oil, and rice bran oil and should also work with fish oils.

Revankar et al. (1975) winterized sardine oil in solvent. Of several solvents tested, acetone was found to be the most effective. They were able to increase the iodine value from 164 to 217 with a 48% yield.

Contreras et al. (1971) continuously liquid-liquid extracted Chilean anchovy oil with furfural in a column. The oil was dissolved in petroleum naphtha and run through a York extraction column countercurrently to furfural. Two product streams were obtained in their experiments. After distillation to remove furfural, the bottoms extract had an iodine value

(IV) of 196–206, and the raffinate fraction ranged from 105 to 128 iodine value. The starting oil had an iodine value of 180.

Schlenk and Ener (1959) fractionated crude menhaden oil with liquid sulfur dioxide at $-30°C$. The original oil had an IV of 177, the insoluble fraction representing 43.5% of the starting oil had an IV of 112, while the soluble fraction representing 52% of the starting oil had an IV of 210. The color bodies were concentrated in the insoluble fraction of the oil.

Passino (1949) described a patented process (Solexol process) for fractionating fish oil. The process is based on the solubility of the oil in a hydrocarbon solvent, usually propane. The separation of the oil into fractions is controlled by regulating the temperature and pressure. The apparatus consists of several towers. For menhaden and sardine oils, three towers were needed. The oil was first caustic refined and then mixed with liquid (critical) propane. The soaps and color bodies were removed in the first tower; the remaining oil passed into the second tower, where about 20% was removed at the bottom of the tower by adjusting the temperature and pressure. The remaining solution passed to the third tower, where by adjusting conditions a final fraction was obtained. Table 7-9 shows some typical data for the fractionation of sardine, menhaden, and cod-liver oils.

Table 7-9. Composition of Some Fish Oils Fractionated by the Solexol Process

	CRUDE	SEPARATED FRACTIONS			CONCENTRATE
		I	II	III	
Menhaden oil					
Iodine value	184	260	225	165	90
Unsaponifiables	1	0.9	0.8	0.4	6.8
Vitamin A potency	100	—	—	—	800
Color, Gardner	11+	black	10	4	7
Yield, %	—	2	20	68	10
Sardine oil					
Iodine value	185	250	240	160	110
Unsaponifiables	—	—	—	—	—
Vitamin A potency	350	—	—	—	2,100
Color, Gardner	11	black	8	4	5
Yield, %	—	3	35	47	15
Cod-liver oil					
Iodine value	162	—	210	155	82
Unsaponifiables	1.4	—	0.7	1	10
Vitamin A potency	2,000	—	150	150	41,000
Color, Gardner	6	—	9	1	—
Yield, %	—	—	25	71	5

Source: Passino 1949.

While cholesterol was not an issue back then, it would be contained in the unsaponifiable fraction and one can assume that it would move with that fraction.

Dickinson and Meyers (1952) reviewed the status of the Solexol process. In 1952 there were five commercial plants in operation with a sixth under construction. A plant in Simonstown, South Africa, concentrated vitamins A and D from fish liver oils. The plant had a capacity of 5000 lb of feed oil per day. The plant was expanded to include fractionation of 40,000 lb/day of pilchard oil. Bimbo (1986) mentions that oil from this plant was imported, refined, and encapsulated in the United States in 1962–1963. These capsules were marketed by a pharmaceutical company to reduce serum cholesterol. A plant in Port Monmouth, New Jersey, capable of processing 95,000 lb/day of menhaden oil was also in operation. A plant in Europe was under construction capable of processing 154,000 lb/day of whale oil and 121,000 lb/day of herring oil. In general, the process produced a vitamin concentrate fraction, a standard oil fraction light in color with a low IV, a high fraction with a light color and high IV, and a color body fraction, very dark in color and very high in IV. The process also had the capability to fractionate each product into a stearine and olein fraction.

Detergent Fractionation

Young (1978) describes a third method of fractionation, namely detergent fractionation. The detergent process makes use of the fact that when a partially crystallized fat is mixed with a detergent solution, the stearine crystals are wetted by the detergent and pass into suspension in the aqueous phase and the mixture can then be separated by a centrifuge into an oil (olein) and water (stearine) phase. The aqueous phase is next heated to melt the stearin, which is separated from the detergent by a second centrifuge. The detergent is recycled back to incoming crystallized oil via flow meters.

HYDROGENATION

Hydrogenation of a fat is the largest single reaction in the edible-fat industry and consists of the direct addition of hydrogen at double bonds in the fatty acid chains. The degree of hydrogenation in an oil is directly related to its iodine value. Young (1985) recommends that prerefined feedstock for hydrogenation have the following characteristics:

1. FFA—0.15% maximum.
2. Soap—trace.
3. Phosphorous—4 ppm maximum.
4. Sulfur—15 ppm maximum.

According to Allen (1989), there are two reasons to hydrogenate an oil. First, since the number of double bonds is reduced, the opportunity for oxidation is decreased and flavor stability is increased. Second, the physical characteristics are changed so the product has more utility.

Batch hydrogenation equipment is simple. All that is necessary is a vessel that can stand 50–60 psig, an agitator, heating and cooling, a hydrogen inlet, pumps, and pipes. Figure 7-11 shows a typical batch hydrogenation plant flow diagram. Most hydrogenation is done in batch reactors. The feedstock must be refined, bleached, free of soap (less than 25 ppm), and dry. Free fatty acids, soap, and water can all act as poisons that reduce catalyst activity and selectivity. The hydrogen must be dry and as pure as possible. In general, the batch hydrogenator is a cylindrical pressure vessel having a capacity of 5–20 tons. Two or more agitators (turbine type) are fitted to a shaft running the vertical length of the reactor. The interior of the vessel contains coils for heating and cooling the oil. The hydrogenation process is exothermic; water is circulated through the cooling coil to counteract the heat of reaction and later to cool the oil to filtration temperature. The oil can also be cooled by dropping it into a catch tank equipped with a coil and agitator. After cooling, some of the hardened oil is pumped to a precoat tank, filter aid is added, and the mixture is used to precoat the catalyst filter prior to filtration of the remainder of the charge. To remove colloidal nickel, citric acid is added to the oil in the bleach tank, and after reaction, the mixture is bleached or pumped through a post bleach press equipped with paper as the filter medium (Mounts 1980).

Young (1985) estimates that it takes approximately one cubic meter of hydrogen gas at 0°C and 760 mm mercury pressure to reduce the iodine value of one metric ton of fish oil by one unit. He says that the IV reduction rate at the start of hydrogenation of good-quality fish oil with fresh catalyst is around 3 IV units per minute. This heat of reaction raises the temperature of the oil 1.6°C per unit IV drop, necessitating the use of cooling water to maintain the reaction temperature. He also describes the processing steps that take place when the oil leaves the hydrogenator. Essentially, the hydrogenated oil goes through the same type of processing as the raw oil. The oil is neutralized with a 0.05–0.10% phosphoric acid pretreatment to remove colloidal nickel, followed by a weak alkali refining and water washing to remove residual soaps. The oil is then

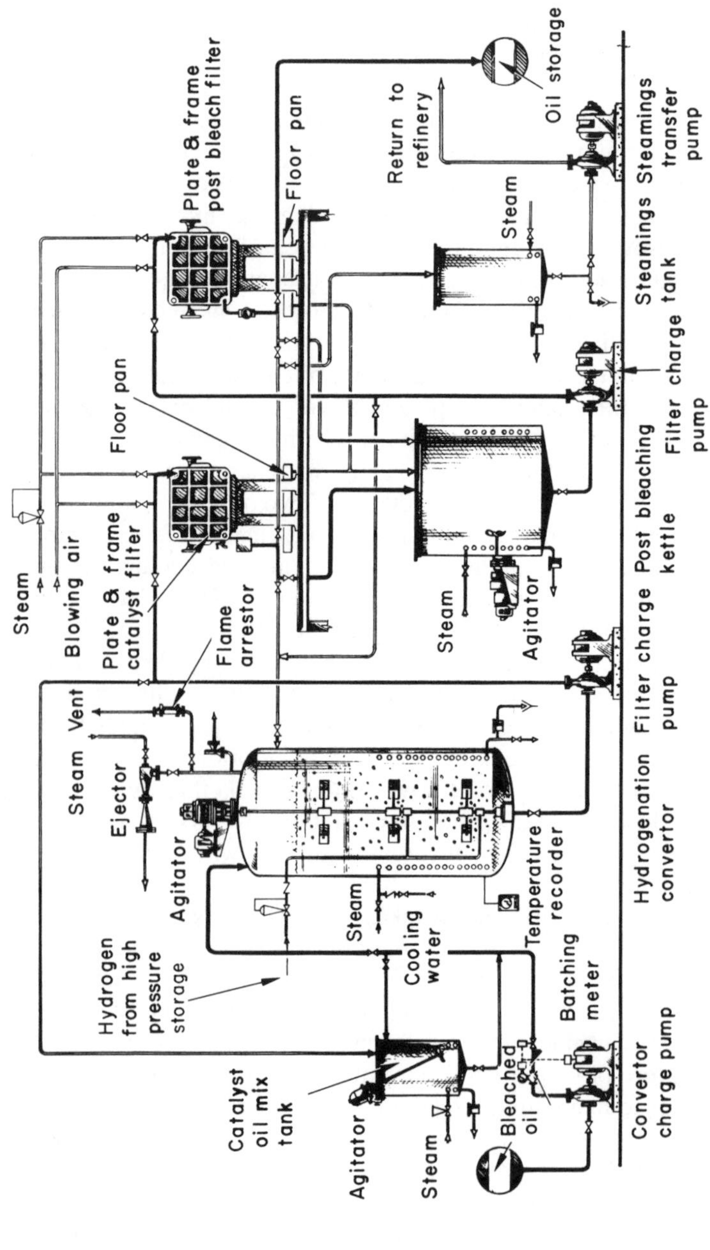

Fig. 7-11. Layout of a hydrogenation plant. (*Source:* Bailey's Industrial Oil and Fat Products, by Daniel Swern. Courtesy Interscience Publishers.)

bleached and filtered as described earlier. An alternative process, called "white filtration," involves the use of 0.01–0.02% citric acid in water to split the nickel soaps and chelate any metals present. The oil is then vacuum dried, bleached, and filtered before blending and deodorization. Hydrogenated fish oil can be deodorized on its own or blended with other oils before deodorization.

Sebedio et al. (1981) evaluated the changes that take place in the fatty acid composition of herring oil during partial hydrogenation under commercial conditions. Sebedio and Ackman (1983A, B) evaluated the change in fatty acids during the partial hydrogenation of menhaden oil. Samples were taken at the starting iodine value of 159 and at intervals down to an IV of 84.5. Partial hydrogenation resulted in the disappearance of the pentaenoic and hexaenoic fatty acids, a decrease in tetraenes, and an increase in trienes, dienes, and monoenes. There was no change in the level of saturated fatty acids. The change in the fatty acid composition of menhaden oil grouped by level of unsaturation over the course of the reaction is seen in Table 7-10.

Young (1985B) mentions that hydrogenation has had the greatest effect on the interchangeability of oils because the process has resulted in the production of a very large number of alternatives to naturally occurring hard fats. Over 1 million tons of fish oil per year, which in its extracted state contains fatty acids with up to six double bonds in the chains, have been made available to the edible-oil industry. By virtue of their wide triglyceride composition resulting from fatty acid chain lengths from C14 to C24 in significant quantities, hardened fish oils possess useful crystal-stabilizing properties and assist in the creaming performance of bakery products. Young (1986C) outlined the solid fat indices of partially hydro-

Table 7-10. Change in Fatty Acid Type in Grams/100 Grams of Menhaden Oil During Hydrogenation

	IODINE VALUES							
	159[a]	150	140	131.5	120.5	96.5	90	84.5
Saturate	41.6	40.7	41.7	42.1	43.1	41.8	43.2	43.8
Monoene	24	25.1	25.9	26.3	29	33.7	33.1	34.2
Diene	3.9	4.2	5.1	7.7	8	10.5	10.5	13.2
Triene	4.2	4.8	6.1	8.9	8.7	10.7	10.9	8.3
Tetraene	5.6	5.4	5.7	6.5	6	3	2.1	0.4
Pentaene + Hexaene	21.2	19.8	15.3	8.8	4.9	0.1	trace	trace

Source: Sebedio and Ackman 1983A.
[a]Starting oil.

genated fish oil over the range of melting points commercially important in Europe; these appear in Table 7-11. For melting points below 38°C, the fats possess relatively steep solid fat curves and are very useful for retail margarines and as the middle-melting components of industrial cake and creaming products. The higher-melting-point hardened fish oils have flat curves at lower temperatures and melt more rapidly above 30°C. This property is of use for increasing the plastic range of shortenings and for producing the desired toughness and plasticity in puff pastry fats. He described the wide range of uses for partially hydrogenated fish oils in Europe and South America, and these are outlined in Table 7-12. Young (1986B) described the commercial blends of fish oil and a variety of vegetable oils used in the United Kingdom in a wide range of baking fats. Four major partially hydrogenated marine oils are used up to 60% in blends with palm oil, lard, tallow, and liquid vegetable oils. These blends are outlined in Table 7-13.

DEODORIZATION

Deodorization is the last major processing step in the refining of edible oils. It has the responsibility for removing both the undesirable ingredients occurring in natural fats and oils and those which might be produced by previous processing such as caustic refining, bleaching, hydrogenation, or even storage conditions. It is this unit process that finally establishes the oil characteristics of "flavor and odor" that are most readily recognized by the consumer (Gavin 1978).

Young (1986A) suggests that deodorized hardened fish oil should have

Table 7-11. Solid Fat Index, Melting-Point Ranges, and Iodine Values of Hydrogenated Marine Oils

Slip melting point range, °F	79/82	86/90	90/93	93/97	97/100	104/108	109/113	115/118
Iodine value range, WIJS	95/100	78/85	75/83	72/80	68/75	50/60	40/45	35/40
TEMP., °F			SOLID FAT INDEX BY DILATATION					
50	19	39	40	44	50	59	67	>69
59	15	33	35	41	47	59	67	73
68	11	26	29	37	43	57	67	74
77	8	16	20	30	34	53	66	73
86	4	5	9	18	22	44	65	68
95	0	0	1	4	9	30	59	CA60
104			0	0	2	12	36	CA40
113				0	0	—	CA20

Source: Young 1986C; Bimbo 1987A.

Table 7-12. Summary of Suggested Uses for Partially Hydrogenated Marine Oils

IODINE VALUE	USES
PHMO 110/120	Salad oil, single-use shallow frying
PHMO 78/85	Economic replacement for brush-hydrogenated soybean oil
PHMO 75/83	Margarine, shortening (both table and industrial), bread fats and emulsions
PHMO 72/80	Deep-fat frying blends, margarine, shortening (both table and industrial), biscuit cream filling fat, puff pastry compound fats
PHMO 72/75	Danish pastry
PHMO 68/75	Bread fats and emulsions
PHMO 60/72	Shortenings for biscuit dough
PHMO 50/60	Baking fats, bread fats and emulsions, industrial cake and creaming margarine, retail shortening, puff pastry compound fats
PHMO 45/55	Industrial puff or flaky pastry margarines
PHMO 35/40	Baking fats, stick table margarines, bread fats and emulsions, high-speed dough mixing, industrial cake and creaming margarines, retail shortening, puff pastry compound fats
PHMO 30/40	Baked products eaten when hot
PHMO 18/25	Antistaling agent in bread dough
PHMO 3 MAX	Glyceryl monostearate emulsifiers

Source: Young 1986A; Bimbo 1987A.

characteristics as outlined in Table 7-14. Steam deodorization is possible because of the great differences in volatility between the triglycerides and the substances that give oils and fats their natural flavors and odors (Mattil 1964). It is essentially a process of steam distillation where the volatile compounds are stripped from the nonvolatile oil. Deodorization also destroys peroxides in the oil and removes any aldehydes or other volatile products that may have resulted from atmospheric oxidation. Hsieh et al. (1989) evaluated the volatile components of crude winterized menhaden oil by dynamic headspace gas analysis. They found many components derived from lipid oxidation, including short-chain saturated and unsaturated aldehydes, ketones, and carboxylic acids. They suggest that the odor-significant volatiles may be used as specific flavor quality markers to determine deodorization efficiency and flavor stability of the oil. Karahadian and Lindsay (1989) evaluated the volatile compounds present in vacuum steam deodorized fish oils oxidized under fluorescent light at room temperature. They found that hexanal,2,4-heptadienals and 2,4-decadienals contributed general oxidized, painty flavors to the oil. Pelura (1987) evaluated the volatiles produced from the deodorization of menhaden oil at 150°C and 250°C and found that at the lower temperature aldehydes and hydrocarbons dominated the volatile compounds, while at the

Table 7-13. Typical Margarine and Shortening Blends Used in the United Kingdom, % of Fat Blend

	PARTIALLY HYDROGENATED MARINE OILS[a]				PALM OIL	LIQ. OIL	TALLOW	LARD
	90/93	93/97	104/108	115/118				
Refrigerator margarine	65	0	0	0	15	20	0	0
Standard cake margarine	45	0	0	5	0	25	25	0
Standard pastry margarine	0	0	0	60	0	10	0	30
Standard cooking margarine	0	40	35	0	0	25	0	0
Puff pastry margarine	0	50	0	15	35	0	0	0
Domestic shortening	55	0	0	5	0	0	0	40
General-purpose shortening	50	0	0	5	40	5	0	0
Bread fat	0	0	0	30	0	0	70	0
Cake shortening	0	25	0	20	15	40	0	0

Source: Young 1986B; Bimbo 1989.
[a]Melting point in degrees fahrenheit.

higher temperature aromatic and other hydrocarbons dominated. He mentions that the aldehydes result from the decomposition of hydroperoxides, while the aromatic compounds at the higher temperature could come from the decomposition of carotenoids. Mattil (1964) suggests that strongly rancid oils cannot be completely reclaimed by deodorization, as such oils will have lost most of their natural stability through oxidation and hence will become rancid a second time with relative ease. There are a number of deodorizer configurations in use today. These are discussed in the following sections.

Batch Deodorizer

The conventional batch deodorizer is a well-insulated, vertical cylinder with dished or cone heads, and internal coils for heating and cooling. The

Table 7-14. Typical Partially Hydrogenated and Deodorized Fish Oil Guideline Specifications

Free fatty acids, %	0.10% maximum
Peroxide value, meq/kg	0
Totox value	$<\frac{1}{2}$ of TV of bleached hydrogenated oil
Color, lovibond $5\frac{1}{4}$-in. scale	3.0 red, 30 yellow maximum
Iron, ppm	0.12
Copper, ppm	0.05
Nickel, ppm	0.20
Flavor and odor	bland

Source: Young 1986A.

capacity usually ranges from 10,000 to 40,000 lb. Sometimes the upper half of the unit is heated to prevent refluxing of the distilled volatiles within the deodorizer. Stripping steam is admitted at the bottom of the vessel through perforated pipe. After deodorization is completed, the oil must be cooled before it is discharged to the atmosphere; this can be done in the deodorizer or externally by pumping it through a heat exchanger. A typical batch deodorizer can be seen in Fig. 7-12.

Semicontinuous Deodorizer

Carlson (1988) mentions that semicontinuous deodorization is characterized by the intermittent movement of a relatively small batch of product through consecutive heating, deodorizing, and cooling stages in the system. The semicontinuous deodorizer consists of a tall cylindrical carbon steel shell containing five stainless steel stages. These deodorizers

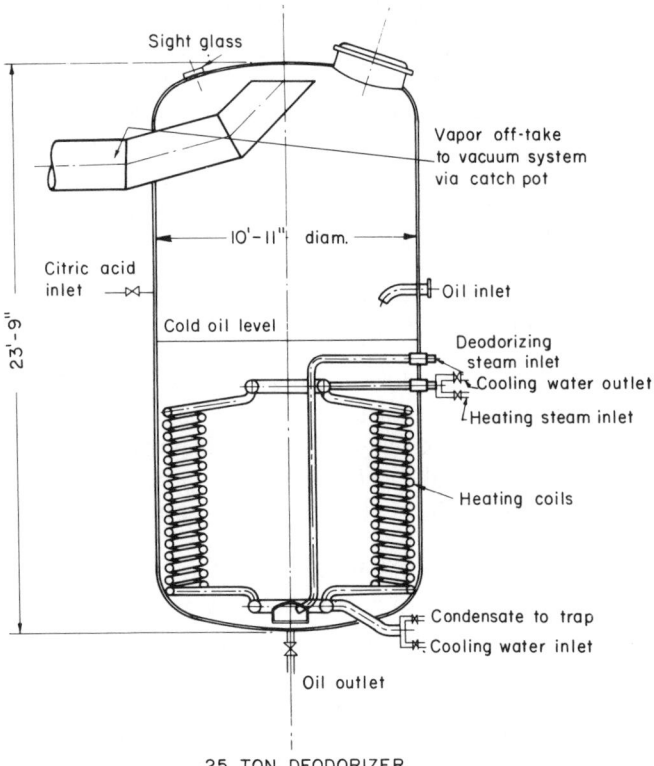

25 TON DEODORIZER

Fig. 7-12. Batch-type deodorizer. (*Source:* Devine and Williams, *Chemistry and Technology of Edible Fats and Oils,* 1961. Courtesy of Pergamon Press Ltd.)

handle batches of oil in a timed sequence of deaerating-heating, holding–steam stripping, and cooling, such that each parcel of oil is subjected to each condition before proceeding to the next step. These systems generally are associated with ease of stock oil change and usually have the lowest contamination of one product into another. The intermittent flow pattern and tray-cycling sequence provides natural break points in the product flow, making stock change simpler and often faster. This type deodorizer can be seen in Fig. 7-13.

Continuous Deodorizer

In the continuous double-shell deodorizer, deodorization is conducted in a series of seven vessels all mounted within but separate from a single outer shell which is maintained under vacuum. The first vessel is maintained at the same vacuum as the deodorizer and is used to deaerate the oil at about 120°F. The oil is circulated through coils in a heat recovery tank, where hot, previously deodorized oil preheats the feedstock. The preheated oil is then pumped to the top tank in the deodorizer, where it is further deaerated. From the top tank the oil flows by gravity to the next tank, where it is heated to deodorization temperature by live steam which is also used to agitate the oil. The oil then flows countercurrently to the stripping steam over a series of stripping trays. The final tray is the heat recovery tray used to preheat the incoming oil. The oil then flows from the heat recovery tank to the cooling tank.

Continuous Thin-Film Deodorizer

The Cambrian Campro deodorizer employs a thin-film concept to strip volatiles from the oil at high transfer rates. The operations of deaerating, heating, deodorizing, heat exchanging, and cooling the oil are carried out within one single rectangular, stainless steel processing tray that is housed in a split, horizontal, cylindrical shell connected to a vacuum exhaust system (Brekke 1980A).

Figure 7-14 shows a schematic diagram of a 500 kg/hr Campro deodorizer for fish oils. The numbers in parenthesis below refer to the numbers on the diagram. Preheated oil is pumped into the deodorizer via the preheated oil inlet (1). The preheated oil is heated to temperature by thermal fluid entering the deodorizer via the thermal fluid inlet (2) and flowing through the heating coils (3) in the heating section (4). The inside tray (12) of the deodorizer is divided into concentric compartments, with the heating section (4) at the outside, the deodorizing section (7) in the middle,

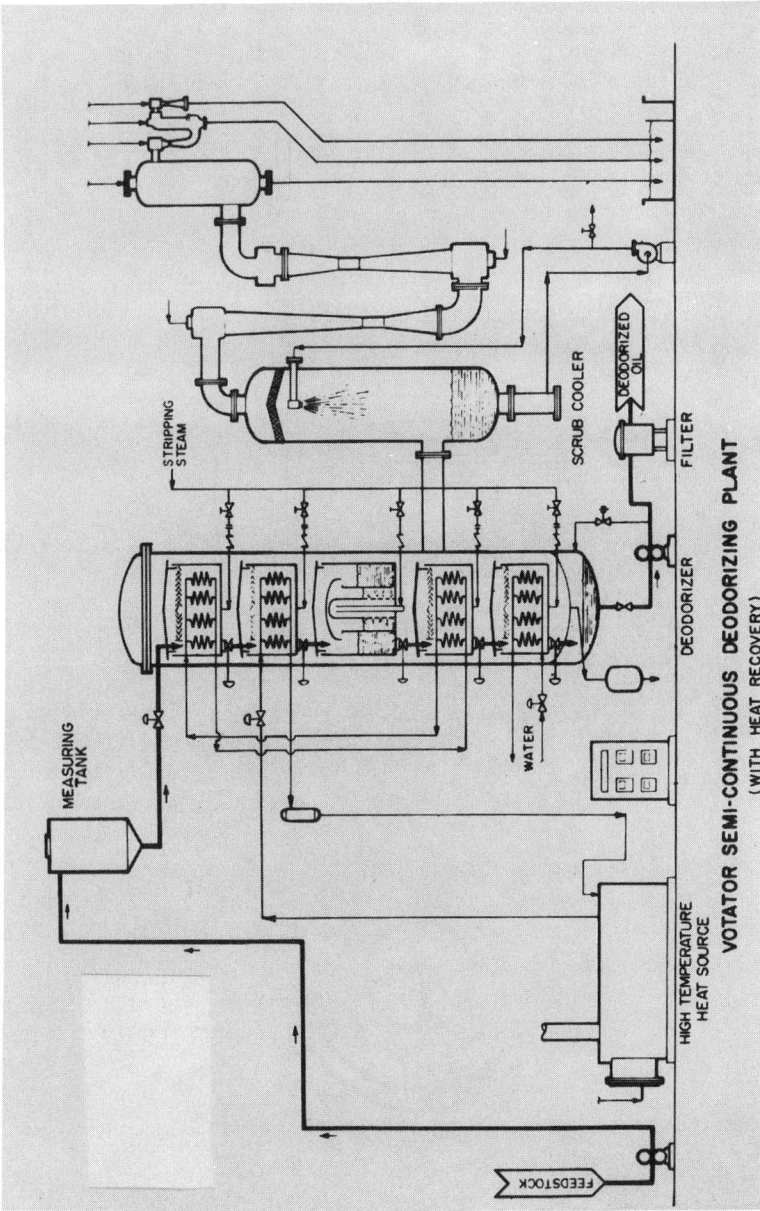

Fig. 7-13. Votator semicontinuous deodorization plant—process flow diagram of the deodorization system. (*Source:* Votator Div., Cherry-Burrel, Louisville, Kentucky.)

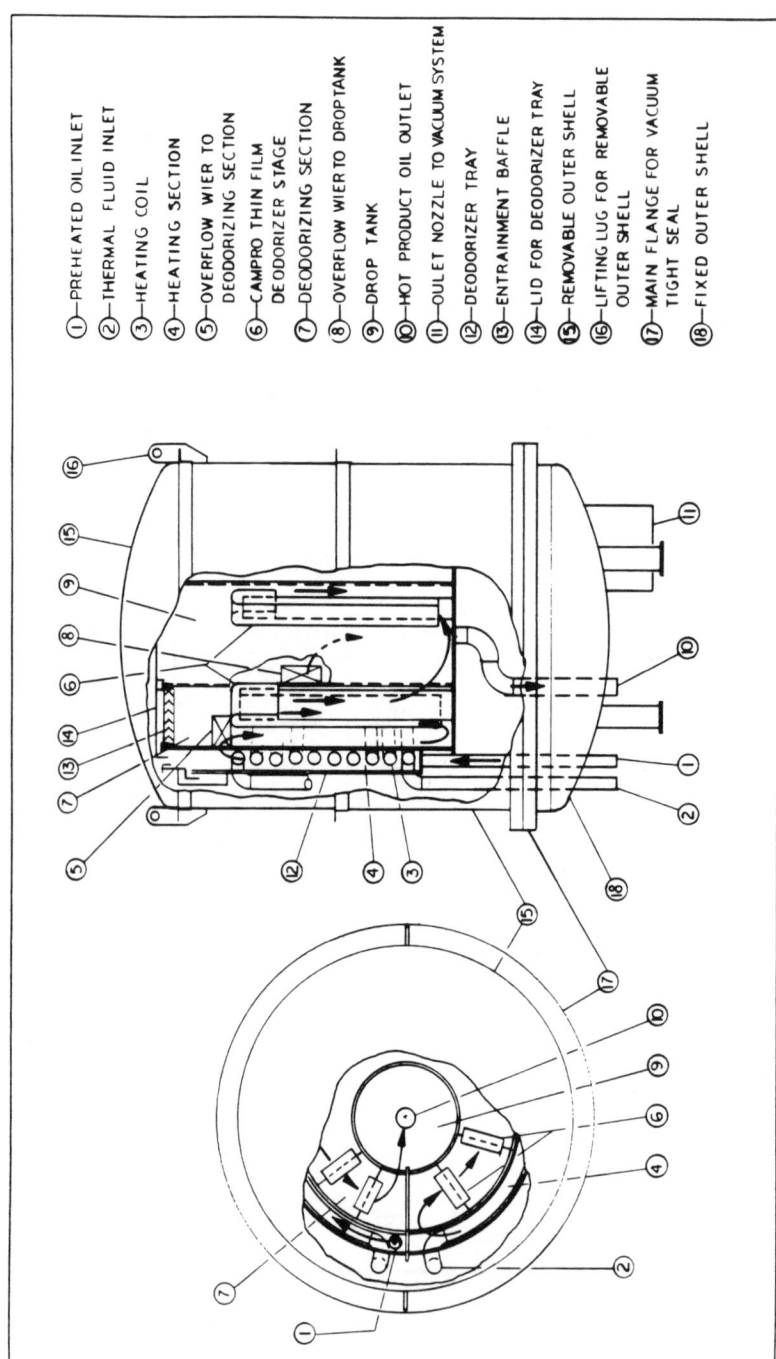

① PREHEATED OIL INLET
② THERMAL FLUID INLET
③ HEATING COIL
④ HEATING SECTION
⑤ OVERFLOW WIER TO DEODORIZING SECTION
⑥ CAMPRO THIN FILM DEODORIZER STAGE
⑦ DEODORIZING SECTION
⑧ OVERFLOW WIER TO DROPTANK
⑨ DROP TANK
⑩ HOT PRODUCT OIL OUTLET
⑪ OULET NOZZLE TO VACUUM SYSTEM
⑫ DEODORIZER TRAY
⑬ ENTRAINMENT BAFFLE
⑭ LID FOR DEODORIZER TRAY
⑮ REMOVABLE OUTER SHELL
⑯ LIFTING LUG FOR REMOVABLE OUTER SHELL
⑰ MAIN FLANGE FOR VACUUM TIGHT SEAL
⑱ FIXED OUTER SHELL

Fig. 7-14. Schematic diagram of the 500 kg/hr Campro deodorizer for fish oils, showing internal details and circular oil path. (*Source:* Cambrian Engineering Group Limited, Mississauga, Ontario, Canada.)

and the drop tank (9) in the center of the tray. The preheated oil enters the tray at the bottom and flows around the heating section, before dropping into the middle deodorizing section via the overflow wier (5). The oil enters into the bottom entrance of the deodorizer stage (6) and is spread into a thin film on the inside surfaces of the stage and forced to flow vertically upward against gravity by the high velocity of the sparge steam. Each stage consists of a rectangular channel formed from two sheets of stainless steel. At the top of the stage, the channel turns downward, forcing the oil from the first stage to drop to the entrance of the second stage, while the vapors flow vertically upward and out of the tray. Thus the oil moves with minimum back-mixing from stage to stage around the middle deodorizing section (7). At the end of the deodorizing section, the oil drops by another overflow wier (8) into the drop tank (9). It exits the deodorizer via the hot product oil outlet (10) and feeds the hot oil transfer pump.

The Campro deodorizer was designed to incur minimal damage to the polyunsaturated fatty acids in fish oil by subjecting the oil to mild temperature exposure. Because of the high intrinsic stripping efficiency of the Campro thin-film deodorizer stage, the volatile materials can be distilled from fish oil at lower temperatures. Also, because of the continuous operation and design features, the residence time at temperature is very short. Before the vapor stream leaves the deodorizer through the outlet nozzle (11), it must pass through the entrainment baffles (13) at the top of the tray (12). The purpose of the entrainment baffles is to control losses of neutral oil in the distillate. The lid (14) for the deodorizer tray ensures that all surfaces in contact with the fish oil are of stainless steel and also prevents condensed fatty acids from refluxing back into the oil. For periodic maintenance, the removable outer shell (15) is taken off by using the lifting lugs (16) after the bolts securing the main flange (17) are removed. On lifting off the removable outer shell, the entire tray assembly, which is mounted to the fixed outer shell (18) is exposed for inspection, cleaning, and maintenance.

Figure 7-15 shows the Campro deodorizing system in its final stages of fabrication. Because all component parts are preassembled and skid mounted, the system is compact and highly portable. It requires only hookup to steam, water, electricity, nitrogen, and instrument air to be fully operational.

Zehnder (1988) mentions that prior to the early 1960s the steam and condensed volatiles from the oil were condensed in the barometric condenser water. This required separation before the water could be pumped to local sewage treatment plants and the fat (when marketable) separated and sold as a feeding fat, pumped into the soapstock, or hauled to land

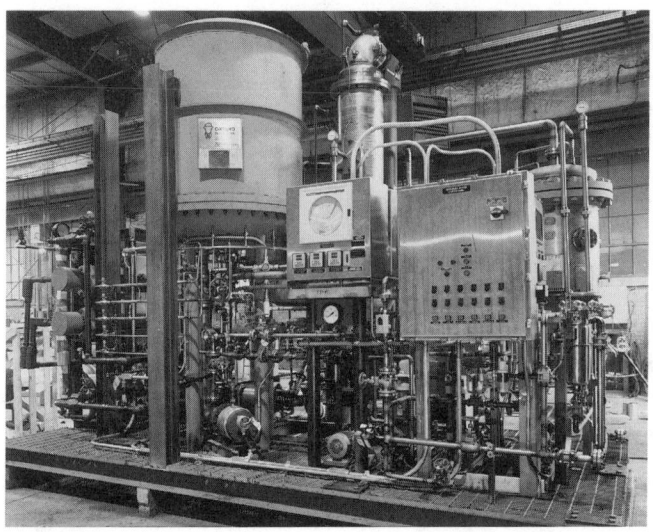

Fig. 7-15. The 500 kg/hr Campro deodorizing/steam refining system for fish oils. The entire system is preassembled and skid mounted, requiring only hookup to plant utilities. (*Source:* Cambrian Engineering Group Limited, Mississauga, Ontario, Canada.)

fills. As environmental pressures increased, distillate recovery systems changed to indirect contact systems, thus separating condensed volatiles and steam from the cooling and barometric condenser water. This change resulted in a distillate rich in tocopherols and other sterols and a market in the pharmaceutical industry.

CHOLESTEROL AND CHLORINATED HYDROCARBON REMOVAL

Steam Deodorization

Addison et al. (1978) evaluated the changes in several chlorinated pesticides and hydrocarbons during the processing of marine oils. They found that the hydrogenation and deodorization steps effectively reduced these compounds to nondetectable levels.

Pelura (1987) evaluated the change in cholesterol and cholesterol esters during vacuum steam deodorization of a refined menhaden oil at various temperatures and found that cholesterol is not significantly distilled at temperatures below 200°C, but at 200°C and higher distillation does occur, with increasing removal from 200° to 250°C. He further mentions that while free cholesterol is distilled, the cholesterol esters are not easily removed. According to his data around 40–50% of the free cholesterol was removed at 200°C for 3 hr, while only 26% of the cholesterol esters were removed at 250°C for 3 hr in a bench scale glass deodorizer. He evaluated the change in chlorinated pesticides and PCBs in menhaden oil at a number of temperatures and found reduction in PCBs, below detectable levels at a temperature of 175°C. He also reports that organochlorine and organophosphorous pesticides are easily removed, even under the mildest conditions.

Vacuum Stripping

Vacuum-stripping technology takes advantage of the fact that each chemical substance has a characteristic vapor pressure. It is this relative difference in vapor pressures that dictates how easily a complex compound can be separated into its constituent components.

The thin-film evaporator/molecular still technique has been successfully used for over 40 years for removal of free fatty acids from fats and oils, distilling of fats and oils, deodorization of oils, and removal of free cholesterol from fats and oils. Ackman (1988) mentions that in his laboratory, an initial oil stripping is used to reduce polychlorinated biphenyls and a final stripping for purification of fish oil concentrates in a short-passage time wiped-wall molecular still. He mentions that the short-passage time limits the thermal abuse possible when other processes are used.

In the National Institutes of Health/Department of Commerce drug master files for fish oil ω3s the process for the production of vacuum-deodorized fish oil is described. Partially refined menhaden oil is fed from 55-gal containers under nitrogen pressure through the first-stage feed pump to the first-stage still body. Rotating Teflon blades spread the oil downwards in a thin film along the inner wall of the still. Figure 7-16 shows a cutaway view of the wiped-film glass molecular still, showing the slotted wiper blades, drive, and internal condenser. The first stage is operated at 100°C and 1 torr vacuum. In this stage, the oil is preheated and degassed; hydroperoxides are decomposed and short-chain volatile compounds are distilled. The volatiles are condensed in a −84°C electric vapor trap. The oil then enters the second stage, where carbon blades wipe the oil into a thin film and move it downwards. In this stage the oil is heated at 260°C at 0.5 torr vacuum. The second stage contains an internal condenser heated to 150°C by circulating heat exchange fluid. In this stage cholesterol, pesticides, and PCBs are volatilized and collected in a trap after the condenser. The nonvolatile triglycerides exit the second stage, pass through a stainless steel heat exchanger and a 150-mm Teflon filter,

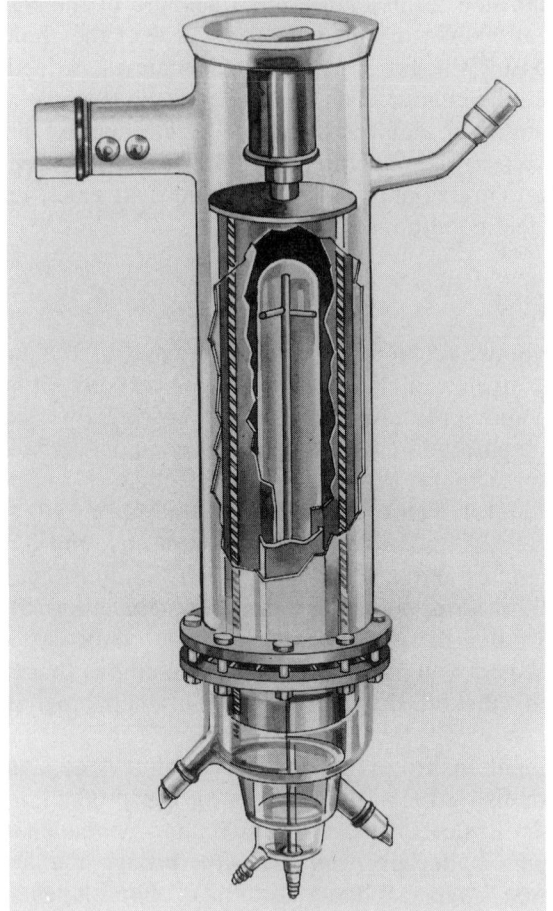

Fig. 7-16. Cutaway view of the Pope Scientific, Inc., wiped-film glass molecular still, showing slotted wiper blades, drive, and internal condenser. Upper ports are feed in and vapor out. Lower ports are distillate and residue out and condensor in/out. (*Source:* Pope Scientific, Inc., Menomonee Falls, Wisconsin.)

and after cooling are collected in inert gas purged containers (U.S. Dept. of Commerce 1989 in press). Figure 7-17 shows the two-stage continuous wiped-film still system.

Vacuum Stripping/Steam Deodorization

Marschner and Fine (1989) described a combination process that not only deodorizes but also removes cholesterol from nonhydrogenated fish oils. The physical process can be used with freshly refined or stored oils

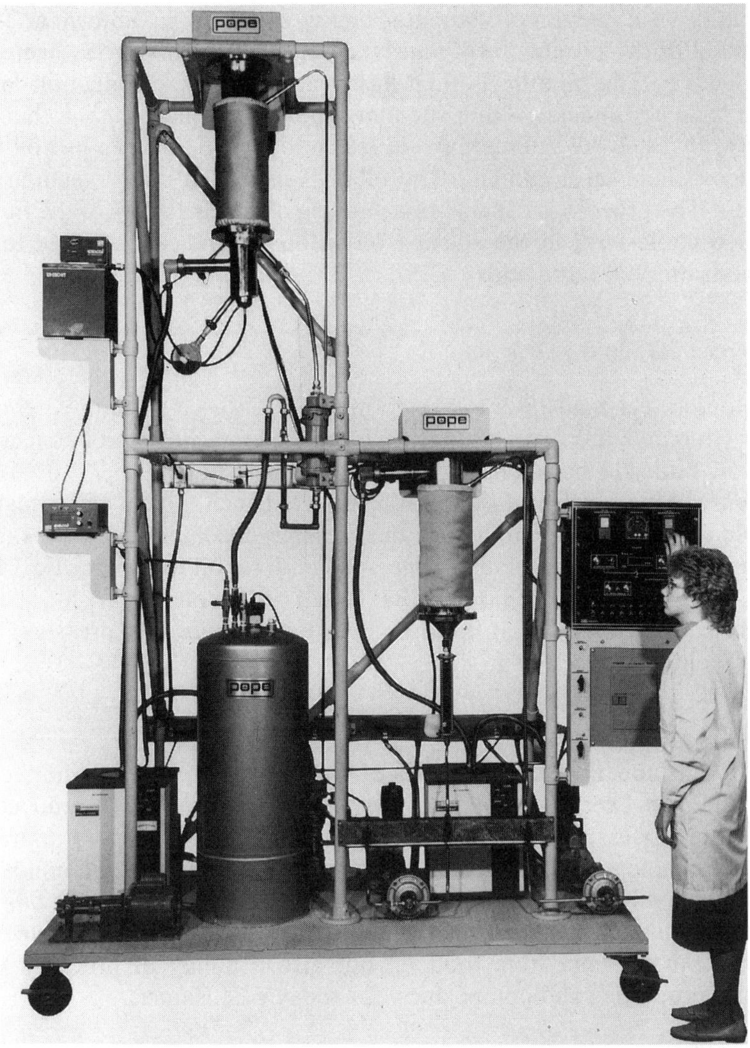

Fig. 7-17. The Pope Scientific, Inc., turnkey two-stage continuous wiped-film still system for fish oil fractionating, deodorizing, and PCB removal. (*Source:* Pope Scientific, Inc., Menomonee Falls, Wisconsin.)

that have oxidized (reverted). The oil is deaerated, mixed with steam, heated, flash vaporized, thin-film stripped with countercurrent steam, cooled, and stored. The final product is clean tasting and free of nonesterified cholesterol.

The researchers describe the process as follows: The fish oil is deaerated to an oxygen level of less than 0.1% dissolved oxygen by subjecting the oil to vacuum with or without sparging with inert gas. Steam at 2–5% is added to the oil under 1–7 mm vacuum and the mixture is heated to 450°–480°F. The mixture is then flash vaporized by introduction into a flash chamber under 1–7 mm vacuum. The fish oil phase is then thin-film stripped with 2–5% countercurrent steam to provide a clean fish oil with reduced cholesterol content. The oil is then cooled under vacuum and stored. The process is capable of removing as much as 98% of the nonesterified cholesterol in the starting oil without significant damage to the polyunsaturated fatty acids.

Supercritical Fluid Extraction

Supercritical fluid (SCF) extraction has been used to remove cholesterol from milk fats. Single-stage SCF reduced the cholesterol concentration in butterfat by 15%, while a multistage unit reduced it 30%. An increase in the number of stages of contact between solvent and feedstock would make it possible to reduce the cholesterol content by 90% (Anonymous 1989). Krukonis (1989) subjected cod-liver oil to supercritical fluid processing in order to remove PCBs. Based on laboratory bench tests, the PCBs can be removed at quite modest temperature and pressure with little yield loss of the fish oil.

SUMMARY

Fish oils contain the same types of compounds present in other edible fats and oils. These compounds or impurities are removed or reduced by the same processes that are used with edible vegetable oils and/or animal fats. Technology has kept pace with current health issues and concerns, and by a combination of "old" processes and new concepts, fish oils can be made suitable for use in many food applications, thus supplying not only another competitive food oil but also a family of products with unique properties and composition for today's consumer.

REFERENCES

Ackman, Robert G. 1988. The year of the fish oils. Oils and Fats Group International Lecture. *Chem. Ind.* 7 March 1988:139–145.

Addison, R. F., et al. 1978. Behavior of DDT, polychlorinated biphenyls (PCBs), and dieldrin at various stages of refining of marine oils for edible use. *J. Am. Oil Chemists' Soc.* 55:391–394.

Allen, D. A. 1989. Hydrogenation—A user's view. Paper read at the 80th Annual Conference of the AOCS, 3–6 May 1989, Cincinnati, Ohio.

Anonymous 1987. Pope Wiped Film Stills—Introduction and Description of Basic Technology. Menomonee Falls: Bulletin No. 1. Pope Scientific Inc.

Anonymous 1989. Supercritical extraction holds promise for cholesterol free butter. *Food Eng.* February 1989:83–86.

Barlow, S. M. 1988. The challenges to the world fish oil industry. *N-3 News: Unsaturated Fatty Acids and Health* 3:(2)1–3.

Bimbo, A. P. 1986. Use of fish oils: Task for new technology. *N-3 News: Unsaturated Fatty Acids and Health* 1(3):1–4.

Bimbo, A. P. 1987A. The emerging marine oil industry. *J. Am. Oil Chemists' Soc.* 64:706–715.

Bimbo, A. P. 1987B. Marine oils—Perspectives on the U.S. industry. Paper read at the American Institute of Baking Technical Seminar Fish Oil (Omega-3 Fatty Acids) and Other Unconventional Oils, 11–12 May 1987, Manhattan, Kansas.

Bimbo, A. 1988. Fish oils: Future challenges and opportunities. In *Seafood Technology— Preparing for Future Opportunities,* ed. Marvin Kragt and Donn Ward, pp. 167–203. Chicago: Institute of Food Technologists.

Bimbo, A. 1989A. Fish oils as foods: Challenges and opportunities. In *Fats and Oils in Bakery Products,* ed. Okkyung Kim Chung, pp. 282–308. St. Paul: American Association of Cereal Chemists.

Bimbo, A. P. 1989B. Technology of production and industrial utilization of marine oils. In *Marine Biogenic Lipids, Fats and Oils,* vol. II, ed. R. G. Ackman, pp. 401–433. Boca Raton, Fla.: CRC Press.

Bimbo, A. P. 1989C. Recent advances in upgrading industrial fish to value added products. In *New Technologies for Value-Added Products from Protein and Co-Products,* ed. Lawrence A. Johnson, Symposium III Changing Resources and Needs. Champaign, Ill.: American Oil Chemists' Society.

Brekke, O. L. 1980A. Oil degumming and soybean lecithin. In *Handbook of Soy Oil Processing and Utilization,* ed. D. L. Erickson et al., pp. 71–88. St. Louis: American Soybean Association; and Champaign, Ill.: American Oil Chemists' Society.

Brekke, O. L. 1980B. Bleaching. In *Handbook of Soy Oil Processing and Utilization,* ed. D. L. Erickson et al., pp. 105–130. St. Louis: American Soybean Association; and Champaign, Ill.: American Oil Chemists' Society.

Brekke, O. L. 1980C. Deodorization. In *Handbook of Soy Oil Processing and Utilization,* ed. D. L. Erickson et al., pp. 155–191. St. Louis: American Soybean Association; and Champaign, Ill.: American Oil Chemists' Society.

Carlson, K. F. 1988. Deodorization options and trends. *J. Am. Oil Chemists' Soc.* 65:306–313.

Carr, Roy A. 1988. Degumming and refining of vegetable oils. Paper read at the AOCS Northeast Section Symposium on Processing, 11 April 1988, Newark, N.J.

Chang, S. S. 1967. Processing of fish oils. In *Fish Oils,* ed. M. E. Stansby, pp. 206–221. Westport, Conn.: AVI Publishing Co.

Contreras R., Oscar, Migliardo O., Aldo and Raffo R., Andres 1971. Continuous fractionation of Chilean anchovy oil with furfural. *J. Am. Oil Chemists' Soc.* 48:98–100.

Deffense, Etienne. 1985. Theory and practice of fractionation. Paper read at Society of Chemical Industry: Oils and Fats Group Teach-In on Fat Modification, 5 December 1985, Chester, England.

Deffense, E. 1987. The Tirtiaux physical refining process. In *One Dimension Ahead.* Fleurus, Belgium: S. A. Fractionnement Tirtiaux. 32 pp.

Dickinson, N. L., and Meyers, J. M. 1952. Solexol fractionation of menhaden oil. *J. Am. Oil Chemists' Soc.* 29:235–239.

Dijkstra, A. J., and Opstal, M. V. 1989. The total degumming process. *J. Am. Oil Chemists' Soc.* 66:1002–1009.

Eckert, C. A., Van Alsten, J. G., and Stoicos, T. 1986. Supercritical fluid processing. *Environ. Sci. Technol.* 20:319–325.

Elson, C. M., and Ackman, R. G. 1978. Trace metal content of a herring oil at various stages of pilot-plant refining and partial hydrogenation. *J. Am. Oil Chemists' Soc.* 55:616–618.

Elson, C. M., Bem, E. M., and Ackman, R. G. 1981. Determination of heavy metals in a menhaden oil after refining and hydrogenation using several analytical methods. *J. Am. Oil Chemists' Soc.* 58:1024–1026.

FAO. 1977. Dietary fats and oils in human nutrition. Report of an expert consultation. *FAO Food and Nutrition Paper No. 3*. Rome: Food and Agriculture Organization of the United Nations. 94 pp.

Fernandez, Carmen. 1986. Refinement of fish oil for human consumption: Engineering investigations. Dissertation submitted to the University of Washington. 350 pp.

Gavin, Arnold M. 1978. Edible oil deodorization. *J. Am. Oil Chemists' Soc.* 55:783–791.

Hilditch, T. P. 1949. The refining of fats. In *The Industrial Chemistry of the Fats and Waxes*, 3rd ed., pp. 236–261. London: Bailliere, Tindall and Cox.

Hsieh, Thomas C. Y., et al. 1989. Characterization of volatile components of menhaden fish (*Brevoortia tyrannus*) oil. *J. Am. Oil Chemists' Soc.* 66:114–117.

IAFMM, 1988. *Digest of Selected Statistics*. Compiled for the 28th Annual Conference, Lima, Peru.

Karahadian, C., and Lindsay, R. C. 1989. Evaluation of compounds contributing characterizing fishy flavors in fish oils. *J. Am. Oil Chemists' Soc.* 66:953–960.

Kokubu, K., Hayashi, S., and Kodama, K. 1984. Purification method for marine oils. Japanese Patent No. S58-883410.

Krukonis, V. J. 1989. Supercritical fluid processing of fish oils: Extraction of polychlorinated biphenyls. *J. Am. Oil Chemists' Soc.* 66:818–821.

Lee-Poy, F. 1987. Cost-effective in-plant treatment for finished, deodorized fish oil. In *Rendering Profits*, pp. 47–80. Anchorage: Alaska Fisheries Development Foundation, Inc.

Letan, A., and Koslowsky, L. 1975. Fractionation of edible oils from isopropanol. *La Rivista Italiana Delle Sostanze Grasse LII*, Luglio, pp. 217–220.

Marschner, S., and Fine, J. 1989. Process for deodorizing and reducing cholesterol in fats and oils by employing flash vaporization and thin film steam stripping. U.S. Patent No. 4,804,555.

Mattil, K. F. 1964. Deodorization. In *Bailey's Industrial Oil and Fat Products*, 3d ed., ed. Daniel Swern, pp. 897–930. New York: Interscience.

Mounts, T. L. 1980. Refining. In *Handbook of Soy Oil Processing and Utilization*, ed. D. L. Erickson et al., pp. 89–103. St. Louis: American Soybean Association; and Champaign, Ill.: American Oil Chemists' Society.

National Fish Meal and Oil Association (NFMOA). 1986. Petition to the Food and Drug Administration Requesting Affirmation of Menhaden Oil and Partially Hydrogenated Menhaden Oil as Generally Recognized as Safe for Use in Foods.

National Institutes of Health/Department of Commerce. 1989. Drug master files for fish oil omega 3s, Biomedical Test Materials Program.

Nilsson, L., Brimberg, U., and Haraldson, G. 1989. Experience of pre-refining of vegetable oils with acids. Paper read by K. Carlson at the 80th Annual Conference of the AOCS, 6 May 1989, Cincinnati, Ohio.

Noguchi, Y., and Hibino, H. 1982. Separation of highly unsaturated fatty acids. Japanese Patent No. S57-124434.

Norris, F. A. 1982. Refining and bleaching. In *Bailey's Industrial Oil and Fat Products*, vol. 2, 4th ed., ed. Daniel Swern, pp. 253–314. New York: Wiley.

Passino, H. J. 1949. Drying oils. The solexol process. *Ind. Eng. Chem.* 41:280–287.

Pelura, Timothy J. 1987. The effect of deodorization time and temperature on the chemical, physical and sensory characteristics of menhaden oil. Dissertation submitted to the Graduate School—New Brunswick Rutgers, the State University of New Jersey. 273 pp.

Revankar, G. D., et al. 1975. Solvent winterisation of sardine oil. *J. Oil Technologists' Assoc. India* July/September:85–87.

Sano, Y. 1984. Concentration of polyunsaturated triglycerides. Japanese Patent No. S58-104566.

Schlenk, H., and Ener, Marita A. 1959. Solubility and fractionation of lipids in sulfur dioxide. *J. Am. Oil Chemists' Soc.* 36:145–149.

Sebedio, J-L., and Ackman, R. G. 1983A. Hydrogenation of a menhaden oil: I. Fatty acid and C20 monoethylenic isomer compositions as a function of the degree of hydrogenation. *J. Am. Oil Chemists' Soc.* 60:1986–1991.

Sebedio, J-L., and Ackman, R. G. 1983B. Hydrogenation of a menhaden oil: II. Formation and evolution of the C20 dienoic and trienoic fatty acids as a function of the degree of hydrogenation. *J. Am. Oil Chemists' Soc.* 60:1992–1996.

Sebedio, J-L., et al. 1981. Alteration of long chain fatty acids of herring oil during hydrogenation on nickel catalyst. *J. Am. Oil Chemists' Soc.* 58:41–48.

Spinelli, J., Stout, V. F., and Nilsson, W. B. 1987. Purification of fish oils. U.S. Patent No. 4,692,280.

Stirton, A. 1964. Fractionation of fats and fatty acids. In *Bailey's Industrial Oil and Fat Products,* 3rd ed., ed. Daniel Swern, pp. 1005–1037. New York: Interscience.

Takao, Masayasu. 1985. Refined fish oils and the process for production thereof. U.S. Patent No. 4,554,107.

U.S. Dept. of Commerce. 1989. Biomedical test materials program: Production methods and safety manual, ed. J. Joseph. NOAA Technical Memorandum NMFS CL-693.

U.S. Food and Drug Administration. 1989. Substances affirmed as generally recognized as safe: Hydrogenated and partially hydrogenated menhaden oils. Notice. *Federal Register* 54(178):38219–38223.

Ward, J. 1989. "Super refining tm" a large scale chromatographic process for the production of high purity lipids. Unpublished paper. Croda Inc., New York.

Weiss, T. J. 1983. Basic processing of fats and oils. In *Food Oils and Their Uses,* 2nd ed., pp. 65–98. Westport, Conn.: AVI Publishing Co.

Young, F. V. K. 1978. Processing of oils and fats. *Chem. Ind.* 16 September 1978:692–703.

Young, F. V. K. 1985A. The Refining and Hydrogenation of Fish Oil. Fish Oil Bulletin 17. International Association of Fish Meal Manufacturers. 27 pp.

Young, F. V. K. 1985B. Interchangeability of fats and oils. *J. Am. Oil Chemists' Soc.* 62:372–376.

Young. F. V. K. 1986A. *The Chemical and Physical Properties of Hydrogenated Fish Oils for Margarine and Shortening Manufacturers.* Fish Oil Bulletin 19, International Association of Fish Meal Manufacturers. 18 pp.

Young, F. V. K. 1986B. Formulation in a multi-feedstock situation. Paper read at the AOCS Short Course No. 2 on Hydrogenation, May 1986, Honolulu, Hawaii.

Young, F. V. K. 1986C. *The Use of Hydrogenated Fish Oils in Margarines, Shortenings and Compound Fats.* Fish Oil Bulletin 20. International Association of Fish Meal Manufacturers. 8 pp.

Young, F. V. K. 1986D. *The Chemical and Physical Properties of Crude Fish Oils for Refiners and Hydrogenators.* Fish Oil Bulletin 18. International Association of Fish Meal Manufacturers. 19 pp.

Zehnder, C. T. 1988. Deodorization and physical refining. Paper read at the AOCS Northeast Section Symposium on Processing, 11 April 1988, Newark, N.J.

Chapter 8
LIPID METABOLISM IN FISH

Diana H. Greene

INTRODUCTION

Recent research has added a great deal of information to our understanding of lipid metabolism in fish. The rapid expansion of aquaculture as a worldwide industry, refinements in analytical techniques using gas chromatography, and medical discoveries detailing the therapeutic effects of fish oils in the treatment of cardiovascular disease have all served to promote research in this field.

When the original chapter on this topic (Stansby 1967, ch. 21) was written, very little was known about the details of lipid metabolism in fish. The last few decades, however, have supplied evidence to support the assumption that the pathways of lipid biosynthesis and oxidation in fish are essentially the same as those known from mammalian systems. Most of this biochemical information has been obtained from research with rainbow trout (*Salmo gairdneri*). Additional studies with different species also suggest that lipid metabolism in fish is a dynamic process, since these organisms must constantly adjust membrane composition in order to maintain homeostasis against changes in water temperature. Environmental conditions such as salinity and the available food supply likewise play a role in directing the pathways of lipid metabolism. In short, many more factors than heredity dictate which fatty acids each species will require and how those fatty acids will be utilized under any given circumstance.

The following discussion will cover recent discoveries about enzymes involved in lipid-related pathways in both marine and freshwater fish, the fatty acid requirements of cultured and wild fish, and the effects of temperature and environmental changes on lipid metabolism.

GENERAL LIPID METABOLISM

The most obvious difference between fish and mammals lies in their ability to desaturate and elongate fatty acids. While mammals are only capable of modifying fatty acids of the $\omega9$ and $\omega6$ families (Fig. 8-1), early studies with rainbow trout demonstrated that fish could also elongate and

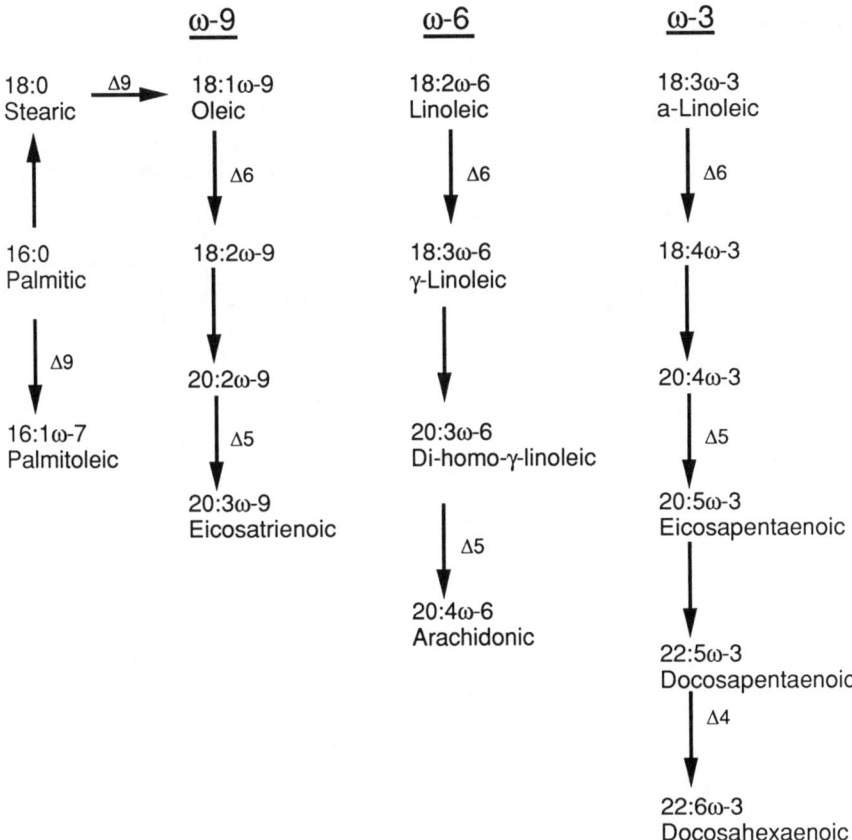

Fig. 8-1. Elongation and desaturation pathways in the biosynthesis of polyunsaturated fatty acids.

desaturate fatty acids of the ω3 family. This capability suggested the presence of unique digestive and biosynthetic enzymes in fish and a major role for the ω3 fatty acids in fish nutrition.

Lipogenesis

Key enzymes in the synthesis of lipids (Fig. 8-2) have been identified in numerous species. Acetyl-CoA, the fundamental building block of all endogenously formed lipids, is generated by ATP citrate lyase. The activity of this enzyme has been identified in rainbow trout (Henderson and Sargent 1981), coho salmon (*Oncorhynchus kisutch*) (Lin et al. 1977A, B,

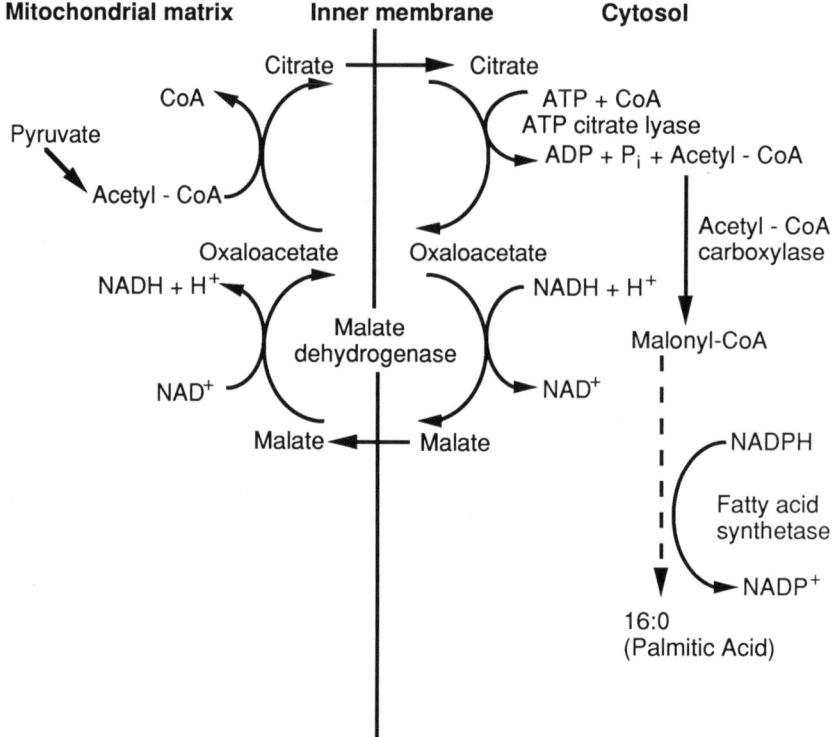

Fig. 8-2. Key enzymatic pathways in the biosynthesis of fatty acids.

C), and European eel (*Anguilla anguilla*) (Abraham et al. 1984). Cytosolic acetyl-CoA is formed in turn from mitochondrial acetyl-CoA, which is the product of pyruvate metabolism. Since pyruvate is the end product of carbohydrate metabolism, one might expect high-carbohydrate diets to enhance the fatty acid enzymes. This was found to be the case in salmon and catfish (Likimani and Wilson 1982). When these fish were fed high-carbohydrate diets, increases in fatty acid synthetase and malate dehydrogenase were observed. Conversely, when salmon (Lin et al. 1977B, C), catfish (Likimani and Wilson 1982), yellowtail (*Seriola quinqueraldiata*) (Shimeno et al. 1981), and trout (Jurss et al. 1985) were fed high fat diets, they exhibited depressed activity of enzymes involved in the production of nicotinamide adenine dinucleotide (reduced form) (NADPH), which serves as an electron donor in the subsequent elongation of fatty acids by enzymes of the fatty acid synthetase complex.

Acetyl-CoA must first be transformed into malonyl-CoA before its incorporation into fatty acids. This is accomplished by the enzyme acetyl-

CoA carboxylase. Abraham et al. (1984) had observed a direct correlation between the reduced activity of this enzyme and a decrease in fatty acid synthesis in response to fasting in eels. More recently, McKim and coworkers (1989) isolated the enzyme from trout liver hepatocytes.

Long-term feeding and short-term radiolabel studies have both shown that the majority of lipogenic activity in fish tissue occurs in the liver. Lin et al. (1977C) reported that fatty acid synthesis proceeded 30 times faster in salmon liver than in adipose tissue. Further, dietary lipids that evoked enzyme activity changes in the liver had no effect on lipogenic enzymes in the adipose tissue of either salmon (Lin et al. 1977B) or catfish (Likimani and Wilson 1982). Similarly, the enzyme response to a high-carbohydrate diet was significantly delayed in catfish adipose tissue compared to hepatic tissue.

Pathways for the incorporation of de novo and dietary fatty acids into triacylglycerols and phospholipids have been delineated by experiments with rainbow trout. Glycerol-3-phosphate is the structural unit from which all further mono-, di-, and triacylglycerols and polar lipids are derived. The enzymes glycerol-3-phosphate acyl-transferase and phosphatidate phosphatase are involved in adding fatty acids to the glycerol-3-phosphate backbone. The activities of both enzymes were confirmed in rainbow trout in an early study by Holub et al. (1975A). When trout hepatocytes were incubated with radiolabeled glycerol-3-phosphate and an activated fatty acid, palmitoyl-CoA, 23% of the recovered radioactivity was found in the neutral lipid fraction and 77% in the phospholipid fraction.

The polar lipid phosphatidylcholine (PC) (lecithin) is formed from 1,2-diacylglycerol and CDP-choline by the action of the enzyme phosphocholine phosphotransferase. Holub et al. (1975B) confirmed the presence of this enzyme in rainbow trout. When hepatocytes were incubated with radiolabeled CDP-choline, 1,2-diacylglycerol and Mg^{2+}, the researchers recovered radioactivity as phosphatidylcholine. Alternatively, new species of PC can be formed by attaching a different acyl group at the sn-2 position of lysolecithin (1-acyl-sn-glycerol-3-phosphoryl choline). This is accomplished by lysolecithin transferase, which was shown to be active in rainbow trout liver microsomes when they were incubated with lysolecithin and radiolabeled CoA-activated fatty acids (Holub et al. 1976).

Dietary Lipid Metabolism

Long-chain polyunsaturated fatty acids predominate in marine and freshwater food chains. Hydrolysis of dietary triacylglycerols in mammals is normally mediated by pancreatic lipase, which hydrolyzes the acyl groups at the *sn*-1 and *sn*-3 positions on the glycerol backbone, leaving the 2-monoacylglycerol intact. Polyunsaturated fatty acids, particularly of the ω3 family, have an affinity for the *sn*-2 position of triacylglycerols. Since many fish species also have a dietary requirement for these fatty acids, it has been suggested that fish might possess unique lipases that are capable of hydrolyzing fatty acids at the *sn*-2 position.

Patton et al. (1975) evaluated the action of intestinal juice preparations from anchovy (*Engraulis mordax*), striped bass (*Morore saxatilis*), jack mackerel (*Trachurus symmetricus*), Pacific mackerel (*Scomber japonicus*), and pink salmon (*Oncorhynchus gorbuscha*) on a synthetic triacylglycerol, racemic 1-palmitate-2-oleate-3-stearate. All of the fish preparations released oleic acid from the *sn*-2 position. In contrast, when pig lipase was added to the same substrate, only 16:0 and 18:0 were released. Oleate was left intact as a monoacylglycerol. The fish intestinal juices also hydrolyzed both ω6 and ω3 long-chain fatty acyl groups from methyl esters to a greater extent than pig lipase. These results suggest the presence of a nonspecific lipase capable of hydrolyzing acyl groups at all three positions on the glycerol backbone. Lie and Lambertsen (1985) reported that the enzymes in cod digestive juice preferentially hydrolyzed polyunsaturated fatty acids. Such nonspecific hydrolysis, however, has not been observed in all fish species. Tocher and Sargent (1984B) reported that rainbow trout intestinal extracts released oleic acid from only the *sn*-1 and *sn*-3 positions of glycerol trioleate, consistent with the behavior of pig pancreatic lipase.

Pancreatic lipases in mammalian digestive systems are known to be assisted by the protein colipase, which serves as a common point of attachment for pancreatic lipase and triacylglycerols. Evidence for its presence in dogfish (*Squalus acanthius*), trout, hagfish, rayfish, and Greenland shark has appeared in the literature (Tocher and Sargent 1984B). Sternby et al. (1984) purified the protein from dogfish pancreas and found it to be highly homologous with mammalian and avian colipases.

A large proportion of the long-chain fatty acids available to fish in the marine food web occur in the form of wax esters. Mammals generally are incapable of digesting wax esters, while fish possess the enzyme wax ester hydrolase, which readily hydrolyzes these ester bonds. The proportion of dietary lipid that is in the form of wax esters varies greatly from species to species. The anchovy, for example, consumes over 70% of its diet by dry weight as wax ester, while reef fish normally ingest only limited quantities of wax esters (Patton and Benson 1975). Under experimental conditions, however, both types of fish displayed similar competence in digesting wax esters. Sargent et al. (1979) likewise reported that rainbow trout, which do not normally encounter wax esters in wild diets, are capable of assimilating wax esters as efficiently as herring, which rely heavily on copepods that are rich in 20 : 1 and 22 : 1 esters. The differences observed between these different species in the natural state, however, were explained by anatomical differences. There appeared to be a close correlation between the number of pyloric caeca in fish such as herring, anchovy, chub mackerel, and yellowtail (Mankura et al. 1984), which feed on diets rich in wax esters, and the quantity of wax ester that can be retained long enough to be assimilated. Species such as reef fish, flatfish, and bream, in which pyloric caeca are absent or very few, cannot retain dietary wax esters in the intestine long enough to effect any appreciable assimilation.

In mammals, liberated dietary fatty acids are reassembled into triacyl-glycerols inside the intestinal villi, then packaged into chylomicrons or very-low-density lipoproteins (VLDL) for delivery to peripheral tissues. These structures provide an amphiphilic layer of phosphatidylcholine, cholesterol, and apoproteins, which facilitate the transport of hydrophobic lipids through the aqueous lymph and blood stream. Early studies on lipid absorption in rainbow trout (Robinson and Mead 1973) and carp (Kayama and Iijima 1976) failed to provide evidence for this transport system in fish. However, more recent radiolabel experiments with trout have demonstrated that long-chain fatty acids are rapidly esterified to TAGs, followed by the appearance of chylomicrons and VLDLs (Sire and Vernier 1981; Sire et al. 1981). In addition, the trout intestinal epithelial cells synthesized different sizes of chylomicrons, depending on the type of dietary fat ingested. The largest chylomicrons, up to 650 nm, appeared after ingestion of long-chain ω3 fatty acids, while palmitic acid was incorporated into particles in the VLDL range.

Very-low-density lipoprotein, low-density lipoprotein (LDL), and high-density lipoprotein (HDL), which are well characterized in mammals, have also been identified in trout (Black and Skinner 1986), catfish (McKay et al. 1985), and carp (Nakagawa 1979; Iijima et al. 1985). Starvation studies with rainbow trout (Black and Skinner 1986) and catfish (McKay et al. 1985) showed that in fish, as in other animals, VLDLs and LDLs are primarily carriers of triacylglycerol, while HDLs are primarily associated with cholesterol and phospholipid transport. Amino acid analysis of protein fractions isolated from carp (Nakagawa 1979) and catfish (McKay et al. 1985) lipoproteins also revealed a high degree of homology between the fish and mammalian apoproteins.

ESSENTIAL FATTY ACIDS

Fish do not normally utilize carbohydrates, but rely on protein and lipid to meet the energy demands of growth and reproduction. For this reason, the formulation of artificial diets for hatcheries and commercial aquaculture has been an active area of research. Pioneering studies at Oregon State University demonstrated that trout in particular require dietary ω3 long-chain fatty acids to support normal growth. Prior to this work, the only fatty acids generally considered essential for higher organisms were linoleic acid (18:2) and arachidonic acid (20:4), both of the ω6 family. However, it appears that the ability to elongate and desaturate fatty acids varies greatly among fish, thus affecting specific dietary requirements. As a result, there has been a great deal of experimental repetition in determining the essential fatty acid (EFA) requirements of fish on a species-by-species basis. The following section summarizes the data obtained for five commercially important fish—trout, salmon, carp, catfish, and tilapia.

Rainbow Trout

Castell and co-workers (1972B) observed that when rainbow trout were fed fat-deficient diets, several degenerative disorders appeared. These included tail fin erosion, swollen pale livers, myocarditis, and the "shock" or "fainting" syndrome. The last symptom is characterized by rapid swimming in response to any stress introduced to the culture tank, followed by loss of consciousness. The swollen liver is in part due to an increase in the neutral to polar lipid ratio and reflects the overall increase in moisture content observed in fish kept on EFA-deficient diets (Castell et al. 1972A, B; Takeuchi and Watanabe 1976). The liver disorders resulting from fat-deficient diets were reversed, however, by adding between 0.5% linolenate and 1% linolenic acid to the diet (Castell et al. 1972A, B). In contrast, neither 1% linoleic acid (18:2ω6) nor 5% oleic acid (18:1ω9) was effective in restoring trout livers to a normal condition. Subsequent experiments comparing linolenate, soybean, and cod-liver oils have repeatedly documented the effectiveness of ω3 fatty acids in reducing the lipid level in the liver and high tissue moisture (Takeuchi and Watanabe 1976; Watanabe et al. 1974A, C).

Trout readily convert linolenic acid to eicosapentaenoic (20:5ω3) and docosahexaenoic acid (22:6ω3), the two fatty acids normally found in the highest concentration in trout tissues. As a result, trout raised for two generations with linolenic acid as the sole source of EFA were found to have normal kidney, heart, and liver tissues (Yu et al. 1979). When ω3 fatty acids are undersupplied, however, the trout overproduce eicosatrienoic acid (20:3ω9), which is the longest-chain fatty acid that can be synthesized endogenously, in order to compensate for the lack of PUFAs in the diet. Hepatic degeneration usually becomes evident when the 20:3ω9/22:6ω3 ratio of the tissue exceeds 0.4. The addition of linolenate to the diet at 0.83% to 1.66% by weight has generally been regarded as optimum for maintaining the ratio below 0.4 (Watanabe et al. 1974B).

In trout, as in mammals, fatty acids of the $\omega 6$ and $\omega 3$ families compete with each other for the desaturation and elongation enzymes necessary to convert dietary lipids to longer-chain, more highly unsaturated derivatives (Yu and Sinnhuber 1976; Yu et al. 1979). Linoleic acid in the form of both triacylglycerol and ethyl ester was shown to improve the growth of trout fed diets that contained less than 0.5% linolenate, but when linolenate was increased to 0.5% and 1.0% of the diet, linoleate depressed fish growth (Yu and Sinnhuber 1975, 1976). Consequently, these researchers strongly suggested that $\omega 3$ fatty acids do not improve the growth rate or feed conversion efficiency of trout diets that are already adequate in $\omega 3$ fatty acids.

Radiolabel studies have shown that trout convert precursor $18:3\omega 3$ to the more highly unsaturated $22:6\omega 3$ more rapidly and efficiently than any other species studies. Owen et al. (1975) reported that trout converted 70% of dietary $18:3\omega 3$ to $22:6\omega 3$, while turbot (*Scophthalmus maximus*) did not convert any of the labeled precursor to longer-chain derivatives. Similarly, trout far surpassed ayu (*Plecoglossus altivelis*), eel (*Anguilla japonica*), red sea bream (*Chrysophrys major*), rockfish (*Sebasticus marmoratus*), globefish (*Fugu rubripes rubripes*), and prawn (*Penaeus japonicus*) in its ability to convert injected $18:3\omega 3$ to $20:5\omega 3$, $22:5\omega 3$, and $22:6\omega 3$ combined (Kanazawa et al. 1979). These results suggest that the biological requirement is for the longer-chain, more highly unsaturated derivatives of linolenic acid. Experiments with diets containing $20:5\omega 6$ and $22:6\omega 3$ enriched oils in excess of 1%, however, have suggested that there might be an upper limit to the level of $\omega 3$ fatty acids that will promote healthy growth (Takeuchi and Watanabe 1976). Recent studies comparing the effects of animal fats and vegetable oils with salmon oil in trout diets have provided further evidence that high levels of the highly unsaturated $\omega 3$ fatty acids may result in less than optimum growth (Greene and Selivonchick 1989).

Salmon

Chum (*Oncorhynchus keta*), coho (*O. kisutch*), and chinook (*O. tshawytscha*) salmon, like rainbow trout, have a dietary requirement for the $\omega 3$ fatty acids. However, these fish do not have the same capacity for chain elongation and desaturation of $18:3\omega 3$ as rainbow trout but require a certain level of $20:5\omega 3$ and $22:6\omega 3$ preformed in the diet (Yu and Sinnhuber 1979; Takeuchi et al. 1979; Takeuchi and Watanabe 1982). The growth efficiency of short-term diets combining $18:2\omega 6$ and $18:3\omega 6$ has been reported as comparable to diets containing highly unsaturated fatty acid mixtures. However, the higher tissue levels of $20:3\omega9$ in coho salmon raised on the linoleic/linolenic acid mixture suggested that the nutritional needs of the fish were better supplied by the preformed poly-unsaturates (Takeuchi and Watanabe 1982; Takeuchi et al. 1979).

Since salmon farming has become a commercially important industry, considerable research effort has been directed toward formulating diets that meet both the nutritional requirements of the fish and economic considerations. Coho, chinook, and Atlantic salmon (*Salmo salar*) have demonstrated good growth on a variety of high-lipid diets when the basal EFA requirements were met by a marine oil and the remainder of the dietary lipid was supplied by beef tallow, linseed oil, or soybean oil (Hardy et al. 1987; Mugrditchian et al. 1981; Yu and Sinnhuber 1981). Hardy and co-workers (1987) further investigated the effects of different marine oils in diets to supply the basal EFA requirements for Atlantic salmon and found that menhaden oil at 7% of an 18% lipid diet promoted greater weight gain than herring oil added at the same level and resulted in higher tissue levels of the $\omega3$ fatty acids.

Carp

The essential fatty acid deficiency symptoms reported for rainbow trout on diets containing less than 1% linolenate have also been reported for carp (*Cyprinus carpio*). Reduced growth, fin erosion, swollen pale fatty livers, and high levels of moisture in the muscle tissue were apparent in carp when linoleate was less than 1% of diets that were relatively low in total lipid (1.5–9.1%) (Csengeri et al. 1978). Carp fed low-linolenate diets also lost balance when the tank water temperature dropped below 8–10°C (Farkas et al. 1980), while carp raised on diets incorporating 7% fish oil survived at temperatures as low as 4.5°C (Viola et al. 1988).

Linolenate appears to play a vital role in lipogenesis in carp, and consequently affects membrane adaptation to changes in temperature. Farkas et al. (1978) observed an inverse relationship between $18:1\omega9$ in tissue triacylglycerols and $18:3\omega3$ in the diet, suggesting that linolenate might regulate the fatty acid synthetase and stearyl-CoA desaturase enzymes. Data in support of this hypothesis was obtained by feeding carp diets containing linolenate at 0.5%, 1.0%, and 11.4%, then injecting them with radiolabeled acetate, the prerequisite for acetyl-coA. Carp fed 0.5% linolenate rapidly incorporated the sodium acetate. Approximately half of the radioactivity recovered from carp on the high-linolenate diets was incorporated into PUFAs, while the major product of fatty acid biosynthesis in fish on the low-linolenate diets was oleic acid.

While early studies based on weight gain and feed conversion ratios suggested an essential requirement for both ω3 and ω6 fatty acids (Takeuchi and Watanabe 1977; Watanabe et al. 1975), observations on fish behavior at lowered temperatures point more clearly to linolenate as the essential fatty acid for carp. The ability to synthesize polyunsaturated fatty acids becomes critically important at low temperatures when a higher degree of phospholipid unsaturation is required in order to maintain a fluid environment for enzymes located in the cell membranes. Farkas et al. (1980) reported that fish mortalities occurred at temperatures below 8–10°C because the carp were unable to increase production of long-chain polyunsaturated fatty acids. This failure to adjust lipid biosynthesis in response to temperature was only evident in fish on low-linolenate diets. Since previous experiments adding linoleic acid to diets did not affect fatty acid synthesis, Farkas and co-workers (1978) concluded that the ω3 fatty acid plays a more essential role in carp nutrition than 18 : 2ω6.

Catfish

It has generally been assumed that since catfish normally inhabit warmer water than trout they have little or no requirement for ω3 fatty acids. Diets formulated with beef tallow and olive oil that contained only ω6 and ω9 fatty acids outperformed diets containing linolenic acid-rich linseed oil in promoting growth of channel catfish fingerlings. Yet in two separate feeding trials (Stickney and Andrews 1971A, B), menhaden oil performed as well as beef tallow and outperformed safflower oil, suggesting there may be a role for ω3 fatty acids in catfish nutrition. Yingst and Stickney (1979, 1980) demonstrated that fingerlings grew better when fed fish oil at 5% of the diet than when soybean oil was used as the dietary lipid. Catfish fry also had greater weight gains and a higher survival rate on fish oil than soybean oil diets (Gatlin and Stickney 1982).

An experiment feeding fish oil, soybean oil and beef tallow, each at 6, 8, 10, 12 and 14% of the diet to larger catfish (10–12 grams) further substantiated the value of long chain ω3 fatty acids in catfish diets (Gatlin and Stickney 1982). The researchers determined 10% lipid to be optimum and observed no significant differences in weight gain among fish on the three diets at this level of added lipid. However, fish raised on the fish oil had the lowest level of whole-body moisture and retained the highest total lipid. In contrast, catfish on the beef tallow diet deposited more protein and less lipid, which would appear to be the more economic conversion, since most of the fat deposited by catfish is visceral.

Tilapia

Research with tilapia has emphasized that this warm-water species may have a greater requirement for the $\omega6$ fatty acids than the $\omega3$ fatty acids. Comparing the effects of $18:2\omega6$, $18:3\omega3$, $20:4\omega6$, and $20:5\omega3$ at varying levels in diets for *Tilapia zilli*, Kanazawa et al. (1980) observed that the $\omega6$ fatty acids at either 0.5% or 1.0% of the diet promoted greater weight gains, feed conversion, and protein efficiency ratios than the $\omega3$ fatty acids. Increased levels of $20:4\omega6$ and $22:6\omega3$ in polar lipids indicated that the tilapia were unable to elongate and desaturate both $\omega6$ and $\omega3$ precursor fatty acids, but growth parameters did not provide evidence for an $\omega3$ requirement.

Tilapia nilotica similarly gained the most weight on diets containing 0.5% and 1.0% methyl linoleate ($18:2\omega6$) compared to $18:1\omega9$ and $18:3\omega3$ methyl esters at the same levels (Takeuchi et al. 1983). Depressed growth on all tilapia species has resulted from diets containing up to 1% $18:3\omega3$ methyl esters, while diets incorporating menhaden and catfish oil have promoted superior growth. On the basis of these results, Stickney and Wurts (1986) suggested that $18:3\omega3$ in particular is implicated in growth reduction and not the $\omega3$ fatty acids in general.

THERMAL ADAPTATION

Our understanding of lipid metabolism in fish has been greatly enhanced by thermal acclimation studies, and the research literature on this topic has been extensively reviewed (Hazel 1984; Greene and Selivonchick 1987; Henderson and Tocher 1987). As the ambient temperature decreases, it becomes necessary for these organisms to modify the lipid composition of cell membranes in order to maintain a constant fluid matrix for enzymes associated with the membranes. Conversely, higher temperatures require an increase in phospholipid saturation to counteract excessive fluidity. By changing assay temperature or altering the rearing temperature in growth experiments it has been possible to monitor patterns of lipid modification and mobilization.

Most of the work in this field has been conducted with rainbow trout, but certain basic features of temperature acclimation appear to be common to many species. The three primary means by which fish modify phospholipids are: (1) change in acyl chain composition, (2) rearrangement of fatty acids esterified to the phospholipid backbone, and (3) change in phospholipid class. These modifications, in turn, are dependent on changes in enzyme activity. The following section briefly reviews these two aspects of temperature compensation.

Phospholipids

Hazel and co-workers (Hazel 1979; Hagar and Hazel 1985) observed all three of the changes outlined above in trout liver phospholipids when the acclimation temperature was lowered from 20°C to 5°C. There was a general increase in polyunsaturated fatty acids and a decrease in saturated fatty acids. The increase in phospholipid unsaturation was due primarily to increases in $20:3\omega3$, $20:4\omega3$, $22:6\omega3$, and $20:4\omega6$, while the loss of $16:0$ accounted in large part for the decrease in saturation. The proportion of phosphatidylethanolamine (PE) increased at the expense of sphingomyelin and cardiolipin. Hui et al. (1981) suggested that PE counteracts the condensing effects of cold temperature by forming a wedge in the membrane bilayer. Within the PE fraction there was also an increase in the esterification of $22:6\omega3$ at the sn-2 position.

Green sunfish (*Lepomis cyanellus R.*) also increased the proportion of PE in liver phospholipids when the acclimation temperature was lowered from 25°C and 15°C to 5°C (Christiansen 1984). The decrease in saturated fatty acids, however, was balanced by an increase in monounsaturated fatty acids. Similar increases in PE and monounsaturates were observed in carp liver mitochondrial membranes at 10°C (Wodtke 1978). In contrast to trout, the level of $\omega3$ fatty acids, especially $22:6\omega3$, decreased with cold acclimation. Miller et al. (1976) observed similar decreases in $22:6\omega3$ in goldfish at 5°C. Docosahexaenoic acid decreased more than 20% in PE isolated from goldfish brain, synaptosomes, and myelin tissues. However, later studies (Farkas et al. 1980) have illustrated that, for carp at least, increases or decreases in $22:6\omega3$ in response to cold exposure are related to prior dietary history. The researchers observed that carp reared on sufficient linolenic acid immediately increased the level of PUFAs and $22:6\omega3$ in both total lipid and phospholipid, while fish that were fed diets deficient in linolenic acid decreased the level of $22:6\omega3$ in liver phospholipids.

Tilapia differ from salmonids and carp in their pattern of fat deposition and mobilization, which limits the temperature range that will support growth. Experiments have shown that *Oreochromis niloticus* and *Oreochromis* hybrids (*aureus* × *niloticus*), for example, do not store excess lipid in the musculature, but rely on visceral deposits (Anderson et al. 1984; Viola et al. 1988; Viola and Amedan 1980). Further, these fish were incapable of mobilizing stored visceral lipid at low temperature, resulting in mortality between 8°C and 6.5°C. Carp, which can mobilize lipids from both muscular and visceral deposits, were able to survive to 4.5°C under the same conditions (Viola et al. 1988). Sluggish lipid mobilization at low temperature was also reported for *Tilapia niloticus* (Satoh et al. 1984).

Desaturase and Phospholipase Activity

Acyl modifications of both phospholipids and neutral lipids at low temperature ultimately rely on a broad spectrum of enzymes. Of these, the enzymes involved in acyl transfer and desaturation have received the most research attention.

The acyl chain changes reported for rainbow trout hepatocytes as a result of cold acclimation agree with in vitro experiments with trout liver phospholipase A_2. Hazel (1979) observed decreases in $18:1\omega9$ and $18:2\omega6$ at the sn-2 position of trout liver PC after changing the water temperature from 20°C to 5°C. Neas and Hazel (1984) later reported that the enzyme isolated from trout acclimated to 5°C preferred to hydrolyze $18:1$ from PC, accounting for the decrease in this fatty acid in trout membranes at low temperature. The same enzyme from trout acclimated to 20°C preferred to hydrolyze $18:0$ when assayed at 5°C, possibly explaining the decrease in saturation observed at low temperature.

Comparison of Δ^9, Δ^6, and Δ^5 desaturase activities in trout liver at 5°C and 10°C demonstrated higher activity of all enzymes at 5°C, and significantly higher activity of Δ^5 desaturase (Hagar and Hazel 1985). The specific enhancement of this desaturase was also observed in *Pimelodus maculatus* (Ninno et al. 1974). In trout there also appeared to be a certain cooperation among enzymes to produce $22:6\omega3$ at low temperature. At 5°C, most of the $22:5\omega3$ formed by hepatocytes was converted to $22:6\omega3$. Sellner and Hazel (1982) also observed that the Δ^6 desaturase preferred $18:3\omega3$ as a substrate over $18:2\omega6$ and $18:1\omega9$, regardless of temperature.

ENVIRONMENTAL FACTORS AFFECTING LIPID COMPOSITION

The characteristic fatty acid composition of each genus and species is a complex response to food availability, water salinity, water temperature, and stage of development, migration, starvation, or spawning.

The Food Chain

The marine food chain above 30°N latitude is particularly rich in $\omega3$ fatty acids, and this is extensively reflected in the fatty acid composition of fish inhabiting northern waters (Ackman 1982). In North Atlantic and Pacific fish, $20:5\omega3$ and $22:6\omega3$ comprise approximately 90% of total PUFAs, while $18:2\omega6$ plus $20:4\omega6$ generally add up to less than 2% of total fatty acids (Ackman and McLeod 1988). Consequently, in these fish the $\omega6/\omega3$ ratio is quite low (generally 0.15 ± 0.1) compared to 0.38 to

0.93 in fish taken from Australian waters (Sinclair et al. 1983). Arachidonic acid appears to be a major fatty acid in the southern latitude food chain, and it has been measured at levels as high as 16% in Australian fish (Gibson 1983). In fish that contain high proportions of 20:4ω6 in total body lipids, the major long-chain ω3 is 22:6ω3 (Sinclair et al. 1986). Conversely, as the habitat moves farther south, from 10°S Australia to 70°N Antarctica, for example, the content of 20:4ω6 in fish lipids decreases, but the content of 20:5ω3 increases.

Water Salinity

Fresh water and salt water also evoke specific lipid patterns, particularly in respect to phosphatidylcholine. In the guppy (*Poecilia reticulata*), adaptation to seawater brought about an increase in PC in gill, digestive tract, and muscle tissues, and the PC fraction was itself enriched in 22:6ω3. The level of 22:6ω3 in the phospholipid fraction of saltwater-adapted guppies increased at the expense of 20:4ω6 compared to freshwater guppies (Daikoku et al. 1982). In eels likewise, 20:4ω6, which is the most abundant PUFA in the gills of freshwater animals, was replaced by 22:6ω3 when the eels were transferred to salt water (Thomson et al. 1977). Transfer of trout to seawater also effected an increase in the 22:6ω3 level of PC isolated from intestinal membranes (LeRay et al. 1984).

The Natural Habitat

A recurring theme among studies investigating the lipids of wild freshwater fish compared to those of cultured fish has been the greater role of ω6 fatty acids in fish consuming wild diets and the appearance of 18:3ω3 as a major ω3 fatty acid. In two separate studies profiling carp lipids, the 20:4ω6 levels of both dorsal muscle (Suzuki et al. 1986) and adipose tissue (Csengeri et al. 1978) were significantly higher in the wild carp, as was 18:3ω3 in the adipose tissue. Wild American eels also had lower total lipid than cultured, although the 20:4ω6 and 18:3ω3 contents were 2 and 4.3 times higher, respectively (Otwell and Richards 1981/1982). Less total lipid in wild fish compared to cultured has been observed for other species, including red sea bream (Morishita et al. 1988), ayu (Hirano and Suyama 1983), and coho salmon (Yamaguchi et al. 1988). Conversely, docosahexaenoic acid was almost twice as high in the neutral and polar fractions of cultured eels (Otwell and Richards 1981/1982). Dorsal muscle extracts of Japanese eels showed the same higher percentages of 18:3ω3 and 20 : 4ω6 and lower 22 : 6ω3 in the wild eels compared to cultured. Wild rainbow trout also deposited significantly more 18 : 3ω3 and less 22 : 6ω3 in dorsal muscle lipids than their cultured counterparts, which converted almost all dietary 18 : 3ω3 to 22 : 6ω3 (Suzuki et al. 1986).

Another freshwater species, ayu, likewise deposited more 18 : 3ω3 and 20 : 5ω3 in total, neutral, and phospholipids in the wild than under culture conditions at all seasons of the year (Hirano and Suyama 1983). The level of 22 : 6ω3 in the PE fraction, however, was twice as high in cultured ayu compared to wild (Ohshima et al. 1982).

Similar patterns have been observed in wild Atlantic salmon compared to cultured fish from two different hatchery stations (Ackman and Takeuchi 1986). Linolenic acid and arachidonic acid were higher in the total lipid, phospholipid, and triacylglycerol fractions of wild salmon compared to hatchery fish. Conversely, 22 : 6ω3 in the phospholipid fraction was approximately 30% lower in wild than in cultured salmon. Comparison of wild and cultured coho salmon showed a greater proportion of polar lipid in the muscle of wild fish and a correspondingly lower percentage of tricylglycerols. Levels of 20 : 1 and 22 : 1, representing dietary wax esters, were approximately threefold higher in the wild coho (Yamaguchi et al. 1988).

Spawning

Lipid adaptations to periods of feeding and spawning have also been observed. In the course of mobilizing lipid stores during spawning migration, chum salmon, for example, tend to concentrate 22 : 6ω3 in the outer muscle layer (Suzuki et al. 1988). Whole-body PC analysis has also shown that spawning migration is attended by very specific rearrangements of the acyl configurations on the PC backbone (Takahashi et al. 1985). During the feeding migration, 16 : 0/22 : 6 is the dominant PC in both males and females. In the seagoing phase of spawning migration, 16 : 0/22 : 6 tends to decrease and 16 : 0/20 : 5 increases in females, while both 16 : 0/ 20 : 5 and 16 : 0/22 : 6 continue to increase in males. During river migration, the percentages of 16 : 0/22 : 6 and 16 : 0/20 : 5 PC species decline precipitously. Post spawning, the 16 : 0/22 : 6 species of PC again dominates the muscle of both male and female chums.

Docosahexaenoic acid has been identified as the main PUFA of all lipoprotein classes in immature and spawning male trout. Very-low-density lipoproteins and LDLs were highest in the serum of immature trout, while HDLs comprised more than half the total lipoproteins in the spawning trout (Fremont and Marion 1982). Docosahexaenoic acid is also the major PUFA in the roes of cod (*Gadus morhua*), Atlantic herring, haddock (*Melanogrammus aeglefinus*), saithe (*Pollachius virens*), whiting (*Merlangus merlangus*), sand eel (*Ammodytes lancea*), and capelin (*Mallotus villosus*), pointing to a variety of roles for 22 : 6ω3 in the reproductive processes of fish (Tocher and Sargent 1984A). The appearance of 20 : 4ω6 as the dominant fatty acid in the phosphatidylinositol (PI) fraction of most of these roes, however, strongly suggests a distinct metabolic need for this fatty acid as well. The affinity of 20 : 4ω6 for PI has also been observed in the chloride cells of eel gills, where it appears to function as a precursor fatty acid in the regulation of salt secretion by prostaglandins (Bell et al. 1983).

CONCLUSION

Extensive research with many different fish from varied latitudes and geographical locations has demonstrated more similarities than differences between fish and mammals in terms of lipid pathways and basic enzymes. The ω3 fatty acids are now recognized as playing an essential role in cold-water fish. The hierarchy between ω3 and ω6 fatty acids in fish that inhabit warmer waters is far less clear. Current in vitro evidence has demonstrated that most fish are capable of at least limited elongation and desaturation for both ω3 and ω6 fatty acids. Environmental studies, on the other hand, have shown that diet and life-style influence the interplay of the enzymes involved in the metabolism of these two fatty acid systems, perhaps more than genetic predisposition. There is still great potential for research exploring the unique lipid adaptations to diet and other factors of the habitat among the freshwater and marine fish.

REFERENCES

Abraham, S., Heinz, J. M., Hansen, H. J. M., and Hansen, J. N. 1984. The effect of prolonged fasting on total lipid synthesis and enzyme activities in the liver of the European eel (*Anguilla anguilla*). *Comp. Biochem. Physiol.* 79B:285–289.

Ackman, R. G. 1982. Fatty acid composition of fish oils. In *Nutritional Evaluation of Long Chain Fatty Acids in Fish Oil*, ed. S. M. Barlow and M. E. Stansby, pp. 25–88. London: Academic Press.

Ackman, R. G., and McLeod, C. 1988. Total lipids and nutritionally important fatty acids of some Nova Scotia fish and shellfish food products. *Can. Inst. Food Sci. Technol. J.* 21:390–398.

Ackman, R. G., and Takeuchi, T. 1986. Comparison of fatty acids and lipids of smolting hatchery-fed and wild Atlantic salmon *Salmo salar*. *Lipids* 21:117–120.

Anderson, J., Jackson, A. J., Matty, A. J., and Capper, B. S. 1984. Effects of dietary carbohydrate and fibre on the tilapia *Oreochromis niloticus* (Linn.). *Aquaculture* 37:303–314.

Bell, M. V., Simpson, C. M. F., and Sargent, J. R. 1983. (n-3) and (n-6) polyunsaturated fatty acids in the phosphoglycerides of salt-secreting epithelia from two marine fish species. *Lipids* 18:720–726.

Black, D., and Skinner, E. R. 1986. Features of the lipid transport system of fish as demonstrated by studies on starvation in the rainbow trout. *J. Comp. Physiol.* B156:497–502.

Castell, J. D., Sinnhuber, R. O., Lee, D. J., and Wales, J. H. 1972A. Essential fatty acids in the diet of rainbow trout. Physiological symptoms of essential fatty acid deficiency. *J. Nutr.* 102:87–92.

Castell, J. D., Sinnhuber, R. O., Wales, J. H., and Lee, D. J. 1972B. Essential fatty acids in the diet of rainbow trout (*Salmo gairdneri*). Growth, feed conversion and some gross deficiency symptoms. *J. Nutr.* 102:77–85.

Christiansen, J. A. 1984. Changes in phospholipid classes and fatty acids and fatty acid desaturation and incorporation into phospholipids during temperature acclimation of green sunfish *Lepomis cyanellus* R. *Physiol. Zool.* 57:481–492.

Csengeri, I., Farkas, T., Majoros, F., Oláh, J., and Szalay, M. 1978. Effect of feeds on the fatty acid composition of carp (*Cyprinus carpio* L.) *Aquacultura Hungarica* (Szarvas) I:24–34.

Daikoku, T., Yano, I., and Masui, M. 1982. Lipid and fatty acid compositions and their changes in the different organs and tissues of guppy, *Poecilia reticulata* on sea water adaptation. *Comp. Biochem. Physiol.* 73A:167–174.

Farkas, T., Csengeri, I., Majoros, F., and Oláh, J. 1978. Metabolism of fatty acids in fish II. Biosynthesis of fatty acids in relation to diet in the carp. *Cyprinus carpio* Linnaeus 1758. *Aquaculture* 14:57–65.

Farkas, T., Csengeri, I., Majoros, F., and Oláh, J. 1980. Metabolism of fatty acids in fish III. Combined effect of environmental temperature and diet on formation and deposition of fatty acids in the carp, *Cyprinus carpio* Linnaeus 1758. *Aquaculture* 20:29–40.

Fremont, L., and Marion, D. 1982. A comparison of the lipoprotein profiles in male trout (*Salmo gairdneri*) before maturity and during spermiation. *Comp. Biochem. Physiol.* 73B:849–855.

Gatlin, D. M. III, and Stickney, R. R. 1982. Fall-winter growth of young channel catfish in response to quantity and source of dietary lipid. *Trans. Am. Fish. Soc.* 111:90–93.

Gibson, R. A. 1983. Australian fish—An excellent source of both arachidonic acid and ω-3 polyunsaturated fatty acids. *Lipids* 18:743–752.

Greene, D. H. S., and Selivonchick, D. P. 1987. Lipid metabolism in fish. *Prog. Lipid Res.* 26:53–85.

Greene, D. H., and Selivonchick, D. P. 1989. Effects of dietary vegetable, animal and marine lipids on muscle lipid and hematology of rainbow trout (*Salmo gairdneri*). *Aquaculture,* in press.

Hagar, A. F., and Hazel, J. R. 1985. The influence of thermal acclimation on the microsomal fatty acid composition and desaturase activity of rainbow trout liver. *Mol. Physiol.* 7:107–118.

Hardy, R. W., Scott, T. M., and Harrell, L. W. 1987. Replacement of herring oil with menhaden oil, soybean oil or tallow in the diets of Atlantic salmon raised in marine netpens. *Aquaculture* 65:267–277.

Hazel, J. R. 1979. The influence of thermal acclimation on membrane lipid composition of rainbow trout liver. *Am. J. Physiol.* 236:R91–R101.

Hazel, J. R. 1984. Effects of temperature on the structure and metabolism of cell membranes in fish. *Am. J. Physiol.* 246:R460–R470.

Henderson, R. J., and Sargent, J. R. 1981. Lipid biosynthesis in rainbow trout fed diets of different fat content. *Comp. Biochem. Physiol.* 69C:31–37.

Henderson, R. J., and Tocher, D. R. 1987. The lipid composition and biochemistry of freshwater fish. *Prog. Lipid Res.* 26:281–347.

Hirano, T., and Suyama, M. 1983. Fatty acid composition and its seasonal variation of lipids of wild and cultured ayu. *Bull. Jap. Soc. Sci. Fish.* 49:1459–1464.

Holub, B. J., Connor, J. T. H., and Slinger, S. J. 1975A. Incorporation of glycerol-3-phosphate into the hepatic lipids of rainbow trout, *Salmo gairdneri*. *J. Fish. Res. Board Can.* 33:61–64.

Holub, B. J., Nilsson, K., Piekarski, J., and Slinger, S. J. 1975B. Biosynthesis of lecithin by the CDP-choline pathway in liver microsomes of rainbow trout, *Salmo gairdneri*. *J. Fish. Res. Board Can.* 32:1633–1637.

Holub, B. J., Piekarski, J., Cho, C. Y., and Slinger, S. J. 1976. Incorporation of fatty acids into phosphatidylcholine by acyl-CoA: 1-acyl-*sn*-glycero-3 phosphorylcholine acyltransferase in liver of rainbow trout, *Salmo gairdneri*. *J. Fish. Res. Board Can.* 33:2821–2826.

Hui S. W., Stewart, T. P., Yeagle, P. L., and Albert, A. D. 1981. Bilayer to nonbilayer transition in mixtures of phosphatidylethanolamine and phosphatidylcholine: Implications for membrane properties. *Arch. Biochem. Biophys.* 207:227–240.

Iijima, N., Kayama, M., Okazaki, M., and Hara, I. 1985. Time course changes of lipid distribution in carp plasma lipoprotein after force feeding with soybean oil. *Bull. Jap. Soc. Sci. Fish.* 51:467–471.

Jurss, K., Bittorf, T., and Vokler, T. 1985. Influence of salinity and ratio of lipid to protein in diets on certain enzyme activities in rainbow trout (*Salmo gairdneri* Richardson). *Comp. Biochem. Physiol.* 81B:73–79.

Kanazawa, A., Teshima, S. I., and Ono, K. 1979. Relationship between essential fatty acid requirements of aquatic animals and the capacity for bioconversion of linolenic acid to highly unsaturated fatty acids. *Comp. Biochem. Physiol.* 63B:295–298.

Kanazawa, A., Teshima, S., Sakamoto, M., and Awal, M. A. 1980. Requirements of *Tilapia zillii* for essential fatty acids. *Bull. Jap. Soc. Sci. Fish.* 46:1353–1356.

Kayama, M., and Iijima, N. 1976. Studies on lipid transport mechanism in the fish. *Bull. Jap. Soc. Sci. Fish.* 43:987–996.

LeRay, C., Chapelle, S., Duportail, G., and Florentz, A. 1984. Changes in fluidity and 22:6(n-3) content in phospholipids of trout intestinal brush-border membranes related to environmental salinity. *Biochim. Biophys. Acta* 778:233–238.

Lie, Ø, and Lambertsen, G. 1985. Digestive lipolytic enzymes in cod (*Gadus morhua*): Fatty acid specificity. *Comp. Biochem. Physiol.* 80B:447–450.

Likimani, T. A., and Wilson, R. P. 1982. Effects of diet on lipogenic enzyme activities in channel catfish hepatic and adipose tissue. *J. Nutr.* 112:112–117.

Lin, H., Romsos, D. R., Tack, P. I., and Leveille, G. A. 1977A. Influence of dietary lipid on lipogenic enzyme activities in coho salmon. *J. Nutr.* 107:846–854.

Lin, H., Romsos, D. R., Tack, P. I., and Leveille, G. A. 1977B. Effects of fasting and feeding various diets on hepatic lipogenic enzyme activities in coho salmon. *J. Nutr.* 107:1477–1483.

Lin, H., Romsos, D. R., Tack, P. I., and Leveille, G. A. 1977C. Influence of diet on *in vitro* and *in vivo* rates of fatty acid synthesis in coho salmon. *J. Nutr.* 107:1677–1682.

Mankura, M., Kayama, M., and Saito, S. 1984. Wax ester hydrolysis by lipolytic enzymes in pyloric caeca of various fishes. *Bull. Jap. Soc. Sci. Fish.* 50:2127–2131.

McKay, M. C., Lee, R. F., and Smith, M. A. K. 1985. The characterization of the plasma lipoproteins of the channel catfish *Ictalurus punctatus*. *Physiol. Zool.* 58:693–704.

McKim, J. M., Schaup, H. W., Marien, K., and Selivonchick, D. P. 1989. Isolation and identification of acetyl-CoA carboxylase from rainbow trout (*Salmo gairdneri*) liver. *Lipids* 24:187–192.

Miller, N. G. A., Hill, M. W., and Smith, M. W. 1976. Positional and species analysis of membrane phospholipids extracted from goldfish adapted to different environmental temperatures. *Biochim. Biophys. Acta* 445:644–654.

Morishita, T., Uno, K., Matsumoto, Y., and Takahaski, T. 1988. Comparison of the proximate compositions in cultured red sea bream differing the localities and culture methods, and of the wild fish. *Nippon Suisan Gakkaishi* 54:1965–1970.

Mugrditchian, D. S., Hardy, R. W., and Iwaoka, W. T. 1981. Linseed oil and animal fat as alternative lipid sources in dry diets for chinook salmon (*Oncorhynchus tshawytscha*). *Aquaculture* 25:161–172.

Nakagawa, H. 1979. Biochemical studies on carp plasma protein—III. *Bull. Jap. Soc. Sci. Fish.* 45:219–224.

Neas, N. P., and Hazel, J. R. 1984. Temperature-dependent deacylation of molecular species of phosphatidylcholine by microsomal phospholipase A$_2$ of thermally acclimated rainbow trout, *Salmo gairdneri*. *Lipids* 19:258–263.

Ninno, R. E., DeTorrengo, M. A. P., Castuma, J. C., and Brenner, R. R. 1974. Specificity of 5- and 6- fatty acid desaturases in rat and fish. *Biochim. Biophys. Acta* 360:124–133.

Ohshima, T., Widjaja, H. D., Wada, S., and Koizumi, C. 1982. A comparison between cultured and wild ayu lipids. *Bull. Jap. Soc. Sci. Fish.* 48:1795–1801.

Otwell, W. S., and Rickards, W. L. 1981/1982. Cultured and wild American eels, *Anguilla rostrata*: Fat content and fatty acid composition. *Aquaculture* 26:67–76.

Owen, J. M., Adron, J. W., Middleton, C., and Cowey, C. B. 1975. Elongation and desaturation of fatty acids in turbot (*Scophthalmus maximus* L.) and rainbow trout (*Salmo gairdneri* Rich.). *Lipids* 10:528–531.

Patton, J. S., and Benson, A. A. 1975. A comparative study of wax ester digestion in fish. *Comp. Biochem. Physiol.* 52B:111–116.

Patton, J. S., Nevenzel, J. C., and Benson, A. A. 1975. Specificity of digestive lipases in hydrolysis of wax esters and triglycerides in anchovy and other selected fish. *Lipids* 10:575–583.

Robinson, J. S., and Mead, J. F. 1973. Lipid absorption and deposition in rainbow trout (*Salmo gairdneri*). *Can. J. Biochem.* 51:1050–1058.

Sargent, J. R., McIntosh, R., Bauermeister, A., and Blaxter, J. H. S. 1979. Assimilation of the wax esters of marine zooplankton by herring (*Clupea harengus*) and rainbow trout (*Salmo gairdneri*). *Marine Biology* 51:203–207.

Satoh, S., Takeuchi, T., and Watanabe, T. 1984. Effects of starvation and environmental temperature on proximate and fatty acid compositions of *Tilapia nilotica*. *Bull. Jap. Soc. Sci. Fish.* 50:79–84.

Sellner, P. A., and Hazel, J. R. 1982. Desaturation and elongation of unsaturated fatty acids in hepatocytes from thermally acclimated rainbow trout. *Arch. Biochem. Biophys.* 213:58–66.

Shimeno, S., Hosokawa, H., Takeda, M., Takayama, S., Fukui, A., and Sasaki, H. 1981. Adaptation of hepatic enzymes to dietary lipid in young yellowtail. *Bull. Jap. Soc. Sci. Fish.* 47:63–39.

Sinclair, A. J., O'Dea, K., and Naughton, J. M. 1983. Elevated levels of arachidonic acid in fish from northern Australian coastal waters. *Lipids* 18:877–881.

Sinclair, A. J., O'Dea, K., and Naughton, J. M. 1986. Polyunsaturated fatty acid types in Australian fish. *Prog. Lipid Res.* 25:81–82.

Sire, M.-F., Lutton, C., and Vernier, J.-M. 1981. New views on intestinal absorption of lipids in teleostean fishes: An ultrastructural and biochemical study in the rainbow trout. *J. Lipid Res.* 22:81–94.

Sire, M.-F. and Vernier, J.-M. 1981. Étude ultrastructurale de la synthèse de chylomicrons au cours de l'absorption intestinale des lipides chez la truite. Influence de la nature des acides gras ingérés. *Biol. Cell* 40:47–62.

Stansby, M. E., ed. 1967. Fish Oils; Their Chemistry, Technology, Stability, Nutritional Properties, and Uses. Westport, Conn.: AVI Publishing Co.

Sternby, B., Engström, A., and Hellman, U. 1984. Purification and characterization of pancreatic colipase from the dogfish (*Squalus acanthius*). *Biochim. Biophys. Acta* 789:159–163.

Stickney, R. R., and Andrews, J. W. 1971A. Combined effects of dietary lipids and environmental temperature on growth, metabolism and body composition of channel catfish (*Ictalurus punctatus*). *J. Nutr.* 101:1703–1710.

Stickney, R. R., and Andrews, J. W. 1971B. Effects of dietary lipids on growth, food conversion, lipid and fatty acid composition of channel catfish. *J. Nutr.* 102:249–258.

Stickney, R. R., and Wurts, W. A. 1986. Growth response of blue tilapias to selected levels of dietary menhaden and catfish oils. *Prog. Fish. Cult.* 48:107–109.

Suzuki, H., Chung, B. S., Isobe, S., Hayakawa, S., and Wada, S. 1988. Changes in ω-3 polyunsaturated fatty acids in the chum salmon muscle during spawning migration and extrusion cooking. *J. Food Sci.* 53:1659–1661.

Suzuki, H., Okazaki, K., Hayakawa, S., Wada, S., and Tamura, S. 1986. Influence of commercial dietary fatty acids on polyunsaturated fatty acids of cultured freshwater fish and comparison with those of wild fish of the same species. *J. Agric. Food Chem.* 34:58–60.

Takahashi, K., Egi, M., and Zama, K. 1985. Changes in molecular species of fish muscle phosphatidylcholine of chum salmon during migration. *Bull. Jap. Soc. Sci. Fish.* 51:1487–1493.

Takeuchi, T., Satoh, S., and Watanabe, T. 1983. Requirement of *Tilapia nilotica* for essential fatty acids. *Bull. Jap. Soc. Sci. Fish.* 49:1127–1134.

Takeuchi, T., and Watanabe, T. 1976. Nutritive value of ω-3 highly unsaturated fatty acids in pollock liver oil for rainbow trout. *Bull. Jap. Soc. Sci. Fish.* 42:907–919.

Takeuchi, T., and Watanabe, T. 1977. Requirement of carp for essential fatty acids. *Bull. Jap. Soc. Sci. Fish.* 43:541–551.

Takeuchi, T., and Watanabe, T. 1982. Effects of various polyunsaturated fatty acids on growth and fatty acid composition of rainbow trout. *Salmo gairdneri,* coho salmon *Oncorhynchus kisutch,* and chum salmon *Oncorhynchus keta. Bull. Jap. Soc. Sci. Fish.* 48:1745–1752.

Takeuchi, T., Watanabe, T., and Nose, T. 1979. Requirement for essential fatty acids of chum salmon (*Oncorhynchus keta*) in freshwater environment. *Bull. Jap. Soc. Sci. Fish.* 45:1319–1323.

Thomson, A. J., Sargent, J. R., and Owen, J. M. 1977. Influence of acclimatization temperature and salinity on fatty acid composition in the gills of the eel (*Anguilla anguilla*). *Comp. Biochem. Phyisol.* 56B:223–228.

Tocher, D. R., and Sargent, J. R. 1984A. Analyses of lipids and fatty acids in ripe roes of some northwest European marine fish. *Lipids* 19:492–499.

Tocher, D. R., and Sargent, J. R. 1984B. Studies on triacylglycerol, wax ester and sterol ester hydrolases in intestinal caeca of rainbow trout (*Salmo gairdneri*) fed diets rich in triacylglycerols and wax esters. *Comp. Biochem. Phyisol.* 77B:561–571.

Viola, S., and Amidan, G. 1980. Observations on the accumulation of fat in carp and *Sarotherodon* (Tilapia) fed oil-coated pellets. *Bamidgeh* 32:33–40.

Viola, S., Mokady, S., Behar, D., and Cogan, U. 1988. Effects of polyunsaturated fatty acids in feeds of tilapia and carp. 1. Body composition and fatty acid profiles at different environmental temperatures. *Aquaculture* 75:127–137.

Watanabe, T., Kobayashi, I., Otsue, O., and Ogino, C. 1974A. Effect of dietary methyl linolenate on fatty acid composition of lipids in rainbow trout. *Bull. Jap. Soc. Sci. Fish.* 40:387–392.

Watanabe, T., Ogino, C., Koshishi, Y., and Matsunaga, T. 1974B. Requirement of rainbow trout for essential fatty acids. *Bull. Jap. Soc. Sci. Fish.* 40:493–499.

Watanabe, T., Takashima, F., and Ogino, C. 1974C. Effect of dietary methyl linolenate on growth of rainbow trout. *Bull. Jap. Soc. Sci. Fish.* 40:181–188.

Watanabe, T., Takeuchi, T., and Ogino, C. 1975. Effect of dietary methyl linoleate and linolenate on growth of carp—II. *Bull. Jap. Soc. Sci. Fish.* 41:263–269.

Wodtke, E. 1978. Lipid adaptation in liver mitochondrial membranes of carp acclimated to different environmental temperatures—phospholipid composition, fatty acid pattern and cholesterol content. *Biochim. Biophys. Acta* 529:280–291.

Yamaguchi, T., Sato, Y., Ito, M., Moritani, N., and Hata, M. 1988. The lipid and fatty acid compositions in tissues of cultured and wild coho salmon *Oncorhynchus kisutch. Nippon Suisan Gakkaishi* 54:1601–1605.

Yingst, W. L. III, and Stickney, R. R. 1979. Effects of dietary lipids on fatty acid composition of channel catfish fry. *Trans. Am. Fish. Soc.* 108:620–625.

Yingst, W. L. III, and Stickney, R. R. 1980. Growth of caged channel catfish fingerlings reared on diets containing various lipids. *Prog. Fish Cult.* 42:24–26.

Yu, T. C., and Sinnhuber, R. O. 1975. Effect of dietary linolenic and linoleic acids on growth and lipid metabolism of rainbow trout (*Salmo gairdneri*). *Lipids* 10:63–66.

Yu, T. C., and Sinnhuber, R. O. 1976. Growth response of rainbow trout (*Salmo gairdneri*) to dietary ω9 and ω6 fatty acids. *Aquaculture* 8:309–317.

Yu, T. C., and Sinnhuber, R. O. 1979. Effect of dietary ω3 and ω6 fatty acids on growth and feed conversion efficiency of coho salmon (*Oncorhynchus kisutch*). *Aquaculture* 16:31–38.

Yu, T. C., and Sinnhuber, R. O. 1981. Use of beef tallow as an energy source in coho salmon (*Oncorhynchus kisutch*) rations. *Can. J. Fish. Aqua. Sci.* 38:367–370.

Yu, T. C., Sinnhuber, R. O., and Hendricks, J. D. 1979. Reproduction and survival of rainbow trout (*Salmo gairdneri*) fed linolenic acid as the only source of essential fatty acids. *Lipids* 14:572–575.

Chapter 9
NUTRITIONAL VALUE OF FISH OIL AS ANIMAL FEED

Neva L. Karrick

INTRODUCTION

Fish oils have been incorporated into animal feeds for many years. They have growth-promoting effects, are a cheap source of energy, and often contain significant amounts of vitamins A and D. They are also used because of the benefits of their broad spectrum of fatty acids. The interest in polyunsaturated fatty acids in human diets has led to the use of fishery products and fish oils to change the lipid composition of fats in poultry, cultured fish, and some red meats. Considerable work has been done on the problems and limitations related to incorporation of highly unsaturated fats and oils as well as on measures to prevent problems and to ensure optimum utilization.

GROWTH

Fish oils support growth of animals at least equal to that of any other source of fat in the diet. This was often considered surprising by those who equate the presence of the classical essential fatty acids (EFA) as necessary for growth. For a long time only linoleic, linolenic, and arachadonic acids were thought to have essential fatty acid activity. As techniques to study lipids were refined, other members of the linoleic and linolenic families of fatty acids were also shown to be active, particularly in promoting growth.

The amounts of linoleic and linolenic acids are low in fish oils, but the amount of the linolenic acid family is high. The reason for the growth-promoting activity of fish oils can be seen in Table 9-1 by comparing the amounts of the total linoleic plus linolenic acid series in fish oils with the amount of the linoleic acid in tallow, which is often used to supply the fat in animal diets.

Table 9-1. Amounts of Linoleic and Linolenic Family Fatty Acids in
Marine and Animal Oils and Fats

FAT OR OIL	LINOLEIC SERIES, %	LINOLENIC SERIES, %	TOTAL, %
Menhaden	2	31	33
Herring	2	17	19
Tuna	5	33	38
Tallow	2	<1	<3

The growth-promoting activity of the linolenic acid series from fish oils was demonstrated in nutritional studies by Privett et al. (1959). They fed EFA-deficient rats supplements of C_{16}, C_{18}, C_{20}, and C_{22} fatty esters fractionated from tuna oil and compared results with a supplement of ethyl linoleate. The supplements did not cure dermal symptoms, but all except the C_{16} fraction had growth-promoting activity equivalent to the ethyl linoleate.

These data on linolenic acid series were supported in nutritional studies by Privett et al. (1960), who also showed that menhaden, herring, and tuna oils fed to EFA-deficient rats at a 10% level in the diet not only stimulated growth but also cured dermal symptoms.

Linoleic acid metabolism was depressed when large quantities of the linolenic acid series were present (Aaes-Jørgensen 1967). Studies on several species of fish have shown that the linolenic acid series have an essential fatty acid role (Castell et al. 1972A, B, C; Sinnhuber 1969; Lee et al. 1967). The actual quantities required vary with different species of fish. The requirement of the longer-chain, more highly unsaturated fatty acids ($C_{20}:5\omega3$ and $C_{22}:6\omega3$) as opposed to linolenic acid also varies with species, but the requirement has been shown by a number of researchers (Kanazawa 1985).

Coefficients of digestibility of marine oils reflect their feeding and their growth-promoting values. Analyses by different laboratories on different animals report high values for fish oils (Artman 1964; Deuel 1954; Leoschke 1959; Reder 1942). Thomasson (1955; 1956A, B) studied the rate of intestinal absorption of oils and fats and found that, although a correlation apparently exists between rate of absorption and growth action, some oils do not conform to this relation and that longevity of the animals may be as important as either absorption or growth action in evaluation of the oils. Absorption of whale oil was similar to lard but less than butterfat, corn oil, soybean oil, or coconut oil. Steenbock et al. (1936) compared rate of absorption of fats from the alimentary canal of rats and reported that halibut liver oil, cod-liver oil, and butter oil were absorbed more rapidly than lard, corn oil, or partially hydrogenated fats.

The digestion and absorption of fish oils are confirmed by the often-made observations that addition of fish oils in the diet of different animals is reflected in the composition of their fats (Ault et al. 1960; Century, et al. 1961; Edwards and Marion 1963; Feigenbaum and Fisher 1959).

Metabolizable energy and feed efficiency of fish oils are high. Renner and Hill (1958) reported that the metabolizable energy value of menhaden oil for chicks is 3700 calories per pound (cal/lb). Tallow has a value of 2900 cal/lb. Artman (1964) studied fats as energy sources for chicks and found that menhaden oil supported good growth and had good feed efficiency, high metabolizable energy value, and digestibility when the oil was fed at levels less than 12%. March et al. (1965A, B) found that the metabolizable energy of herring oil was 1502 cal/lb of diet when the oil was added at a level of 10% in the diet.

FAT-SOLUBLE VITAMINS

Vitamins A and D

Many species of fish store large amounts of vitamins A and D in their livers. The actual amounts of these vitamins vary tremendously, not only among different species (Bills et al. 1935) but also among different fish within the species. This variation within species depends on age, sex, and size. After vitamin A was synthesized and produced commercially, production of the liver oils for vitamins A and D became a minor industry in North America. A market still exists, however, because liver oils may be incorporated into animal feeds. Other oils, although they are not fed for this purpose, also contribute vitamins A and D to the diet. Menhaden oil, for example, contains 200–500 units of vitamin A per gram and 50–100 units of vitamin D per gram.

Both body oils and liver oils from fish have been fed to furnish vitamins A and D to poultry, swine, cattle, and fur-bearing animals. Much of the nutritional research in the 1920s and 1930s on fish oils were aimed at determining the value of fish oils for this purpose. A voluminous literature exists on this topic, but no attempt is made here to include it because excellent reviews have already been written on the use of fish oils as sources of these vitamins, on the requirements of various animals, and on the metabolism and nutritional value of vitamins A and D (Bills 1954; Cruickshank 1962; Deuel 1951, 1954, 1957; Goodwin 1954; Lambertsen and Braekkan 1956; Moore 1953, 1957; Olson 1964).

Vitamin E

Fish oils contain varying amounts of vitamin E. Einset and co-workers (1957) reported the following amounts in commercial fish oils: herring 140, menhaden 70, and tuna 160 micrograms per gram of oil. The variation of the vitamin E content may be a partial explanation of differences in the stability of various oils. Vitamin E is not a chemical antioxidant but plays a role in vivo in intracellular protection (Privett and Cortesi 1972).

Adequate vitamin E is critical in diets because of the diseases that result from its deficiency and because higher dietary levels of polyunsaturated acids increases the requirement of some animals for vitamin E. The protective effects of vitamin E in animals are related to the dietary form of the tocopherol, as well as the presence or absence of selenium and ascorbic acid (vitamin C) (Halver 1985).

Many species of animals develop nutritional muscular dystrophy from a vitamin E deficiency. Species differences are apparent, and requirements for vitamin E vary both among species and according to the polyunsaturation of the fats in their diets. Mattill and Golumbic (1942) found that muscular dystrophy induced by cod-liver oil was the same as nutritional muscular dystrophy produced in animals by lack of vitamin A. Mattill (1938, 1940) previously questioned the direct toxic action of cod-liver oil and showed that vitamin E was oxidized in the presence of unsaturated fatty acid undergoing oxidation. Vitamin E will prevent nutritional muscular dystrophy in fish and may also improve the hatchability of fish eggs (Halver 1989).

Vitamin E deficiency in chicks results in encephalomalacia. Hammond (1941) related outbreaks of encephalomalacia in chicks with a factor in cod-liver oil that destroyed, inactivated, or prevented utilization of vitamin E and resulted in exudative diathesis on chicks. Dam (1943, 1944) found that when no fat was added to the diet the former was never produced and the latter rarely. When linseed oil, lard, or 5% cod-liver oil or its fatty acids was added, both conditions were produced. Dam and Granados (1945) reported that the causative factor(s) was concentrated in the fraction with an iodine value of 283. The importance of adequate vitamin E on the diet has been demonstrated many times for a broad spectrum of animals (Blaxter et al. 1953A, C, 1962; Brown 1953; Budowski et al. 1979; Bunnell et al. 1954, 1956; Cormier 1948; Dam 1964; Dam et al. 1958; Griffiths 1961; Halver 1982; Jensen et al. 1955, 1956; Maplesden and Loosli 1960; Moore et al. 1959; Moore and Sharman 1961; Scott 1951, 1953; Singsen et al. 1954A, B, 1955A, B; Watanabe 1982).

OXIDATION OF FISH OILS

Most nutritional problems attributed to fish oils are related to their oxidation. Oxidation can occur in the diet itself and cause destruction of vitamins and possibly loss of amino acids. It may also occur in vivo, particularly in cases of vitamin E deficiency as discussed above. Fish oils or fish oil fatty acids are not of themselves toxic, but oxidized oils cause various symptoms in unprotected animals, including cultured fish (Hung et al. 1981; Lea 1965; Lea et al. 1966; Moccia et al. 1984; Murai and Andrews 1974).

Kaneda et al. (1955) fed ethyl esters of the fatty acids from fish oils with an iodine value of 370 to mice and rats. Every precaution was taken to avoid oxidation of esters. Growth and feed consumption were both good. This led the authors to believe that the toxicity attributed to fish oils was due to autoxidation products. They then let the highly unsaturated material autoxidize at room temperature and found a high level of toxicity in the fraction that would not form urea complexes. Common et al. (1957) also found toxicity in this fraction. After extensive experiments, Kaneda et al. (1955) concluded that peroxides were the most toxic of the autoxidation products. The lethal dose of peroxides was above 278 mg total peroxide per kilogram of fat. These and other workers have shown that high levels of peroxides are damaging to animals and that the level of peroxide rather than the source of oil, whether fish, other animal, or vegetable, is the cause of toxicity. Matsuo (1954A, B) also related toxicity of fish oils to their peroxide content. Ethyl esters with a peroxide value (PV) of 240 mg percent were toxic to rats. These esters then were heated for 120 hr at 212°F, had a PV of 30 mg percent, and were no longer toxic. Matsuo (1960, 1962) reported that oxidized ethyl esters from fish oils were toxic when absorbed through the skin. Groot and Kleinobbink (1953) fed rats a diet containing 10% oxidized cod-liver oil. The rats grew normally when the peroxide value was less than 24 or when the oil had been heated in a vacuum. Decreased growth occurred when the PV was greater than 54. Rasheed et al. (1963) reported that fresh menhaden oil fed to rats at the 10% level supported growth equal to the control diet containing lard. When the oil was oxidized to PV 125 and above, toxic symptoms began to appear. They also added the antioxidants ethoxyquin or vitamin E to the diet along with a menhaden oil with a PV of 60. They found that even under these conditions the antioxidants afforded considerable protection to the rat. Carpenter et al. (1963) fed herring oil with a PV of 142 to chicks at a level of 6% in a diet designed to prevent vitamin deficiencies and found no depression in weight gain or in feed consumption.

Polymerized Oils

The nutritive value of polymerized oils depends on the method of preparation (Common et al. 1957; Kaneda et al. 1955; Raulin and Petit 1962; Witting et al. 1957). In general, oils treated at high temperatures for a long period will be a poor feed additive. Fish oils polymerized under mild conditions have been reported to have good nutritive value (Kaneda 1955; Nicolaysen and Pihl 1953). When polymerized oils have had poor nutritive value, the factors involved have included poor digestibility (Lassen et al. 1949; Raulin and Petit 1962; Raulin et al. 1962) and poor acceptance by the animal (Oldfield and Anglemier 1957). Although the polymerized fish oils cause poor growth in animals, they apparently are not actually toxic. Matsuo (1960) incriminated cyclic monomers formed during heat polymerization as causes of decreased nutritive value.

FISH OILS IN ANIMAL DIETS

All animals can utilize good-quality fish oils for energy and for growth when the oils are included in a balanced diet adequately fortified with vitamins. Fish oils are even being added to attempt to change the fatty acid composition of the fat in edible products. The amount, quality of oil, and conditions of feeding animals that are being grown for food use must be controlled to avoid development of undesirable flavors or a poor product after frozen storage. These requirements apply only to the extracted oil and not to oil in fishery products such as fish flesh or fish meal.

Fish meals are used in feed formulations for poultry and fish and sometimes for cattle, swine, and pets. The high nutritional value of fish meal for these animals indicates that the 5–8% lipid in fish meal is satisfactory. This conclusion has been supported by experimental studies. Scott (1951) extracted oil from sardine meal and from menhaden meal and fed them to turkeys at levels of 1% and 2%. The turkeys did not develop the enlarged hock disorders that they did when 1% and 2% fish liver oils were fed under the same conditions. March et al. (1962) extracted the lipid fraction from herring meal and studied its nutritive value for chicks. The extracted oil showed no toxicity when fed at the 10% level in diets with adequate amounts of vitamins.

When fish meals cause a poor growth rate, the problem is not so much oxidized oils as the results of reaction between fat oxidation products or free radicals and the protein with the result that part of the amino acids become unavailable to the animal. Carpenter et al. (1963) oxidized herring meal, extracted the lipid, and found that the oxidized lipids were not toxic. They repeated the studies on an anchovy meal that was known to have poor nutritional value under practical commercial conditions. The extracted lipid was not toxic to chicks. The experimental conditions in both series were chosen to preclude any effect from vitamin deficiencies. The residual meal did depress the growth of the chick, supporting the above thesis that the oxidizing lipids render some of the amino acids of the protein unavailable.

Poultry

Fish oils in poultry are efficiently utilized by the birds and permit growth. Much work has been done to determine the optimum amount of the oils and the conditions under which they can be incorporated into the diet. The oils must be fresh and have low peroxide values, and oxidation in the diets must be prevented. The principal limitations are the effects on flavor and stability of the carcass and the increased requirement of the chicks for vitamin E.

Artman (1964) obtained good growth and feed efficiency when menhaden oil was fed at 4.5% and 9% in the diet, but 15% oil gave poor results. The breaking point in his test appeared to be about 12%. Both menhaden and soybean oil mixed with tallow (1:1) increased utilization of the tallow. The ability of commercial fish oils to promote growth and feed efficiency in poultry have been reported by other workers (Dansky 1962; Edwards and Marion 1963; Edwards et al. 1961, 1962; March and Biely 1955).

Effects on Poultry Products. The amount of fish oils that can be incorporated into poultry diets is determined by their effect on poultry products. Laying hens can be fed 2–6% fish oil because of the beneficial effect on egg production and hatchability. Broilers should be fed no more than 1% fish oil because larger amounts cause off-flavors and odors in the animal carcasses.

Eggs. Fish oils fed to laying hens have a beneficial effect on egg production. Biely et al. (1954) fed 6% herring oil to layers for 11 months. The birds consumed 8% less feed and egg production was the same. Thus the amount of feed required to produce a dozen eggs was decreased. Edson (1932) found in a three-year study that 2% cod-liver oil increased egg production and hatchability. Increased egg production was also reported by Erikson and Insko (1934) and by Holmes et al. (1937) when 1–2% body oil was fed, and by Kudo (1947) when oil from the waste portion of fish was fed. Antioxidants have been recommended in diets containing 2% fish oil to prevent the destruction of carotenoids and the formation of pale yolks.

"Fishy" flavors are sometimes found in eggs, but these are not related to fish oils. These off-flavors and odors often occur when fishery products have not been included in the diet. In addition, excessive amounts of both fish oils and fish meals have often been fed without causing any "fishy" flavors or odors in the eggs. Vendell and Putman (1945) fed 14 times the recommended amount of a strong-smelling, low-grade sardine oil for 30 days and found that the eggs had no fishy odor or flavor and could not be distinguished from the eggs of chickens on other rations. Nilsen (1954) fed 1%, 2%, and 8% menhaden oil. The eggs were satisfactory except that some of the eggs from chickens fed 8% oil had a slight off-flavor. Koehler and Bearse (1975) reported that 1.5% fish oils caused off-flavors.

Carcass Quality.   Carcass quality is measured by the flavor, color, odor, texture, and moistness of the meat and by its stability during storage. The texture and moistness of poultry fed fish oils are excellent.

Flavor, odor, color, and stability of the carcasses fed fish oils will be adversely affected unless precautions are taken. These changes result from altered depot fat, which, in turn, reflects the composition of the fat in the diet (Cruickshank 1934, 1939; Edwards and Marion 1963; Hilditch et al. 1934; Hilditch 1947; Hite et al. 1949; Klose et al. 1952; Lipstein and Bornstein 1973; Miller and Robisch 1969; Miller et al. 1967; Schuler and Essary 1971; Wessels et al. 1973).

Fishy flavors and odors in poultry flesh have been demonstrated many times (Carrick and Hauge 1926; Carlson et al. 1957; Dansky 1962; Ewing 1943; Hardin et al. 1964). Unsaturated fats other than fish oils can also cause development of these off-flavors (Klose et al. 1951). The recommendation sometimes is made to remove fish oils from the diet for two or three weeks prior to slaughter. It is interesting to note that fishy flavors apparently do not develop from feeding even high levels of fish meals. The problem arises when extracted oils are fed.

Turkeys seem to be more affected by fish oils in the diet than chickens. Asmundson et al. (1938) found fishy flavors in two out of four turkeys fed 1% fish oils. Klose et al. (1953) reported a slight amount of fishy flavors in carcasses from turkeys fed 0.4% sardine oil and an intense fishy flavor from turkeys fed 2% sardine oil.

Marble et al. (1938) also reported fishy flavors and odors in turkeys fed 1% cod liver oil. When the fish oils were removed from the diet eight weeks prior to slaughter, the fishy flavors were not noted. Marsden et al. (1952) found the fishy flavor more persistent when larger amounts of oil were fed. The diets contained 14% whitefish meal plus 0.375% fortified cod-liver oil or 8% sardine meal plus 2% straight cod-liver oil. Fishy flavors persisted for 13 weeks after the fishery products had been removed from the diet.

Stability of Poultry Products. One of the problems of the poultry industry is development of oxidative rancidity during frozen storage of the products. This limiting factor in the stability and storage life of the product is affected by the composition of the depot fat. Stability decreases with an increase in total body fat and/or in the amount of unsaturated fat present. Klose et al. (1952) correlated the induction period of the fat with its fatty acid composition. They compared the induction period of gizzard depot fat from turkeys fed different dietary fats and found the shortest induction period (less stability) in birds fed 2% sardine oil. This confirmed the results of Schreiber et al. (1947) that feeding 2% fish oil for two weeks prior to slaughter decreased the stability of the carcass toward oxidative rancidity.

Swine

Pigs can assimilate fish oils and utilize them for energy, but the amount must be limited to maintain the quality of the carcass since the dietary fats are deposited with little or no change in the animals. Garton and Duncan (1954) fed lard and cod-liver oil to pigs; the cod-liver oil glycerides were isolated almost unchanged from the back fats. Ellis and Isbell (1926) showed that the character and composition of the depot fat of hogs was affected by the fat in the ration and that too much oil in the ration caused soft pork. Brown (1931) fed 14% menhaden oil for five weeks prior to slaughter and found that 2.7% of the highly unsaturated fatty acids was deposited in the fat of the pigs. The fat in the carcasses had a marked yellow color. He concluded that the pig utilizes the more highly unsaturated fatty acids and stores the remainder. Banks and Hilditch (1932) fed 7% fish meal, which was equivalent to 0.7% fish oil, and found that the lard contained 1–2% of the highly unsaturated C_{20} and C_{22} fatty acids. Oleic and linoleic acids appeared to be stored more freely than the highly unsaturated fatty acids.

The British National Institute for Research in Dairying (Anonymous 1934, 1937, 1939) fed swine a diet containing 10% herring meal or an equivalent amount of crude herring oil without producing fishy flavors in either the bacon or the pork. When this was increased by feeding 10% defatted fish meal plus herring oil equivalent to 20% fish meal, the bacon and ham had a definite fishy flavor and the pork was of poor quality. Results indicated that the pork was good if herring oil in the diet did not exceed 0.5%. Fraser et al. (1934) fed ½ to 1 oz of cod-liver oil or sardine oil daily for 130 days. Pigs slaughtered immediately had a fishy taste, but this was prevented by discontinuing the oil for 30 days before slaughter.

Callow and Lea (1939) and Lea (1936) fed 10% cod-liver oil to pigs and, in addition to fishy flavors in the pork fat, found that the fat was more susceptible to oxidation. Husby and Haug (1938) recommended that bacon pigs should not be fed more than 10 g of fish oil per day because the bacon would develop fishiness during storage. They stated that problems of fishy flavors and soft, yellow fat could be eliminated by discontinuing use of all fish ingredients in the diet six weeks before slaughter of the animals.

Garton et al. (1952) studied a pig that had received 50% of crude whale oil from the time it was weaned. Growth and health of the pig were normal. The whale oil fatty acids were deposited in the fat, particularly in the outer back fat, and the fat was a yellowish brown. Fractional crystallization showed that 26% of the fat was similar to whale oil in composition. The whale oil triglycerides appeared to be deposited without any alteration.

Anglemier and Oldfield (1957) fed pilchard oil at levels of 2.75%, 5.5%, and 8.25%. Pigs fed the highest level failed to eat and growth was unsatisfactory. Growth performance and feed efficiency were satisfactory at the two lower levels. The carcass fat of the pigs in all of the diets had a fishy odor and flavor and a yellowish tinge. Oldfield and Anglemier (1957) also investigated the effects of modified menhaden oils on the quality of carcass fats. They fed 5% of crude, of alkali refined and bleached, and of polymerized oils. Carcasses from the pigs fed polyunsaturated oils were not discolored and had improved flavor and odor, but growth of the animals was poor. Possibly oil polymerized under the correct conditions could be both nutritionally adequate and permit good growth.

Since the fat in the carcass of pigs is affected by fish oils in practical rations, the recommended level for feeding fish oils is about 0.5% in the ration. Another precaution is to remove the oil from the diet for a period prior to slaughter. The time recommended varies from two weeks to four months. Removal of fish oil when the pig reaches 100 lb live weight has also been recommended.

Cattle

Unsaturated fats are converted to saturated fats by bacteria in the rumen of adult cattle; thus their fat deposits do not reflect the composition of their diet. Young ruminants do not change composition of dietary fat (Oltjen 1975).

Beard et al. (1935) and Thomas et al. (1934) fed menhaden oil to steer calves and found that the color, firmness, and palatability of the beef fat were not affected. Reports of effects of fish oils on growth are both favorable (Davis and Maynard 1938) and unfavorable (Madsen et al. 1935; Nicholson et al. 1962). Results are related to the amount of oil given (Leach and Golding 1931; Turner et al. 1936), to the rest of the ration, and particularly to the amount of vitamin E in the diet.

A number of reports about detrimental effects of cod-liver oil on calves have appeared in the literature. Blaxter et al. (1953A, B, C) showed that the muscular dystrophy caused by cod-liver oil was due to the unsaturated fatty acids of cod-liver oil and was prevented when the diet contained adequate vitamin E.

Fish oils in the diet of dairy cows can be used to reduce the butterfat content and to increase the amount of unsaturated fatty acids in milk. Brown and Sutton (1931) reported that menhaden oils lowered milk production, the percentage of butterfat, and total butterfat. Small quantities of the highly unsaturated fatty acids passed from the menhaden oil into the butterfat, and analytical constants of the butter changed to those of a mixture of butter and menhaden oil. Effects on milk production and butterfat content have been noted from whale oil (McDowall et al. 1957) and cod-liver oil (Davis and Maynard 1938; Hilditch and Thompson 1936; McCay and Maynard 1935; Mattick 1928; Petersen 1932).

Graham and Cupps (1938) fed herring oil to goats and observed a similar effect on milk production. Hydrogenated herring oil did not reduce the percentage of milk fat. McCay and co-workers (1935, 1938) reported that hydrogenated cod-liver oil, salmon oil, and shark liver oil had little or no effect on milk production. Fountaine and Bolin (1944) and Blaxter et al. (1946) reported that shark liver oil did not affect the milk yield, butterfat production, or health of the cows. Maynard et al. (1936) found that the iodine value of the milk is influenced by the degree of unsaturation of ingested fat.

Cod-liver oil not only lowers the fat content of the milk but also changes the proportion of volatile fatty acids in the rumen: Propionic acid increases, and both acetic acid and butyric acid decrease (Nicholson et al. 1963; Nottle and Rook 1963; Shaw and Ensor 1959).

Mink

Fish oils as such are not incorporated into diets of mink, but fish or fish scraps often constitute a large part of their diet. When the diet consists principally of fish, the fat content is low and lard or tallow is added. In the past, mink often were affected by steatitis or yellow fat disease, but the diseases can be prevented. These conditions resulted from feeding rancid horse meat, linseed oil, or fish or from a diet containing a low level of vitamin E and a large amount of unsaturated fatty acids. Thus the mink rancher prevents the difficulty by adding adequate vitamin E to the diet and feeding nonrancid horse meat or fish (Gorham et al. 1951; Hartsough and Gorham 1958; Lalor et al. 1951).

Pet Foods

Cats also require vitamin E to prevent steatitis if their diets contain large amounts of fish for a long period. The disease is a vitamin E deficiency aggravated by the polyunsaturated fatty acids in the lipids in the fish. Steatitis should no longer be a problem in cat nutrition because vitamin E is routinely added to processed pet foods and recommendations are made that cats be fed a mixed diet.

Fish

The increase in the cultivation of fish has been paralleled by an increase in knowledge about nutritional requirements. Lipids have received significant attention because of their role in the formulation of efficient diets, their protein-sparing action in carnivorous species, their importance in developing new diets that will ensure adequate supplies as production continues to increase, and their role in determining the amount and composition of fatty acids in the edible product.

Carnivores such as salmonids utilize lipids for energy; higher lipid levels in the diet can permit lower levels of protein in the diet. The lipid component in the diet must contain fatty acids for optimum growth and feed conversion. The effects of the level of lipids in the diet vary with environmental conditions such as temperature and salinity as well as with the size of the fish and the amount of lipid in the diet (Castell 1979; Legler 1985; Takeuchi 1979; Watanabe 1982).

The composition of both carnivores and plant-eating fish can, within limits, be tailored to the composition desired for use in human diets. Although dietary lipids do not change the composition of the phospholipids in fish, the diet plus environmental conditions will determine fatty acids in the triglycerides of fat depots. The alteration in composition can be done so that flavor and texture are actually improved over other cultured fish and without damage to the storage characteristics of the products (Boggio et al. 1985; Hardy et al. 1987; Henderson and Sargent 1985; Sargent et al. 1989).

SUMMARY

Fish oils contain a broad spectrum of fatty acids that are well utilized by animals. They can be used to alter the fatty acid composition of fats in many species. Fish oils of good quality permit good growth, are highly digestible, and furnish significant levels of metabolizable energy. The vitamin E requirement for most animals is increased when fish oils are added to their diet. When the animals fed fish oils are to be used for food, the amount of fish oil must be adjusted to avoid the occurrence of fishy flavors. On the other hand, fish being farmed require fatty acids in their diet to avoid symptoms of deficiency in essential fatty acids.

REFERENCES

Aaes-Jørgensen, E. 1967. Fish oils as a source of essential fatty acids. In *Fish Oils*, ed. M. E. Stansby. Westport, Conn.: Avi Publishing Co.

Anglemier, A. F., and Oldfield, J. E. 1957. Feeding of various levels of pilchard oil to swine. *J. Animal Sci.* 16:922–926.

Anonymous. 1934, 1937, 1939. Fishy flavor in foodstuffs. *Univ. of Reading Natl. Inst. Res. Dairying Ann. Repts.* for years ending Sept. 30, 1934, Sept. 30, 1937, Sept. 30, 1939.

Artman, N. R. 1964. Interactions of fats and fatty acids as energy sources for the chick. *Poultry Sci.* 43:994–1004.

Asmundson, V. S., Jukes, T. H., Fyler, H. M., and Maxwell, M. L. 1938. Effect on certain fish meals and fish oils in the ration on the flavor of the turkey. *Poultry Sci.* 17:147–151.

Ault, W. C., Riemenschneider, R. W., and Saunders, D. H. 1960. Utilization of fats in poultry and other livestock feeds. Agriculture Research Service, Utilization Research Dept. No. 2.

Banks, A., and Hilditch, T. P. 1932. The body fats of the pig. II. Some aspects of the formation of animal depot fats suggested by the composition of their glycerides and fatty acids. *Biochem. J.* 26:298–308.

Beard, F. J., Schulz, J. A., and Culbertson, C. G. 1935. Effect of ingested menhaden and coconut oils upon firmness of beef fat. *Am. Soc. Animal Prod. Rec. Proc. 28th Ann. Mtg.* 1935:286–290.

Biely, J., March B. E., and Silvertrini, D. A. 1954. Fat studies in poultry I. Herring oil, santomerse-80, and thyroprotein in the laying ration. *Poultry Sci.* 33:1130–1135.

Bills, C. E. 1954. The vitamins D. In *The Vitamins*, vol. II, ed. W. H. Sebrell, Jr., and R. S. Harris. New York: Academic Press.

Bills, C. E., McDonald, F. G., Massengale, O. N., Imboden, M., Hall, H., Hergert, W. D., and Wallenmeyer, J. C. 1935. A taxonomic study of the distribution of vitamins A and D in 100 species of fish. *J. Biol. Chem.* 109:vii.

Blaxter, K. L. 1962. Muscular dystrophy in farm animals: Its cause and prevention. *Proc. Nutr. Soc.* 21:211–216.

Blaxter, K. L., Kon, S. K., and Thompson, S. Y. 1946. Effect of feeding shark-liver oil to cows on yield and composition and on vitamin A and carotene contents of the milk. *J. Dairy Res.* 14:225–230.

Blaxter, K. L., Brown, F., and MacDonald, A. M. 1953A. Nutrition of the Ayrshire calf. XIII. The toxicity of unsaturated acids of cod liver oil. *Brit. J. Nutr.* 7:287–298.

Blaxter, K. L., Brown, F., and MacDonald, A. M. 1953B. The nutrition of the young Ayrshire calf. XIV. Some effects of natural and synthetic antioxidants on the incidence of muscular dystrophy induced by cod liver oil. *Brit. J. Nutr.* 7:337–349.

Blaxter, K. L., Wood, W. A., and MacDonald, A. M. 1953C. The nutrition of the young Ayrshire calf. *Brit. J. Nutr.* 7:34–50.

Boggio, S. M., Hardy, R. M., Babbitt, J. K., and Brannon, E. L. 1985. The influence of dietary lipid source and alpha tocopherol acetate level on product quality of rainbow trout (*Salmo gairdneri*). *Aquaculture* 51:13–24.

Brown, F. 1953. Occurrence of vitamin E in cod and other fish oils. *Nature* 171(4357):90.

Brown, J. B. 1931. The nature of the highly unsaturated fatty acids stored in the lard from pigs fed on menhaden oil. *J. Biol. Chem.* 90:133–139.

Brown, J. B., and Sutton, T. S. 1931. Effect of feeding menhaden fish oil on secretion of milk and composition of butterfat in the dairy cow. *J. Dairy Sci.* 14:125–135.

Budowski, P., Bartow, G., Dror, Y., and Frankel, E. N. 1979. Lipid oxidation products and chick nutritional encephalopathy. *Lipids* 14:768–772.

Bunnell, R. H., Matterson, L. D., Singsen, E. P., and Eaton, H. D. 1956. Studies on encephalomalacia in the chick. V. The effect of fish oil and diphenyl-*P*-phenylenediamine on the vitamin metabolism of the chick. *Poultry Sci.* 35:436–451.

Bunnell, R. H., Matterson, L. D., Singsen, E. P., Potter, L. M., Kozeff, A., and Jungherr, E. L. 1954. Studies on encephalomalacia in the chick. III. The influence of feeding or injecting various tocopherols or other antioxidants on the incidence of encephalomalacia. *Poultry Sci.* 33:1046.

Callow, E. H., and Lea, C. H. 1939. The effect of olive oil and cod liver oil in the pig's diet on the quality of pork, sausages, bacon, and hams and the influence of diet on the susceptibility of the pig's fat to oxidation. *Rept. Food Invest. Board.* (*Gr. Brit.*) 1939: 35–38.

Carlson, D., Potter, L. M., Matterson, L. D., Singsen, E. P., Gilpin, G. L., Redstrom, R. A., and Dawson, E. H. 1957. Palatability of chickens fed diets containing different levels of fish oil or tallow. *Food Technol.* 11:615–620.

Carpenter, K. J., Lea, C. H., and Parr, L. J. 1963. Chemical and nutritional changes in stored herring meal. IV. Nutritional significance of oxidation of the oil. *Brit. J. Nutr.* 17:151–169.

Carrick, C. W., and Hauge, S. M. 1926. The effect of cod liver oil upon flavor in poultry meat. *Poultry Sci.* 5:213–215.

Castell, J. D. 1979. Review of lipid requirements of finfish. In *Finfish Nutrition and Fishfeed Technology*, vol. I, ed. J. E. Halver and K. Leios. Proc. World Symposium on Finfish Nutrition and Fishfeed Technology, Hamburg, 20–23 June 1979, pp. 59–82.

Castell, J. D., Lee, D. J., and Sinnhuber, R. O. 1972A. Essential fatty acids in the diet of rainbow trout (*Salmo gairdneri*). Lipid metabolism and fatty acid composition. *J. Nutr.* 102:93–100.

Castell, J. D., Sinnhuber, R. O., Lee, D. J., and Wales, G. H. 1972B. Essential fatty acids in the diet of rainbow trout (*Salmo gairdneri*): Physiological symptoms of EFA deficiency. *J. Nutr.* 102:87–92.

Castell, J. D., Sinnhuber, R. O., Wales, H., and Lee, D. J. 1972C. Essential fatty acids in the diet of rainbow trout (*Salmo gairdneri*): Growth, feed conversion and some gross deficiency symptoms. *J. Nutr.* 102:77–86.

Century, B., Witting, L. A., Harvey, C. C., and Horwitt, M. K. 1961. Composition of skeletal muscle lipids of rats fed diets containing various oils. *J. Nutr.* 75:341–346.

Common, R. H., Crampton, E. W., Farmer, F., and DeFrietas, A. S. W. 1957. Studies to determine the nature of the damage to the nutritive value of menhaden oil from heat treatment. *J. Nutr.* 62:341–347.

Cormier, M., 1948. Antivitamin action of fish liver oils. *Bull. Soc. Chim. Biol.* 30:921–940.

Cruickshank, E. M. 1934. Studies in fat metabolism in the fowl. I. Composition of egg fat and depot of the fowl as affected by ingestion of large amounts of different fats. *Biochem. J.* 28:963–977.

Cruickshank, E. M. 1939. Effect of cod liver oil and fish meal on flavor of poultry products. *Proc. 7th World's Poultry Congr.*, pp. 539–542.

Cruickshank, E. 1962. Fat soluble vitamins. In *Fish as Food*, vol. 2, ed. G. Borgstrom. London: Academic Press.

Dam, H. 1943. Effect of cod liver oil and rancidity on certain vitamin E deficiency symptoms. *Proc. Soc. Exp. Biol. Med.* 52:285–287.

Dam, H. 1944. Studies on vitamin E deficiency in chicks. *J. Nutr.* 27:193–211.

Dam, H. 1964. Relation between vitamin E and polyunsaturated acids (in German). *Fette, Seifen, Anstrichmittel* 66:899–903.

Dam, H., and Granados, H. 1945. Role of unsaturated fat acids in changes of adipose and dental tissues in vitamin E deficiency. *Science* 102:327–328.

Dam, H., Nielsen, G. K., Prange, I., and Søndergaard, E. 1958. Exudative diatheses produced by vitamin E deficient diets without polyenoic fatty acids. *Experentia* 14:291–292.

Dansky, L. M. 1962. The growth promoting properties of menhaden fish oil as influenced by various fats. *Poultry Sci.* 41:1352–1354.

Davis, G. K., and Maynard, L. A. 1938. Cod liver tolerance in calves. *J. Dairy Sci.* 21:145–152.

Deuel, H. J., Jr. 1951. *The Lipids—Their Chemistry and Biochemistry*, vol. 1: *Chemistry*. New York: Interscience.

Deuel, H. J., Jr. 1954. Nutritional significance of the fats. In *Progress in the Chemistry of Fats and Other Lipids*, vol. 2, ed. R. T. Holman, W. O. Lundberg, and T. Malkin. New York: Academic Press.

Deuel, H. J., Jr. 1957. *The Lipids—Their Chemistry and Biochemistry*, vol. III: *Biochemistry*. New York: Interscience.

Edson, A. W. 1932. Cod liver oil in winter ration of pullets. Results of a 3-year study of effects on egg production and hatching power of eggs laid. *Minn. Agr. Expt. Sta. Bull.* 286:3–12.

Edwards, H. M., Jr., and Marion, J. E. 1963. Influence of dietary menhaden oil on growth rate and tissue fatty acids of the chick. *J. Nutr.* 81:123–130.

Edwards, H. M., Jr., Marion, J. E., and Driggers, J. C. 1961. Effect of deutectomy and dietary supplementation with various fats on chick growth. *Poultry Sci.* 40:1937.

Edwards, H. M., Jr., Marion, J. E., and Driggers, J. C. 1962. Fat and fatty acid requirements of poultry. *Proc. 12th World's Poultry Congr.*, 182–186.

Einset, E., Olcott, H. S., and Stansby, M. E. 1957. Oxidative deterioration in fish and fishery products. IV. Progress in studies concerning oxidation of extracted oils. *Com. Fish. Rev.* 19(5A):35–37.

Ellis, N. R., and Isbell, H. S. 1926. Soft pork studies. II. Influence of the character of the ration upon the composition of the body fat of hogs. *J. Biol. Chem.* 69:219–238.

Erikson, S. E., and Insko, W. M., Jr. 1934. Effect of cod-liver oil on the iron and copper contents of egg yolk. *Ky. Agr. Expt. Sta., 46th Ann. Rept.*, pp. 53–55.

Ewing, W. R. 1943. *Handbook of Poultry Nutrition.* South Pasadena, Calif.: W. R. Ewing.

Feigenbaum, A. S., and Fisher, H. 1959. The influence of dietary fat on the incorporation of fatty acids into body and egg fat of the hen. *Arch. Biochem. Biophys.* 79:302–306.

Fountaine, F. C., and Bolin, D. W. 1944. Milk and butterfat production responses to shark-liver oil in the ration. *J. Dairy Sci.* 27:155–158.

Fraser, E. B., Stothart, J. H., and Gutteridge, H. S. 1934. Fish meals and oils: Feeding value for livestock and poultry. *Dom. Can. Dept. Agr. Pamphlet* 163:7–10.

Garton, G. A., and Duncan, W. R. H. 1954. Dietary fat and body fat: The composition of the back fats of pigs fed on a diet rich in cod-liver oil and lard. *Biochem. J.* 57:120–125.

Garton, G. A., Hilditch, T. P., and Meara, M. L. 1952. Composition of depot fat of a pig fed on a diet rich in whale oil. *Biochem. J.* 50:517–524.

Goodwin, T. S. 1954. *Carotenoids: Their Comparative Biochemistry.* New York: Chemical Publishing Co.

Gorham, J. R., Baker, G. A., and Norris, B. 1951. Observations on the etiology of yellow fat disease in mink; preliminary report. *Vet. Med.* 46:100–102.

Graham, W. R., Jr., and Cupps, P. T. 1938. Action of herring oil before and after hydrogenation on yield and fat percentage of milk of the goat. *J. Dairy Sci.* 21:45–48.

Griffiths, T. W. 1961. Studies on the requirement of the young chick for vitamin E. 2. The effects of different sources and levels of dietary lipids and live-weight gain and body vitamin E storage. *Brit. J. Nutr.* 15:271–279.

Groot, E. H., and Kleinobbink, H. J. 1953. Influence of heating cod-liver oil to 230° on growth of young rats. *Voeding* 14:123–136.

Halver, J. E. 1982. The vitamins required for cultivated salmonids. *Comp. Biochem. Physiol.* 73B(1):43–50.

Halver, J. E. 1985. Recent advances in vitamin nutrition and metabolism in fish. In *Nutrition and Feeding in Fish,* ed. C. B. Cowey, A. M. Mackie, and J. G. Bell, pp. 415–429. New York: Academic Press.

Halver, J. E. 1989. *The Vitamins in Fish Nutrition,* 2nd ed., ed. J. E. Halver, pp. 31–109. San Diego, Calif.: Academic Press.

Hammond, J. C. 1941. A factor in cod liver oil that hinders the utilization of vitamin E by chicks. *Poultry Sci.* 20:369–371.

Hardin, J. O., Milligan, J. L., and Sidwell, V. D. 1964. The influence of solvent extracted fish meal and stabilized fish in broiler rations on performance and on the flavor of broiler meat. *Poultry Sci.* 43:858–860.

Hardy, R. W., Scott, T. M., and Harrell, L. W. 1987. Replacement of herring oil with menhaden oil, soybean oil or tallow in the diets of Atlantic salmon raised in marine net-pens. *Aquaculture* 65:267–277.

Hartsough, G. R., and Gorham, J. 1958. *The Blue Book of Fur Farming.* Milwaukee, Wis.: Editorial Service Co.

Henderson, R. J., and Sargent, J. R. 1985. Fatty acid metabolism in fish. In *Nutrition and Feeding in Fish,* ed. C. B. Cowey, A. M. Mackie, and J. G. Bell, pp. 349–364. New York: Academic Press.

Hilditch, T. P. 1947. *The Chemical Constitution of Natural Fats.* New York: Wiley.

Hilditch, T. P., Jones, E. C., and Rhead, A. J. 1934. The body fats of the hen. *Biochem. J.* 28:786–795.

Hilditch, T. P., and Thompson, H. M. 1936. Effect of certain ingested fatty oils upon composition of cow milk fat. *Biochem. J.* 30:677–692.

Hite, J. P., Kloxin, S. E., and Kummerow, F. A. 1949. Fat rancidity in eviscerated poultry. IV. Effect of variations in dietary fat, ethanolamine, and choline on the characteristics of fat extracted from turkeys. *Poultry Sci.* 28:249–253.

Holmes, A. D., Tripp, F., and Campbell, P. A. 1937. Influence of fat-soluble vitamins on egg production and eggshell composition. *Poultry Sci.* 16:404–415.

Hung, S. J. O., Cho, C. Y., and Slinger, S. J. 1981. Effect of oxidized fish oil, DL-alpha tocopherol acitate and ethoxyquin supplementation on the vitamin E nutrition of rainbow trout (*Salmo gairdneri*) fed practical diets. *J. Nutr.* 111:648–657.

Husby, M., and Haug, K. 1938. Influences of animal feeding material on meat quality of pigs. *Norg. Landbruks* 2:1–8.

Jensen, L. S., Carver, J. S., and McGinnis, J. 1955. Vitamin E, diphenyl-*p*-phenylene-diamine, and fish liver oil in turkey reproduction. *Poultry Sci.* 34:1203.

Jensen, L. S., Carver, J. S., and McGinnis, J. 1956. Effects of vitamin E, *N,N'*-diphenyl-*p*-phenylenediamine, and fish liver oil on reproduction in turkeys. *Proc. Soc. Exptl. Biol. Med.* 91:386–388.

Kanazawa, A. 1985. Essential fatty acid and lipid requirement of fish. In *Nutrition and Feeding in Fish,* ed. C. B. Cowey, A. M. Mackie, and J. G. Bell, pp. 281–298. New York: Academic Press.

Kaneda, T., Sakai, H., Ishii, S., and Arai, K. 1955. *Studies on the Nutritive Value of Marine Animal Oils* (in Japanese). Bulletin 12. Tokai Regional Fisheries Research Laboratory.

Klose, A. A., Hanson, H. L., Mecchi, E. P., Anderson, J. H., Streeter, I. V., and Lineweaver, H. 1953. Quality and stability of turkeys as a function of dietary fat. *Poultry Sci.* 32:82–88.

Klose, A. A., Mecchi, E. P., Behman, G. A., Lineweaver, H., Kratzer, F. H., and Williams, D. 1952. Chemical characteristics of turkey carcass fat as a function of dietary fat. *Poultry Sci.* 31:354–359.

Klose, A. A., Mecchi, E. P., Hanson, H. L., and Lineweaver, H. 1951. The role of dietary fat in the quality of fresh and frozen storage turkeys. *J. Am. Oil Chemists' Soc.* 28:162–164.

Koehler, H. H., and Bearse, G. E. 1975. Egg flavor quality as affected by fish meals or fish oils in laying rations. *Poultry Sci.* 54:881–889.

Kudo, K. 1947. Nutritive value of inedible portion of fish in poultry feeding (in Japanese). *Nippon Chikusangaku Kaiho* 28:36–39.

Lalor, R. J., Leoschke, W. L., and Elvehjem, C. A. 1951. Yellow fat in mink. *J. Nutr.* 45:183–188.

Lambertsen, G., and Braekkan, O. R. 1956. Studies on the vitamin A components of fish livers: Determination and origin. In *Biochemical Problems of Lipids,* ed. Popjack and Le Breton. New York: Interscience.

Lassen, S., Bacon, E. K., and Dunn, H. J. 1949. The digestibility of polymerized oils. *Arch. Biochem.* 23:1–7.

Lea, C. H. 1936. Influence of cod liver oil in the diet on susceptibility to oxidation of fat of pig. *Dept. Sci. Ind. Res. Rept. Food Invest. Board,* pp. 73–75.

Lea, C. H. 1965. Chemical and nutritive aspects of oxidized and heated fats. *Chem. Ind.* 6:244–248.

Lea, C. H., Parr, L. J., L'Estrange, J. L., and Carpenter, K. J. 1966. Nutritional effects of autoxidized fats in animal diets. 3. The growth of turkeys on diets containing autoxidized fish oil. *Brit. J. Nutr.* 20:123–133.

Leach, T. A., and Golding, N. S. 1931. Preliminary report of substitution of pilchard oil for butterfat in milk for calf feeding. *Sci. Agr.* 12:204–205.

Lee, D. J., Roehm, J. N., Yu, T. C., and Sinnhuber, R. O. 1967. Effect of ω-3 fatty acids on the growth rate of rainbow trout (*Salmo gairdneri*). *J. Nutr.* 92:93–98.

Legler, C. 1985. *Digestion, Absorption and Transport of Lipids in Nutrition and Feeding in Fish,* ed. C. B. Cowey, A. M. Mackie, and J. G. Bell, pp. 229–333. New York: Academic Press.

Leoschke, W. L. 1959. Digestibility of animal fats and proteins by mink. *Am. J. Vet. Res.* 20:1086–1089.

Lipstein, B., and Bornstein, S. 1973. The effect of dietary fish oil soapstock on the performance, carcass fat and flavour of broilers. *Brit. Poultry Sci.* 14:279–289.

Madsen, L. L., McCay, C. M., Maynard, L. A., Davis, G. K., and Woodward, J. C. 1935.

Synthetic diets for herbivora, with special reference to toxicity of cod liver oil. N.Y. Agr. Exptl. Sta. Mem. No. 178, 55 pp.

Maplesden, D. C., and Loosli, J. K. 1960. Nutritional muscular dystrophy in calves. II. Addition of selenium and tocopherol to a basal dystrophogenic diet containing cod liver oil. *J. Dairy Sci.* 43:645–653.

Marble, D. R., Hunter, J. E., Knandel, H. C., and Dutcher, R. A. 1938. Fish flavor and odor in turkey meat. *Poultry Sci.* 17:49–53.

March, B. E., and Biely, J. 1955. Fat studies in poultry. 3. Folic acid and fat tolerance in the chick. *Poultry Sci.* 34:39–44.

March, B. E., Biely, J., Claggett, F. E., and Tarr, H. L. A. 1962. Nutritional and chemical changes in the lipid fraction of herring meals with and without antioxidant treatment. *Poultry Sci.* 41:873–880.

March, B. E., Biely, J., Tarr, H. L. A., and Claggett, F. G. 1965A. Favourable effect of antioxidants on metabolizable energy and protein value of British Columbia herring meal. Fisheries Research Board Can. Circular No. 34.

March, B. E., Biely, J., Tarr, H. L. A., and Claggett, F. 1965B. The effect of antioxidant treatment on the metabolizable energy and protein value of the meal. *Poultry Sci.* 44:679–685.

Mardsen, S. J., Alexander, L. M., Schopmeyer, G. E., and Lamb, J. C. 1952. Starting diet as a factor in edible quality of turkey. *Poultry Sci.* 31:451–458.

Matsuo, N. 1954A. Toxicity of fish oil (in Japanese). *J. Biochem (Japan)* 41:481–487.

Matsuo, N. 1954B. Toxicity of fish oil (in Japanese). II. *J. Biochem. (Japan)* 41:647–652.

Matsuo, N. 1960. Toxicity of fish oil. XI. Toxicity of heat-polymerized oil (in Japanese). *Yukagaku* 9:37–41.

Matsuo, N. 1962. Nutritional effects of oxidized and thermally polymerized fish oils. In *Symposium on Foods: Lipids and Their Oxidation*, ed. H. W. Schultz. Westport, Conn.: Avi Publishing Co.

Mattick, E. C. V. 1928. Chemical composition of the milk of cows receiving cod-liver oil. *Biochem. J.* 22:144–149.

Mattill, H. A. 1938. Vitamin E and nutritional muscular dystrophy in rabbits. *Proc. XVI Intern. Physiol. Congr.* 2:112–113.

Mattill, H. A. 1940. Muscular dystrophy in rabbits and the autoxidation of animal fats. *J. Nutr.* 19:13.

Mattill, H. A., and Golumbic, C. 1942. Vitamin E, cod liver oil, and muscular dystrophy. *J. Nutr.* 23:625–631.

Maynard, L. A., McCay, C. M., and Madsen, L. L. 1936. Influence of food fat of varying degrees of unsaturation upon blood lipids and milk fat. *J. Dairy Sci.* 19:49–53.

McCay, C. M., and Maynard, L. A. 1935. Effect of ingested cod-liver oil, shark-liver oil, and salmon oil on composition of blood and milk of lactating cows. *J. Biol. Chem.* 109:29–37.

McCay, C. M., Paul, H., and Maynard, L. A. 1938. Influence of hydrogenation and of yeast in counteracting cod-liver oil injury in herbivora and the influence of salmon oil on fat secretion. *J. Nutr.* 15:367–375.

McDowall, F. A., Patchell, M. R., and Reid, C. S. W. 1957. Bloat in cattle. V. Effects of whale oil on production and composition of milk, on flavor of milk and butter, and on properties of butterfat. *New Zealand J. Sci. Technol.* 38A:1036–1053.

Miller, D., Gruger, E. H. Jr., Long, K. C., and Knoble, G. M. Jr. 1967. Effect of refined menhaden oils on the flavor and fatty acid composition of broiler flesh. *J. Food Sci.* 32:342–345.

Miller, D., and Robisch, P. 1969. Comparative effect of herring, menhaden and safflower oils on broiler tissues. Fatty acid composition and flavor. *Poultry Sci.* 48:2146–2157.

Moccia, R. D., Hung, S. S. O., Slinger, S. J., and Ferguson, H. W. 1984. Effect of oxidized fish oil, vitamin E and ethoxy grain on the histopathology and haematology of rainbow trout (*Salmo gairdneri*). *J. Fish Dis.* 7:269–282.

Moore, T. 1953. The fat-soluble vitamins. In *Biochemistry and Physiology of Nutrition*, vol. I., ed. G. H. Bourne and G. W. Kidder. New York: Academic Press.

Moore, T. 1957. Vitamin A. Amsterdam: Elsevier.

Moore, T., and Sharman, I. M. 1961. Prevention of injurious effects of excessive cod-liver oil by its fortification with vitamin E. *Brit. J. Nutr.* 15:297–303.

Moore, T., Sharman, I. M., and Ward, R. J. 1959. Cod-liver oil as source and antagonist of vitamin E. *Brit. J. Nutr.* 13:100–110.

Murai, T., and Andrews, J. W. 1974. Interactions of dietary α-tocopherol, oxidized menhaden oil and ethoxyquin on channel catfish (*Ictalurus punctatus*). *J. Nutr.* 104:1416–1431.

Nicholson, J. W. G., Cunningham, H. M., and Friend, D. W. 1962. Addition of buffers to ruminant rations. II. Additional observations on weight gains, efficiency of gains, and consumption by steers of all-concentrate rations. *Can. J. Animal Sci.* 42:75–81.

Nicholson, J. W. G., Cunningham, H. M., and Friend, D. W. 1963. Addition of buffers to ruminant rations. IV. Effect of addition of sodium bicarbonate, sodium propionate, limestone, and cod liver oil on intrarumen environment. *Can. J. Animal Sci.* 43:309–319.

Nicolaysen, R., and Pihl, A. 1953. Feeding experiments in rats and in man with a commercial heat-treated herring oil. *Tidsskr. Kjemi Bergvesen Met.* 13:5–7.

Nilsen, H. W. 1954. Feeding menhaden oil to growing and laying pullets. *Fish Meal and Oil Industry Yearbook*, pp. 10–11.

Nottle, M. C., and Rook, J. A. F. 1963. The effect of dietary fat on the production of volatile fatty acids in the rumen of the cow. *Proc. Nutr. Soc.* 22(1):vii.

Oldfield, J. E., and Anglemier, A. F. 1957. Feeding of crude and modified menhaden oils in rations for swine. *J. Animal Sci.* 16:917–921.

Olson, J. A. 1964. Biosynthesis and metabolism of carotenoids and retinol (vitamin A). *J. Lipid Res.* 5:281–299.

Oltjen, Robert R. 1975. Manipulations of fatty acids composition of livestock. In *Nutrients in Processed Foods: Fats and Carbohydrates*, ed. P. L. White, D. C. Fletcher, and M. Ellis, pp. 65–75. American Medical Association. Acton, Mass.: Publishing Sciences Group, Inc.

Petersen, W. E. 1932. Effect of cod-liver oil in the ration on the quantity and quality of cow milk. *Dairy Sci.* 15:283–286.

Privett, O. S., Aaes-Jørgensen, E., Holman, R. T., and Lundberg, W. O. 1959. The effect of concentrates of polyunsaturated acids from tuna oil upon essential fatty acid deficiency. *J. Nutr.* 67:423–432.

Privett, O. S., and Cortesi, R. 1972. Observations on the role of vitamin E in the toxicity of oxidized fats. *Lipids* 7:780–787.

Privett, O. S., Pusch, F. J., Holman, R. T., and Lundberg, W. O. 1960. Essential fatty acids properties of tuna, herring, and menhaden oils. *J. Nutr.* 71:66–69.

Rasheed, A. A., Oldfield, J. E., Kaufmes, J., and Sinnhuber, R. O. 1963. Nutritive value of marine oils. I. Menhaden oil at varying oxidation levels with and without antioxidants in rat diets. *J. Nutr.* 79:323–332.

Raulin, J., and Petit, J. 1962. Nutritional value and physiopathological effect of polymerized herring oil. I. Differences between heating in air and heating in inert medium. *Arch. Sci. Physiol.* 16:77–87.

Raulin, J., Richir, C., and Jacquet, R. 1962. Nutritional and pathological effects of nutritional use of fish oil deodorized by heat. *Symp. Substances Etrangeres Aliments 5, Budapest* 1959:227–233.

Reder, R. 1942. Comparative rates of absorption of egg oil and cod-liver oil. *Poultry Sci.* 21:528–531.

Renner, R., and Hill, F. W. 1958. Metabolizable energy values of fats and fatty acids for chickens. *Proc. Cornell Nutrition Conf. for Feed Manuf.*, pp. 95–100.

Sargent, J., Henderson, R. J., and Tocher, D. R. 1989. *The Lipids in Fish Nutrition*, 2nd ed., ed. John E. Halver, pp. 153–218. New York: Academic Press.

Schreiber, M. L., Vail, G. E., Conrad, R. M., and Payne, L. F. 1947. Effect of tissue-fat stability on deterioration of frozen poultry. *Poultry Sci.* 26:14–19.

Schuler, G. A., and Essary, E. O. 1971. Fatty acid composition of lipids from broilers fed saturated and unsaturated fats. *J. Food Sci.* 36:431–434.

Scott, M. L. 1951. Studies on the enlarged hock disorder in turkeys. 3. Evidence of the detrimental effect of fish liver oil and the beneficial effect of dried brewer's yeast and other materials. *Poultry Sci.* 30:846–855.

Scott, M. L. 1953. Prevention of enlarged hock disorder in turkeys with niacin and vitamin E. *Poultry Sci.* 32:670–677.

Scott, P. P., and Humphreys, E. R. 1961. Addition of herring and vegetable oils to diet of cats. *Proc. Nutr. Soc.* 21(1):xiii.

Shaw, J. C., and Ensor, W. L. 1959. Effect of feeding cod liver oil and unsaturated fatty acids on rumen volatile fatty acids and milk fat content. *J. Dairy Sci.* 42:1238–1240.

Singsen, E. P., Bunnell, R. H., Matterson, L. D., Kozeff, A., and Hungherr, E. L. 1955A. Studies on encephalomalacia in the chick. 2. Protective action of DPPD against encephalomalacia. *Poultry Sci.* 34:262–271.

Singsen, E. P., Bunnell, R. H., Matterson, L. D., Kozeff, A., and Jungherr, E. L. 1954A. Studies on encephalomalacia in the chick. I. The influence of a vitamin E deficiency on the performance of breeding hens and their chicks. *Poultry Sci.* 33:192–201.

Singsen, E. P., Potter, L. M., Matterson, L. D., Bunnell, R. H., Kozeff, A., and Jungherr, E. L. 1954B. Studies on encephalomalacia in the chick. 4. The influence of oil in fish meal and oils from various species of fish on incidence of encephalomalacia. *Poultry Sci.* 33:1081.

Singsen, E. P., Potter, L. M., Matterson, L. D., Bunnell, R. H., Kozeff, A., and Jungherr, E. L. 1955B. Studies on encephalomalacia in the chick. 4. Influence of oil in fish meal, oils from various species of fish, and animal fats on the incidence of encephalomalacia. *Poultry Sci.* 34:1075–1079.

Sinnhuber, R. O. 1969. *The Role of Fats in Fish in Research*, ed. O. E. Neuhaus and J. E. Halver, pp. 245–261. New York: Academic Press.

Steenbock, H., Irwin, M. H., and Weber, J. 1936. The comparative rate of absorption of different fats. *J. Nutr.* 12:103–111.

Thomas, B. H., Culbertson, C. C., and Beard, F. 1934. Effect of ingesting soybeans and oils differing widely in their iodine numbers upon firmness of beef fat. *Proc. Am. Soc. Animal Production 27th Ann. Mtg.* 1934:193–194.

Thomasson, H. J. 1955. Biological value of oils and fats. I. Growth and food intake on feeding with natural oils and fats. *J. Nutr.* 56:455–468.

Thomasson, H. J. 1956A. Biological value of oils and fats. IV. Rate of intestinal absorption. *J. Nutr.* 59:343–352.

Thomasson, H. J. 1956B. Biological value of various natural oils and fats. In *Biochemical Problems of Lipids*, ed. Popjack and Le Breton. New York: Interscience.

Turner, W. A., Meigs, E. B., and Converse, H. T. 1936. Toxic effect of cod liver oil in the ration of the rabbit and the calf. *J. Biol. Chem.* 114, civ.

Vendell, J. H., and Putnam, J. N. 1945. Fish oil flavor in eggs. *Poultry Sci.* 24:285–286.

Watanabe, T. 1982. Lipid nutrition. *Fish Comp. Biochem. Physiol.* 73B(1):3–15.
Wessels, J. P. H., Atkinson, A., Van DeMerwe, R. P., and De Jongh, J. H. 1973. Flavor studies with fish meals and with fish oil fractions in broiler diets. *J. Sci. Food Agric.* 24:451–461.
Witting, L. A., Nishida, T., Johnson, O. C., and Kummerow, F. A. 1957. The relationship of pyridoxine and riboflavin to the nutritional value of polymerized fats. *J. Am. Oil Chemists' Soc.* 34:421–424.

Chapter 10
NUTRITIONAL PROPERTIES OF FISH OIL FOR HUMAN CONSUMPTION—EARLY DEVELOPMENTS

Maurice E. Stansby

INTRODUCTION

In very recent years there has been considerable publicity about the value of fish oils in the diet as a means of minimizing certain diseases, especially heart disease. These reports often describe the cause of such effects as being related to the content in the fish oils of $\omega 3$ fatty acids. The general view of many readers of such reports seems to be that such findings of the value of fish oil in the diet are something learned quite recently. Although much of the work, especially that relating to effects of $\omega 3$ fatty acids in fish, is, indeed, relatively quite new, a vast amount of research has been going on for many decades on the value of fish oil to reduce the incidence of certain diseases.

In this chapter this earlier work will be discussed. It will cover research up to the 1970s, at which time the $\omega 3$ fatty acids content of the fish oils was found to be related to some of these effects. The research carried out involving $\omega 3$ fatty acids will be discussed in Chapter 11.

In the earliest time period, the research involved, primarily, comparing the rate at which patients were cured or had symptoms relieved (or in some cases, the mortality rate) when fish oil was fed. In nearly all of this earliest work little was known about why the fish oil gave beneficial results; rather it was assumed that either the fish oil in its entirety or perhaps some unknown component of the fish oil brought about the desirable effect. In these earliest periods nothing was known about vitamins and very little about the makeup of the fish oil itself. Nevertheless in well-planned experiments carried out carefully, important conclusions could be made.

EARLY WORK IN ENGLAND ON COD-LIVER OIL AND ARTHRITIS

Perhaps the best-documented very early experiment involving the effect of fish oil on a disease was carried out at a hospital in Manchester, England, beginning about 1772. The experiments were carried out at the Manchester Infirmary. In 1770 a woman having an extreme degree of rheumatism began coming to the hospital as an outpatient. She was given various treatments, including doses of guaiacum and the rubbing of her joints with cod-liver oil. As had been the previous experience of the hospital, little or no relief of the rheumatism symptoms resulted. After about a year, she asked if she could take the cod-liver oil internally. Although the hospital had no confidence that this would have any effect, she was allowed to do so. Within a few weeks, her symptoms disappeared. The physicians at the hospital still did not believe that the ingestion of cod-liver oil had any effect, feeling rather that, since it was known that rheumatism was often controlled by weather, her improvement was a result of changes in the climatic conditions. About a year later the same woman returned with even worse symptoms of rheumatism. She requested the same treatment of ingesting internally of the cod-liver oil. Again after a short time all her symptoms disappeared.

Dr. Kay, a physician at the hospital, prescribed the use of cod-liver oil for other patients, with equally successful results. Subsequently all physicians at the hospital used this treatment for patients suffering from rheumatism. This remedy was successful in relieving the symptoms of all patients who were so treated.

The usual dose of cod-liver oil employed at the Manchester Infirmary was one to three tablespoons fed two to four times per day. This treatment was given to all rheumatism patients at the Manchester Infirmary over a period of 10 years and resulted in success in all cases. The hospital used either cod-liver oil or, in some cases, ling liver oil which it imported from Newfoundland in 400–525-lb barrels. During the 10 years of the experiment about 600 lb were used for this purpose.

In October 1782, Dr. Thomas Percival, a physician at the Manchester Infirmary, read a paper describing this work before a meeting of the Medical Society of London and Edinburgh held in Paris. The paper was published by the *London Medical Journal* (Percival 1783).

In spite of the highly positive results of this work, the finding did not spread to other areas and, in fact, eventually the study was practically completely forgotten. The reason for this would appear to be related to the nature of the cod-liver oil that was available at that time.

Even today the flavor of cod-liver oil is generally considered unpalatable. The cod-liver oil available in the 1700s was made in quite a different way than that manufactured today. The modern method consists of liberation of the oil by cooking the livers with live steam and then separating the oil. In the late 1700s, cod-liver oil was made by allowing the livers to rot and then separating the oil, which then had a tremendously nauseating flavor.

In the studies made at the Manchester Infirmary, it was stated that the use of cod-liver oil outside a hospital by the general population was not recommended. This was because of the very bad flavor of the oil. In the studies in Manchester it was usually necessary to saponify the cod-liver oil with an alkali to produce a soap that, when flavored with peppermint, could be taken without rejection by most of the patients. After consumption of this cod-liver oil soap, the patients were given lemon juice, which released the oil again.

The saponification process is one that could not be carried out at home by those suffering from arthritis. It would have to be done in a laboratory or a hospital. In all probability this matter prevented any widespread use at that time of cod-liver oil for this purpose. By the time modern-day methods for producing cod-liver oil had been developed, so many decades had elapsed that this Percival treatment for arthritis was completely forgotten.

EARLY WORK ON OTHER MEDICAL USES OF COD-LIVER OIL

Cod-liver oil was used for medical purposes involving such conditions as night blindness and rickets a very long time before anything was known about vitamins. According to Aure (1967), this value of fish liver oil was discovered in the latter half of the eighteenth century. Actually, however, it was known much earlier than that; thus a cure for night blindness by the use of fish bile is mentioned in the Bible, and the use of goat livers for the same purpose was recommended by old Greek, Roman, and Arab physicians (Rosenberg 1942). The general view, however, with few exceptions up until the early 1900s, was that the only nutrients needed by the body were carbohydrates, fats, protein, and salts.

Cod-liver oil was manufactured initially for use for nonmedicinal purposes such as in the tanning of leather and manufacture of soap, starting sometime during the 1700s. Its use for medicinal purposes based on scientific evidence apparently began in the 1780s with the treatment of arthritis (see previous section). Between 1822 and 1824 research was carried out in Germany which showed it was of value in the treatment of rickets (Schütte 1824). These and other studies were included in a British book published in 1841 (Bennett 1841).

Cod-liver oil initially was made for industrial purposes by very crude methods that yielded a dark-colored oil having a vile flavor (see preceding section). As considerable evidence began to accumulate indicating the need for a high-grade medicinal product, much more suitable methods employing fresh cod livers were introduced. In the United States initially the old technique involving rotting of livers was employed. Toward the middle of the nineteenth century, cod-liver oil made by improved procedures was generally imported into this country from Norway. The first modern American plant was built in Provincetown, Massachusetts, in 1849 by N. E. Atwood (Atwood 1883). While early in the eighteenth century the principal uses in the United States for cod-liver oil were in the industrial area, by the start of the twentieth century the medicinal application had become better known and had wider use (Stevenson 1902). Soon thereafter, medicinal cod-liver oil came into widespread use as a general health-promoting medicine even before the discovery of vitamins A and D. Cod-liver oil continued in general use after the discovery of these vitamins until about 1950, when synthetic vitamin concentrates became available.

FISH OIL AND HEART DISEASE

The first suspicion that the consumption of considerable fish in the diet might be beneficial toward diminishing the incidence of atherosclerosis or other cardiac diseases occurred when statistics came out on fatal cardiac diseases in Norway before and after the Nazi occupation during World War II. It appeared that there had been a marked reduction in fatal heart attacks between 1941 and 1946. Strøm and Jensen (1951), after making a thorough examination of such statistics, confirmed that such a decline had occurred. If the average rate of heart fatalities from 1927 to 1940 is arbitrarily indicated as 100, then the rate from 1941 to 1946 was 78.75. After 1946 the rate increased, reaching about 87.5 by the end of 1948. Although Strøm and Jensen could not pinpoint the exact cause of this decline in fatal heart attacks, they felt it was quite possible that the underlying cause might be dietary changes caused by the war. In another paper Strøm (1948) showed that the diet in Norway had changed substantially during the critical period of 1941–1946. On one hand, the consumption of meat and meat products, eggs, whole milk, cream cheese, various fats such as margarine, and vegetables and berries declined substantially. On the other hand, there was a considerable increase in the consumption of fish, skimmed milk, and cereals. Based on the statistics available, however, it was impossible to determine just what was the basic cause for the reduction in fatal heart attacks.

In the late 1940s it became known that high serum cholesterol levels could effect the likelihood of heart attacks, and that such high levels of serum cholesterol could be decreased by the presence of polyunsaturates in the diet. Initially it was assumed that those vegetable oils which are almost completely of the polyunsaturated fatty acid composition were the only oils effective for this purpose. Fish oils, which were known to contain both saturated and polyunsaturated fatty acids, were assumed to be worthless. In the earlier work fish oils were never even tried. Later, however, the work of Bronte-Stewart et al. (1956) showed that fish oils were actually superior to vegetable oils in this respect.

Research of Dr. Averly Nelson

A Seattle physician, Dr. Averly Nelson, carried out a 19-year study on the effects of fish in diet which unfortunately is not widely known. These results are so important that it is worth rather detailed discussion here. Nelson, born in 1914, received a bachelor's degree from the University of Washington followed by a M.D. from the University of Oregon in 1942. He worked for four years in a sanitarium during which time he became interested in the idea of curing of such conditions as heart disease by means of diet. In order to prepare himself for such a career, in 1945 he left his position and enrolled at the University of California at Los Angeles (UCLA) from which he received the degree of Master of Medical Science. This gave him a better background in such fields as nutrition and biochemistry. While at UCLA, he talked to several professors about the then recent indications that the incidence of heart disease had drastically declined in Norway during the several years of World War II when the country was occupied by German forces and when certain foods such as meat were so scarce that the population had to change their diet, using much greater amounts of fish. Nelson was greatly impressed by these discussions.

After he returned to Seattle, Nelson set up practice as a general physician. He gave considerable thought toward specializing in the field of the effect of diet on cardiac conditions. During the next five years, he discussed his ideas with several individuals such as Dr. Lawrence Kinsell, Dr. Morrison, and Dr. Goffman, all of whom had similar ideas. Beginning in 1952, Nelson began practice along the lines of treatment by diet changes of patients who had had one or more heart attacks. Most of his patients were individuals who had been referred to him by other physicians.

Nelson carried out his work from 1952 to 1971. In 1952 there was no evidence indicating that the oil in fish which contained polyunsaturated as

well as saturated fatty acids would be of value in lowering serum cholesterol levels. Nelson, however, was so convinced that this would be the
case that he included as a part of the diet that he recommended to his
heart patients the requirement that at least three meals per week should
include fish as the main course. This idea was confirmed in 1955 with
publication of the Bronte-Stewart et al. (1956) finding that fish oils were
actually considerably more efficient in lowering serum cholesterol levels
than were vegetable oils.

Only about 40% of Nelson's patients were willing and able to adopt and
continue this diet for the 16 to 19 years of the experiment. The remaining
60% of the patients served as controls. The results of this experiment
were indeed quite startling (Table 10-1).

It should be emphasized that all patients in this experiment had had at
least one heart attack before the work began. We can not, therefore,
assume that the same results would have occurred for the general population where many of the individuals had never suffered a heart attack.

It may be asked why only in Nelson's work were such highly successful
results found. The answer lies, to a large extent, in the fact that Nelson
anticipated the possible value of fish fatty acids at a much earlier date than
did anyone else. His work on the project began in 1952, terminating in
1971, with his final paper being published in 1972. Much of his work was
published in relatively obscure journals, although his final paper appeared
in *Geriatrics* (Nelson 1972). Nelson died shortly after the publication of
this final paper. He would likely have seen to it that his results were more
widely known had he not died at that time.

Another very important factor in Nelson's success was his understanding of the need for motivating his patients to adhere to their diet over the
long years that the work lasted. Even with his best efforts, only 39% of his
patients undertook and stayed with the diet over the extended period of

**Table 10-1. Survival of Heart Disease Patients over 16
to 19 Years Comparing Those on a Standard Diet with
Those on a Special Diet Which Included Fish as a
Main Course at Least Three Times per Week**

GROUP	PERCENT SURVIVING
Overall results	
Standard diet (126 patients)	8
High fish diet (80 patients)	36
Results for patients 56–70 years of age	
Standard diet (85 patients)	5
High fish diet (44 patients)	32

time. Dr. Nelson, at the start of the work, had determined by examination of serum cholesterol level data and ratio of serum phospholipid to serum cholesterol that if once per week the patients disregarded their diet and ate whatever they wanted for four successive meals, only a small increase in overall average serum cholesterol levels resulted. This freedom to violate the diet once a week encouraged a much larger percentage of his patients to remain on the diet than would otherwise have been possible. Nelson also employed a full-time dietician and held discussion sessions with his patients at regular intervals to impress upon them the need for following their diet.

Nelson achieved success in getting his patients to adhere to their diet only after a rather detailed regime based on the above-mentioned principles was adopted. New patients first underwent a thorough physical examination including laboratory tests. The patient then attended a $1\frac{1}{2}$- to 2-hour interview with Nelson and his dietician in which the patient was given full information on the importance of the dietary regime and how it would play a major role in minimizing the risk of subsequent atherosclerotic events. A second interview was held after about three weeks. After eight weeks extensive blood lipid tests usually indicated desirable improvement over the initial examination, and these results were discussed with the patient. This bolstered the patient's enthusiasm to continue the diet. After this session, the patient was allowed to consume each week four successive meals without adhering at these meals to his diet. Group lectures were given at periodic intervals over the years to patients and their families.

By following such a program, Nelson still was able to get not quite 40% of his patients to continue his recommended regime over the long years of the diet. It is not surprising, therefore, that others in the medical profession who ordinarily give only cursory advice have not achieved the outstanding success of that reached by Nelson.

An aspect of Nelson's investigation that has not been stressed in the foregoing discussion is the fact that the diet used differs from those in the control group (undieted individuals) not only in the greater consumption of fish but also in other respects. Patients using the prescribed diet, in addition to being required to consume at least three meals per week in which high-fat fish was the main component, also had restrictions limiting fat content and aimed at raising the protein content to some extent. Among such items of the diet were the following:

1. Dairy products: Milk and cheese should be low fat.
2. Meat, lean beef, lamb, veal, chicken, or turkey should be restricted to not more than 6 oz per day. The amount of fish had no limitation.

3. Vegetables and fruit: The patient should have dark green or yellow vegetables, tomatoes, or citrus fruit each day.
4. Bread and cereals: The patient should eat three servings per day of enriched or whole-grain products.
5. Unsaturated fats: A daily intake of three tablespoons of fat, including that used in cooking, is the maximum permitted.
6. A diet high in protein is recommended. The diet should have about 22% protein, 24% fat, and 54% carbohydrate. Protein content can be increased by use of egg whites, defatted wheat germ, low-fat milk powder, gelatin, and low-fat seafood.

It is virtually impossible to estimate what effect the above-mentioned factors would have in comparison to the requirement for the patient to include at least three meals per week containing as the main component high-fat seafood. There can be no doubt that these more general factors played a part in the reduction of fatal heart attacks during the 16–19 years of the experiment. It seems likely, however, that the high-fat seafood may well have been the major factor.

Kromhout-Zutphen Study

In addition to the 19-year study of Averly Nelson, only one other such long-term investigation dealing with the effect of fish in the diet on cardiac fatality has been published. This was a study carried out in the town of Zutphen, Holland, from 1960 to 1980 (Kromhout et al. 1985). This investigation was Holland's contribution to a seven-country study on heart disease (Keys 1980). In Zutphen, a town of about 25,000, a group of 872 middle-aged (40–59 years) men were selected in 1960. None of them had ever had a heart attack. Their diet was carefully studied in 1960. The group was examined with respect to the amount of fish they ordinarily had been eating and five groups were set up with daily average grams of fish consumed: 0, 1–14, 15–29, 30–45, and over 45. Records were also taken on other aspects of their diet in 1960. The fish consumed were found to be two-thirds lean fish and one-third fat fish. After 20 years the number of deaths from coronary heart attack were recorded. It was found that 2.5 times as many individuals who ate no fish died of a heart attack as those who ate 45 g or more per day. Of course such a figure as 45 g of fish per day did not mean that each day this amount of fish was consumed. Rather it was the average amount, which probably indicated that fish may have been consumed at meals over several days of elapsed time. In the report (Kromhout et al. 1985) no data were included on the proportion of lean or fat fish involved except to indicate that overall, two-thirds of the fish consumed were of the lean variety and one-third of the fat variety.

Comparison of Results of Nelson Versus Kromhout

It is difficult to make meaningful comparisons between the results of these two investigations because experimental conditions differed and some data that would make a reliable comparison feasible were not listed in each of these investigations. We do know that all participants in the Averly Nelson investigation had suffered at least one heart attack before the investigation began. In the Kromhout study none of the participants had suffered a heart attack at the start of the investigation. In the Kromhout work those individuals eating no fish had $2\frac{1}{2}$ times as many fatal heart attacks as those eating the most fish (over 45 g per day). For the Averly Nelson study, the corresponding difference was 4 times rather than $2\frac{1}{2}$ times. Those in the Nelson study apparently ate somewhat more fish (about 60 g per day). However, in the Nelson study, all the fish eaten was fat fish, contrasting to only one-third of the fish in the Kromhout study being of the fat variety. All of the information available indicates that it is the fat in the fish that contains components (fatty acids) that are effective in reducing the risk of coronary heart attacks. Therefore the amount of fish oil fat taken by the participants in the two investigations must have been considerably different than the figures 45 g per day versus 60 g per day. If we assume that the lean fish averaged 1.5% fat and the fat fish 7%, the amount of fat consumed would be in the ratio 420 : 150, or almost three times as much for the Nelson participants as for those in the Kromhout group. This difference might at least in part compensate for the more efficient decrease in rate of coronary heart attacks in the Nelson group over that of the Kromhout.

There are other differences in these two investigations that make it difficult to appraise how they compare. In the Nelson project the participants were asked to change their diet by eating more fish than most of them had previously done, whereas in the Kromhout work no difference in diet was suggested. This might have resulted in those in the former group not strictly following the prescribed diet. However, this could not get very far out of line because tests for serum cholesterol levels were run at frequent intervals, and as shown in Nelson's publication, deviations in the diet were readily picked up by such testing. In the Kromhout study, the diet of the participants was not necessarily that which held constant through the entire 20 years of the experiment. Rather it was merely that which pertained in the first year of the study. It seems quite possible that the diet of the participants could have changed over this lengthy period.

Whether or not such a change could have biased the results is impossible to determine.

Probably the best conclusion that can be reached from these two lengthy investigations is that consumption of fish in the diet can reduce the risk of fatal coronary heart attacks and that possibly the success in achieving such an end is greater for individuals who have had previous heart attacks than for average individuals, including many who have not suffered such problems.

EFFECT OF OILS FROM FISH IN REDUCING SERUM CHOLESTEROL IN ANIMALS

As we have just seen, two long-term investigations have been carried out demonstrating that in humans, the incidence of fatal cardiac incidents can be diminished substantially when fish is included in the diet. Such investigations are very time consuming, and we can not expect many to be conducted at such lengths. Many animal feeding tests, on the other hand, have been carried out over much shorter periods of time. Before 1956, as has been stated, no tests were made to determine serum cholesterol level reduction from feeding of fish on fish oil. In fact, it was believed that because fish oils often contained about as much saturated fatty acids as polyunsaturated ones, the use of fish oils would most likely increase rather than decrease serum cholesterol levels. As a result of the paper of Bronte-Stewart et al. (1956), which clearly showed that fish oils were very effective in lowering serum cholesterol levels, in the next 10 years many papers were published confirming these results. During this decade no less than 13 species of fish were shown to possess serum cholesterol-reducing properties (Table 10-2).

Among the investigations looking into what went on with respect to serum cholesterol levels when fish or fish oil was included in the diet, the work of Peifer was the most exhaustive (Peifer 1967). He carried out, at the Hormel Institute under contract from the Bureau of Fisheries Laboratory at Seattle, investigations over a period of nine years on the effects of fish and fish oil on serum cholesterol levels. Two of Peifer's major findings will be mentioned here.

In his research all work was carried out on rats. In most cases the rats were given a pretreatment by a diet containing 10% tallow plus 0.5% cholesterol and 0.5% cholate, which raised their serum cholesterol level prior to testing for effects of fish oil.

In most research carried out by both Peifer and other investigators, the ability of the fish oils to lower serum cholesterol levels in animals was measured by feeding the various oils. Peifer went a step farther. He

Table 10-2. Species of Fish for Which Cholesterol Depressant Effect Has
Been Demonstrated

SPECIES	SOURCE OF OIL	REFERENCE
Cod	liver	Hauge and Nicolaysen 1959; Howe and Bosshardt 1962A,B; Kahn et al. 1963; Kingsbury et al. 1961
Cuttlefish	liver	Kaneda and Alfin-Slater 1963
Dogfish	liver	Peifer et al. 1965; Wood et al. 1961
Halibut	liver	Wood et al. 1961
Menhaden	whole fish	Ahrens et al. 1959; Peifer et al. 1960, 1962, 1965
Mullet	body	Peifer et al. 1962
Ocean perch	body	Peifer et al. 1962
Pilchard	body	Bronte-Stewart et al. 1956
Salmon (coho)	body	Peifer et al. 1962
Sardine	body	Miller et al. 1962
Seal	body	Bronte-Stewart et al. 1956
Tuna	whole fish	Peifer et al. 1960
Whale	body	Malmros and Wigand 1957

compared the effects brought about by the oils to that which took place when the oil in the flesh of the fish was fed. This was done by freeze-drying several different species of fish. Then the freeze-dried fish, the extracted oil, and finally the oil-free flesh were fed and the change in serum lipids determined. As shown in Table 10-3, the change in serum lipids was about the same for either the oil with the fish or for the oil extracted from the same fish. The fish species used in this work were menhaden, silver salmon, mullet, and ocean perch. The first three of these are reasonably oily fish, but the ocean perch is of very low oil content. Yet even under these conditions (where in the case of the ocean perch less than half as much oil was available), about the same change in serum lipids occurred. Feeding of the oil-extracted flesh resulted in no decrease, usually an increase, in the serum lipid content.

Not only does feeding of fish oil affect serum cholesterol levels, but also some of the polyunsaturates are absorbed by the various tissues of the fish. Rats having normal serum cholesterol levels have hearts containing no more than 0.3 mg per gram of hexaene. Rats on a fish diet containing fish oil have 7–17 times this amount (Peifer et al. 1965). The content of pentaenoic acid in the rats' hearts also showed a similar large increase. Since a fish oil diet contains only trace amounts of these fatty acids, it would appear that there is a need for such polyunsaturates in hypercholesterolemic animals and that their body mobilizes them from wherever they are available. With diets containing fish oil, $\omega3$ fatty acids (C22:6, C20:5) are already present. Kingsbury (1964) has found a similar large

Table 10-3. Effects of Fish and Their Component Oils

TREATMENTS	FISH OIL IN DIETS, G/100 G	MARINE OIL-PUFA,[a] IN DIETARY FAT, %	PLASMA LIPIDS, Mg/100 Ml AND % CHANGE			LIVER LIPIDS, G/100 G	
			Mg/100 Ml	TC%	TC/Pl	TC	TC/Pl
Tallow controls	—	—	507	—	2.2	11.3	4.2
Menhaden							
Whole fish	4.9	13	250	−51	1.3	8.5	3.1
Fish oils	4.9	13	223	−56	1.2	8.2	2.7
NL solids	0.0	0	510	0	2.2	10.9	4.1
Silver salmon							
Whole fish	5.3	12	193	−62	1.1	8.1	2.8
Fish oil	5.3	12	162	−68	1.1	10.9	3.4
NL solids	0.0	0	614	+20	2.3	11.7	4.6
Mullet							
Whole fish	3.8	7	359	−49	1.4	7.0	2.5
Fish oil	3.8	7	263	−48	1.3	9.2	3.3
NL solids	0.0	0	563	+12	2.4	10.3	4.1
Ocean Perch							
Whole fish	2.5	5	398	−61	1.3	8.8	2.8
Fish oil	2.5	5	190	−63	1.1	9.9	3.6
NL solids	0.0	0	552	+9	2.2	10.3	3.7

Source: Peifer et al. 1962.
[a]Diets contained 15% fat, most of which was supplied as tallow. NL solids = residual solids after removal of total lipids; PUFA = polyunsaturated fatty acids; Pl = phospholipids; TC = total cholesterol.

increase in these fatty acids in heart tissues of humans who have been on a fish oil diet.

Throughout Peifer's work he has consistently found that the consumption of fish oil in the diet of rats resulted in an immediate gradual reduction of serum cholesterol levels. This contrasts to the initial stationary period, lasting about two weeks, when fatty acids such as linoleic or linolenic acid are fed, after which the serum cholesterol levels start to slowly decline.

EFFECT OF FISH IN DIET ON MULTIPLE SCLEROSIS

It has been suspected for some time that the type of fat in the diet might be important in the disease multiple sclerosis. This idea does not go back hundreds of years such as was the case with arthritis. However, around the middle of this century some observations made on the incidence of multiple sclerosis suggested that excessive consumption of fat from meat in the diet might have a harmful effect. Much of this work stemmed from effort by Swank and co-workers (e.g., Swank and Backer 1950; Swank et al. 1952). These investigators observed that inhabitants of Norway living in the central areas where meat consumption was high had a much greater incidence of multiple sclerosis than those who lived along the coast and who ate considerable quantities of fish and much less meat. These findings received some confirmation by a Norwegian survey made in the early 1960s by Presthus (1962). Swank has recently compiled a 35-year study (Swank 1988) involving more than 100 patients where there is indication that use of a diet with reduced fat intake may slow down somewhat the development of multiple sclerosis. There is also some indication that the use of some polyunsaturated fat is somewhat superior to an all-hard-fat diet.

A paper has appeared (Bernsohn and Stephanides 1967) linking $\omega3$ fatty acids and more specifically docosahexaenoic acid with multiple sclerosis. These authors show that in areas of the world where $\omega3$ fatty acids occur in some quantity in the diet, such as where much fish is eaten or where certain seed products containing linolenic acid are eaten, multiple sclerosis is almost unknown. The disease is most common in areas where very little fatty acids of the $\omega3$ type are found in the diet. Furthermore, Kishimoto et al. (1967) have found that in human subjects who have had multiple sclerosis, the brain, which normally contains considerable $22:6\ \omega3$ fatty acids, contains less than half the normal amount of this fatty acid. In their experiment, they found that the $22:6\ \omega3$ fatty acid content in the average, normal-appearing white matter of the brains of several multiple sclerosis victims averaged 1.5% of total lipids as compared to an average value from control (non-multiple sclerosis patients) of 3.5%.

Bernsohn and Stephanides (1967) have developed the theory that a lack of docosahexaenoic acid or its precursor, linolenic acid, in the diet is one factor in the development of multiple sclerosis. They recognize, of course, that even in areas of high incidence of multiple sclerosis and of low intake of $\omega3$ fatty acids, most individuals do not contract multiple sclerosis. They hypothesize, therefore, that in those individuals in such geographic areas who do develop the disease, in addition to the lack of a safe quantity of $\omega3$ fatty acids in the diet, some other factors such as a faulty enzyme system for the conversion of linolenic acid to docosahexaenoic acid are present. In the presence of adequate dietary $\omega3$ fatty acids, these other factors would not be sufficient to allow the disease to develop. Still to be determined is whether $\omega3$ fatty acid supplementation is effective only at very early ages, while the brain is developing, or to what extent it is important with older individuals. Also, evidence is being sought as to whether supplementation of diets of multiple sclerosis patients with $\omega3$ fatty acids can reverse the trend of the disease. Needless to say, should these findings be positive, the importance of fish in the diet as a source of $\omega3$ fatty acids—and indeed of its high content of the effective component, docosahexaenoic acid—would be much greater than presently recognized.

During the 1960s biochemical studies of the brain, the serum, and the red blood cells of multiple sclerosis patients showed that with such patients the unsaturated fatty acid content was less than with normal individuals (Gerstl et al. 1961; Gul et al. 1970). Thompson (1966) reported that a specific decreased content of linoleic ($\omega6$) acid existed in analyses of tissues of multiple sclerosis patients.

Bernsohn and Stephanides attempted to study the effects of fish oil in the diet upon multiple sclerosis. They conducted a statistical study of the incidence of this disease on two islands off the coast of Scotland. On one of these islands the inhabitants were fishermen. They and their families ate large quantities of fish. On a nearby island the only industry was farming, and very little or no fish was eaten by the inhabitants of this island. Records of cases of multiple sclerosis on these two islands were examined. It was shown that there were more cases of multiple sclerosis on the island where farming was the only industry than on the island occupied by fishermen where commercial fishing was the main industry and a great deal of fish was consumed in the diet. The results of this statistical survey were never published because of the small population involved. It was believed that with a relatively few cases of multiple sclerosis involved, the results might not be of statistical significance.

There is a problem that discourages scientific research on the causes of multiple sclerosis: This disease is one suffered only by humans; no animals ever contract it. With most other diseases, scientific investigation begins with animal studies; the basic ideas are obtained from such animal tests using rats, mice, or sometimes larger animals. The ideas gleaned from these preliminary studies can then be compared to the particular disease occurring with human subjects. Because of this problem, it is very difficult to look into the causes of multiple sclerosis. Many medical institutions are not willing to investigate causes of this disease for this reason. Nevertheless a long-term, modern investigation is currently under way (French 1984).

EFFECTS OF FISH OIL ALKOXYDIGLYCERIDES ON MEDICAL CONDITIONS

In a number of species of fish a considerable portion of the lipid that in most fish occurs primarily as triglycerides is present as alkoxydiglycerides. The presence of such compounds in fish was first reported by Tsujimoto and Toyama (1922). These alkoxydiglycerides, or diacyl glyceryl ethers as they are more generally referred to (sometimes called just glyceryl ethers), occur to the greatest extent in the liver oil and to a lesser extent in the body oil of sharks. They also occur more rarely in the lipids of other species of fish. A very general, long review of the biochemistry of lipids containing ether bonds has been published by Snyder (1969). A shorter review of marine lipids containing the ether bond has also been published (Malins and Varanasi 1972).

Several medical effects have been described for the use of glyceryl ethers from fish lipids following the publication of a Bodman and Maisin (1958) review article. In this paper the idea is advanced that glyceryl ethers such as batyl alcohol occur in embryos at a very early stage before other lipids have appeared. It is suggested that the glyceryl ethers play some role in the subsequent embryonic development to produce other lipids. From these hypotheses, these investigators came to believe that in certain nonhealing wounds, glyceryl ethers might promote healing. In tests with such wounds, mostly connected with surgical operations, they report initiation of healing by the use of an external application of glyceryl ethers to the wound when previous attempts without the use of glyceryl ethers failed to result in healing.

In a very short paragraph, Bodman and Maisin state that "no effect whatever has been observed in the use of glyceryl ethers in the treatment of accidental burns in otherwise fit individuals." This statement is not repeated in the discussion or summary of their paper. As a result of the publication of Bodman and Maisin's paper, pharmaceutical manufacturers (either ignoring or not noticing the very short statement that the results do not apply at all to accidental burns or wounds) began putting out preparations for the healing of burns or wounds with glyceryl ethers as a main ingredient. The myth that glyceryl ethers were of great value in ordinary burn or wound healing was thereby established.

In 1966, the Seattle laboratory of the National Marine Fisheries Service, having great doubt about the efficacy of the use of fish oils for use in an ointment (by then commonly recommended as a sure cure for healing wounds or burns), carried out, on a contract with the Mayo Clinic, work that quite definitely disproved any such beneficial activity. Hairless mice were given burns, and in other cases wounds, under standard conditions and treated using a double-blind system with external applications of fish oil with (1) a high content of glyceryl ethers, (2) no glyceryl ethers, and (3) a high vitamin A content but no glyceryl ethers; and (4) mineral oil disguised to seem to be identical to the fish oil. Another control used was no treatment with oil of any kind. There was no improvement in healing rate for any of the treatments at all. When no oil of any kind was used there was a barely statistically significant increase in healing time over all the other oil treatments (Stansby et al. 1967). In spite of the publication of these results, at least one commercial product with glyceryl ether containing fish oil is still sold with fantastic claims for its healing properties for burns.

Glyceryl ethers are also used for a variety of other medical purposes. Tests conducted by different laboratories, however, do not always agree as to whether the glyceryl ethers serve a useful purpose. Perhaps the leading such use is for the purported value of glyceryl ethers (predominantly selachyl alcohol) when taken internally to reduce undesirable side effects during radiation treatment.

Most of the research on the desirability for the internal taking of selachyl alcohol from fish liver oils containing it as well as batyl alcohol and other glyceryl ethers stems from work by Astrid Brohult. She and coworkers worked at Radiumhemmet in Stockholm, Sweden. This work began in the 1950s and resulted in publication in 1963 of a 99-page report entitled "Alkoxyglycerols and Their Use in Radiation Treatment" (Brohult 1963). As a result of this research, it is our understanding that selachyl alcohol or other glyceryl ether preparations are used routinely at the Radiumhemmet for patients receiving radiation treatment. These findings have been confirmed by workers at other laboratories (e.g., Sviridov et al. 1954; Edlund 1954). On the other hand, in several other laboratories (e.g., Snyder 1969), no such effects could be found. It was Snyder's contention that many of the other reports that seemed to support the view that glyceryl ethers were effective in radioprotection were based on inadequate numbers of subjects to draw significant statistical conclusions.

Evans et al. (1957) reported that batyl alcohol injections could cure cattle that had developed poisoning from consumption of bracken fern. On the other hand, Dalton (1964) was unable to confirm this effect of batyl alcohol.

Abaturova and Shubina (1964) reported a marked depression of carcinoma in rats fed batyl and selachyl alcohol. By contrast, Delmon and Biraben (1966) were unable to obtain any such effect.

Chalmers et al. (1966) patented the use of glyceryl ethers for use in the treatment of inflammatory diseases.

In summary, it would appear that glyceryl ethers have the best documentation for diminishing harmful radiation treatment effects. At the other end of the scale, beneficial effects of the external application of glyceryl ethers to wounds and burns have been generally disproven. The other purported effects for glyceryl ethers require additional research before we can assess their value.

SUMMARY

The use of fish oils for the treatment of diseases goes far back into antiquity. For example, the effective use of fish oils for treating night blindness (now known to be caused by their content of vitamin A) is mentioned in the Bible. It required many centuries for such facts to be fully understood. Perhaps the first usage of fish oil which was tested and reported on the basis of its value for treatment of a disease was the work at the Manchester Infirmary in England based on a 10-year study of the use of cod-liver oil to cure arthritis. This well-documented investigation was reported in the *London Medical Journal* in 1783.

This use of cod-liver oil, although never tested quite as thoroughly as in the study in Manchester, was investigated in the early 1800s with respect to its action in curing rickets and other conditions. This was nearly 100 years before knowledge about vitamins was known. Nevertheless, factories for preparing from fresh fish livers cod-liver oil with a reasonably bland flavor were set up in Norway, Germany, and the United States, and cod-liver oil began to be used as a general medicine to be taken to minimize the chance of acquiring a number of disease conditions.

The use of fish or fish oil in the diet to minimize the chance of acquiring cardiac heart failures awaited the late 1940s and early 1950s before being studied. Spurring interest in this area were two situations. First it was noted that in Norway, the incidence of cardiac disease fell drastically during the German occupation, when the availability of meat decreased and the consumption of fish increased, but rose rapidly at the end of the war, when meat consumption increased. The other situation was connected with the findings, in the late 1940s, that high serum cholesterol levels, which were known to be associated with increased risk of heart failure, could be reduced by consumption of polyunsaturated fat or oil. At first fish oils were considered useless because they contained almost equal proportions of saturated and polyunsaturated fats. In this earlier period it was believed that only certain vegetable oils were suitable. By the mid-1950s, however, research had shown that fish oils were far superior to any vegetable oils in their ability to lower serum cholesterol levels. These findings stimulated the conducting of two 18- to 20-year studies on the effects of fish oils in the diet on heart attack fatalities. One of these studies was carried out in the United States from 1952 to 1970 with about 200 individuals. The other was carried out in Holland from 1960 to 1980 with about 950 individuals. Each of these investigations showed clearly that with increased consumption of fish the risk of fatal heart attacks was decreased.

During the period when these two long-term investigations were under way, it was believed that the reason for the effectiveness of the fish in the diet was based solely on the ability of fish oil to lower serum cholesterol levels. This stimulated the conducting of much shorter-term research, in most cases based on the use of animals such as mice, to find out more about the action of fish oils. These investigations revealed that about three times as much of most polyunsaturated vegetable oils were required to lower serum cholesterol levels by a given amount as was the case with fish oils. Many different fish oils were studied, and all proved highly effective in lowering serum cholesterol levels. It was found that in addition to the consumption of fish oil resulting in decreased serum cholesterol levels, some of the highly polyunsaturated long-chain fatty acids, unique to fish oils, were built up to higher than normal levels in certain tissues such as the heart.

Considerable attention has been given since 1960 to the possibility that consumption of fish oil in the diet might be effective in reducing the occurrence of or curing multiple sclerosis. Quite a few different investigations have dealt with this problem. It is a very difficult matter to investigate, especially since no animals other than humans contract the disease. Beyond the fact that in some countries where fish consumption is low, multiple sclerosis seems to be somewhat higher than average, no great progress has as yet been made.

Glycerol ethers, which occur to a considerable extent in a few species of fish, have been investigated for their effects on several medical conditions. At one time it was quite generally believed that such glyceryl ethers could promote the healing of burns and wounds. A fairly comprehensive investigation between the Mayo Clinic and the National Marine Fisheries Service has proved that this is not true and that neither glyceryl ethers nor fish oils have any such healing properties. Glyceryl ethers from fish oils have been extensively investigated in Sweden as something to be consumed to minimize radiation damage. Apparently this use of glyceryl ethers is being carried out routinely in Sweden. On the other hand, several investigations in other countries have not been able to confirm any such effect. Several other medical effects claimed for glyceryl ethers have been found by others not to be effective. Much more research will be needed before these various claims can be confirmed.

REFERENCES

Abaturova, E. A., and Shubina, A. V. 1964. Effects of batyl and selachyl alcohols in the growth of malignant tumors. *Byul Eksperim Biol. i Med.* 57:81–83.

Ahrens, E. H., Jr., Insull, W., Jr., Hirsch, J., Stoffel, W., Peterson, M. L., Farquahar, J. M., Miller, T., and Thomasson, R. J. 1959. Effect on human serum lipids of a dietary fat, highly unsaturated, but poor in unsaturated fatty acids. *Lancet* i:115–119.

Atwood, N. E. 1883. Unexplained variations in the yield of oil from cod livers. *Bull. U.S. Fish Comm.* 3:431.

Aure, Lars. 1967. Manufacture of fish-liver oil. In *Fish Oils*, ed. Maurice E. Stansby, p. 193. Westport, Conn.: Avi Publishing Co.

Bennett, John Hughes. 1841. *Treatise on the Oleum Jecoris Aselli or Cod Liver Oil.* Edinburg: MacLachlan, Stewart and Co.

Bernsohn, J., and Stephanides, L. M. 1967. Aetiology of multiple sclerosis. *Nature (London)* 215:821–823.

Bodman, J., and Maisin, J. H. 1958. The alpha glyceryl ethers. *Clin. Chim. Acta* 3:253–274.

Brohult, Astrid. 1963. Alkoxyglycerols and their use in radiation treatment. *Acta Radiol., Suppl.* 223:7–99. Stockholm.

Bronte-Stewart, B. A., Antonis, A., Eales, L., and Brock, J. F. 1956. Effects of feeding different fats on serum cholesterol levels. *Lancet* i:521–530.

Chalmers, W., Wood, A. C., Shaw, A. J., and Majnarich, J. J. 1966. Treatment of inflammatory diseases. U.S. Patent 3,294,639, Dec. 27.

Dalton, R. G. 1964. Bracken poisoning. *Vet. Rec., London* 76:411–417.

Delmon, G., and Biraben, J. 1966. Cytostatic activity of an α glyceryl ether against rat carcinoma T8. *Compt. Rend. Soc. Biol.* 160:76–78.

Edlund, T. 1954. Protective effect of *d*,1-α-octadecylglycerol ether in mice given total body x-irradiation. *Nature* 174:1102.

Evans, W. C., Evans, I. A., Edwards, C. M., and Thomas, A. J. 1957. Bracken poisoning of cattle: Therapeutic treatment. *Biochem. J.* 65:6P.

French, J. M. 1984. Max EPA in multiple sclerosis. *Brit. J. Clin. Pract.* 83 #5 Symp. Suppl. 32:117–121.

Gerstl, B., Kahnke, M. J., and Smith, J. K. 1961. Brain lipids in multiple sclerosis and other diseases. *Brain* 84:310.

Gul, S., Smith, A. D., Thompson, R. H. S., Wright, H. P., and Zilka, K. J. 1970. Fatty acid composition of phospholipids from platelets and erythrocytes in multiple sclerosis. *J. Neural Neurosurg. Psychiat.* 33:506.

Hauge, J. G., and Nicolaysen, R. 1959. The serum cholesterol depressive effect of linoleate, linolenic acids and of cod liver oil in experimental hypercholesterolemic rats. *Acta Physiol. Scand.* 45:26–30.

Howe, E. E., and Bosshardt, D. K. 1962A. A study of experimental hypercholesterolemia in the mouse. *J. Nutr.* 76:242–246.

Howe, E. E., and Bosshardt, D. K. 1962B. Effect of thyroid-active substances on plasma cholesterol in the mouse. *J. Nutr.* 77:161–164.

Kahn, S. G., Vandeputte, J., Wind, S., and Yacowitz, H. 1963. A study of the hypocholesterolemic activity of the ethyl esters of the polyunsaturated fatty acids of cod-liver oil in the chicken. I. Effect on serum cholesterol. *J. Nutr.* 80:403–413.

Kaneda, T., and Alfin-Slater, R. B. 1963. A comparison of the effects of the polyunsaturated fatty acids of cuttle fish liver oil and cottonseed oil on cholesterol metabolism. *J. Am. Oil Chemists' Soc.* 40:336–338.

Keys, A. 1980. *Seven Countries: A Multivariate Analysis of Death and Coronary Heart Disease.* Cambridge: Harvard University Press.

Kingsbury, K. J. 1964. Personal communication.

Kingsbury, K. J., Aylott, C., Morgan, D. M., and Emmerson, R. 1961. Effects of ethyl arachidonate, cod-liver oil and corn oil on the plasma cholesterol level. *Lancet* i:739–741.

Kishimoto, Y., Radin, N. S., Tourtellotte, W. W., Parker, J. A., and Itabashi, H. H. 1967. Gangliosides and glycerophospholipids in multiple sclerosis white matter. *Arch. Neurol., Chicago* 16:44–54.

Kromhout, Daan, Bosschieter, Edward B., and Coulander, Cor de Lezenne. 1985. The inverse relation between fish consumption and 20-year mortality from coronary heart disease. *New England J. Med.* 312:1206–1209.

Malins, D. C., and Varanasi, U. 1972. The ether bond in marine lipids. In *Ether Lipids— Chemistry and Biology*, ed. Fred Snyder, pp. 297–312. New York: Academic Press.

Malmros, H., and Wigand, G. 1957. Effects on serum cholesterol of diets containing different fats. *Lancet* ii:1–7.

Miller, S. A., Dymaza, A., and Goldblith, S. A. 1962. Cholesterolemia and cardiovascular sudanophilia in rats fed sardine mixtures. *J. Nutr.* 77:397–402.

Nelson, Averly M. 1972. Diet therapy in coronary disease—Effects on mortality of high protein, high seafood, fat controlled diet. *Geriatrics* 27:103–116.

Peifer, J. J. 1967. Hypercholesterolemic effects of marine oils. In *Fish Oils*, ed. M. E. Stansby, pp. 322–361. Westport, Conn.: Avi Publishing Co.

Peifer, J. J., Janssen, F., Ahn, P., Cox, W., and Lundberg, W. O. 1960. Studies on the distribution of lipids in hypercholesterolemic rats. 1. The effects of feeding palmitate, oleate, linoleate, linolenate, menhaden, and tuna oils. *Arch. Biochem. Biophys.* 86:302–308.

Peifer, J. J., Janssen, F., Muesing, R., and Lundberg, W. O. 1962. The lipid depressant activities of whole fish and their component oils. *J. Am. Oil Chemists' Soc.* 39:292–296.

Peifer, J. J., Lundberg, W. O., Ishio, S., and Warmanen, E. 1965. Studies on distribution of lipids in hypercholesterolemic rats. 3. Changes in hypercholesterolemia and tissue fatty acids induced by dietary fats and marine oil fractions. *Arch. Biochem. Biophys.* 110:270–283.

Percival, Thomas. 1783. Observations on the medicinal uses of the oleum jeconis aselli or cod liver oil in the chronic rheumatism and other painful disorders. *London Med. J.* 3(4):393–401.

Presthus, J. 1962. Report on multiple sclerosis investigations in west Norway. *Acta Psychiat. Neurol. Scand.* (Suppl. 47):88–92.

Rosenberg, H. R. 1942. *Chemistry and Physiology of the Vitamins*, p. 8. New York: Interscience.

Schütte, D. 1824. Beobachtungen über den nutzen des bergen lebertrans (oleum jecoris aselli von gadus aselli L). *Arch. Med. Erfahr.*

Snyder, F. 1969. The biochemistry of lipids containing ether bonds. In *Progress in the Chemistry of Fats and Other Lipids*, vol. 30, pt. 3, ed. Ralph T. Holman, pp. 289–335. Oxford: Pergamon Press.

Stansby, M. E., Zollman, P. E., and Winkleman, R. K. 1967. Efficacy of fish oils in healing wounds and burns. *Fish. Ind. Res.* 3(4):25–46.

Stevenson, Charles H. 1902. Oil from livers of cod and related species. *Report of the Commissioner of Fish and Fisheries*, pp. 216–226.

Strøm, Axel. 1948. Examination into the diet of Norwegian families during the war years 1942–45. *Acta Med. Scand. Suppl.*:1–47.

Strøm, Axel, and Jensen, R. A. 1951. Mortality from circulation diseases in Norway 1940–1945. *Lancet* i:126–129.

Sviridov, N.K., Abaturova, E. A., Shubina, A. V., and Elpt'Evskay, G. N. 1954. *Patogenez Experim Profilactica i Terapiya Luchevykh Porazhenii SB*, p. 254.

Swank, R. L. 1988. Multiple sclerosis: The lipid relationship. *Am. J. Clin. Nutr.* 48:1387–1393.

Swank, R. L., and Backer, J. 1950. Geographic incidence of multiple sclerosis in Norway. *Trans. Am. Neurol. A.* 75:274.

Swank, Lerstad O., Strøm, A., and Backer, J. 1952. Multiple sclerosis in rural Norway: Its geographical and occupational incidence in relation to nutrition. *New England J. Med.* 246:721–728.

Thompson, R. H. S. 1966. Protective effect of d,1-α-octadecylglycerol ether in mice given x-irradiation. *Proc. Royal Soc. Med.* 59:269–276.

Tsujimoto, M., and Toyama, Y. 1922. Unsaponifiable constituents (higher alcohols) of the liver oil of sharks and rays. *Chem. Umschau* 29:27–29, 43–45.

Wood, J. D., Biely, J., and Topliff, J. E. 1961. The effect of diet, age and sex on cholesterol metabolism in white leghorn chickens. *Can. J. Biochm.* 39:1705–1715.

Chapter 11
NUTRITIONAL PROPERTIES OF FISH OIL FOR HUMAN CONSUMPTION— MODERN ASPECTS

Maurice E. Stansby

INTRODUCTION

This chapter, in contrast to Chapter 10, covers more recent work carried out after the mechanism of involvement of ω3 fatty acids became suspected as a possible reason for certain effects of fish oils on diseases. Included in this chapter is a section on mechanism for altering arachidonate through a series of reactions, which was first carried out primarily to account for the action of drugs such as aspirin. A section is included on developments on ω3 action on cardiac diseases, and another section deals with effects on diseases other than those related to heart attacks. Another section of the chapter deals with major meetings at which reports on effects of ω3 fatty acids on disease were presented. Another short section lists several bibliographic reference sources. Finally, short summaries are given regarding our present state of knowledge on ω3 fatty acids, first on cardiac diseases then on other diseases.

RESEARCH ON PROSTANOID MECHANISMS

Preceding the investigations relating to the effects of fish oil ω3 fatty acids on disease was a period of time when intensive research was under way to unravel the facts that would lead to a better understanding of the action of aspirin as well as that of several other related drugs. Linoleic acid, a very common component of much human food, is metabolized to arachidonic acid. In this early work it was assumed that arachidonic acid probably was the starting point for a series of reactions involving various eicosanoids. In 1971, the results of some of this intensive research on aspirin were published simultaneously in two papers. One of these (Smith and Willis 1971), which was carried out with human subjects, showed that volunteers who had taken aspirin ended up with a reduced level of certain prostaglandins. This resulted in a condition where there was a great diminution in aggregation of their blood platelets. These results were bolstered by another paper, by Vane (1971), which gave similar results when guinea pigs were used. The conversion of arachidonate in these animals to prostaglandins was studied when aspirin was present or absent.

In both of these papers the same inhibition of conversion of the arachidonic acid to certain prostaglandins in the presence of aspirin was noted, a condition resulting in a great reduction in levels of blood platelet aggregation. Both of these papers (which were printed on consecutive pages of the same issue of the journal in which they appeared) were the results of long-term research at the Department of Pharmacology, Institute of Basic Medical Research, Royal College of Surgeons of England in London.

The status of knowledge at the stage reached by 1971 was still not at all complete. In particular, the mechanism causing the effect of aspirin was not at all clearly evident. Several series of experiments were carried out at the Chemistry Department of Karolinska Institute in Stockholm, Sweden (Hamberg et al. 1974B, 1975). They reached the conclusion that the type of substances involved in diminishing the degree of platelet aggregation were PGH_2 endoperoxides. However, additional investigation by Moncada et al. (1976), who were carrying out their research at a commercial drug manufacturer's establishment (Welcome Research Laboratories), showed that the component responsible for the antiaggregatory effect on blood platelets was a prostaglandin, which they named PGI_2. It is now more often referred to as prostacyclin (Moncada and Vane 1981).

ω3'S EFFECTS ON CORONARY DISEASES

Until the 1970s it was generally believed that the sole reason fish oils in the diet were effective in alleviating problems in connection with heart disease was their action, like that of other oils containing polyunsaturated fatty acids, toward lowering serum cholesterol levels. Even the possibility that the long-chain polyunsaturated fatty acids of fish oils might have some unknown beneficial effect was never mentioned. An exception occurred in a 1969 review of the nutritional properties of fish oil (Stansby 1969), where on page 88 it says, "Although fish oil polyunsaturated fatty acids in common with any of the omega-3 type lack certain essential fatty acid properties as exemplified by inability for complete curing of dermal symptoms, there is some indication that these same omega-3 fatty acids may, of themselves possess other functions which are lacking in the omega-6 series," and again, on page 89, "If, indeed, the higher members of the omega-3 fatty acid family such as docosahexaenoic acid are needed for some important function, they already occur preformed in fish oils and it is unnecessary for them to be metabolized from linolenic acid. Thus inclusion of fish or fish oils in the diet insures the presence of the higher members of the omega-3 family for whatever benefit they may impart."

Research in Denmark

The first series of investigations that eventually led to work on ω3 fatty acids in fish oil began in 1970. In that year, Dyerberg, Bang, and coworkers at the Aalborg Hospital, Aalborg, Denmark, became interested in ideas they had heard regarding the possible lower death rate occurring for certain diseases in Greenland, which was then a protectorate of Denmark. They began going over old records dealing with the type of food eaten by inhabitants of Greenland and early articles in the literature on death rates from different diseases. Some of these types of study had been carried out long ago. For example, a paper by Krogh and Krogh (1913) discussed a study carried out in 1908 on the diet and metabolism of Greenland Eskimos. Other, somewhat more recent papers along such lines were published by Berthelsen (1940), Gottman (1960), and Anthaud (1970). It appeared that there was sufficient evidence to warrant further investigation not only into the effect of the diet of the inhabitants of Greenland and its effect on disease but also as to the mechanism that caused such effects. Accordingly, workers at the Aalborg Hospital began a long-term study along these lines.

Investigators from Aalborg Hospital made several trips to Greenland and collected typical food samples of what the Eskimos consume. These were examined in Denmark and several papers published. Workers examined the Eskimo food and compared it to that of typical Danes (Bang and Dyerberg 1972; Dyerberg et al. 1975). They noted what had been known for a very long time—that Eskimos are bleeders (Bang and Dyerberg 1980; Norman-Hansen 1911; Meldorf 1904). One individual, the early arctic explorer Peter Freuchen, even suggested that this bleeding tendency might be due to the diet of the Eskimos (Freuchen 1915).

Putting together all these various observations, the group from Aalborg Hospital decided it was quite possible that the ω3 fatty acids in marine oil might act in a manner similar to that which occurs from aspirin and related drugs. After a few preliminary experiments, they carried out a joint investigation with several of the individuals who had been working on the aspirin problem. This project indicated more definitely that this was probably the case (Dyerberg et al. 1978).

Research in Japan

Another situation analogous to that of the Greenland Eskimo diet and its effect on heart disease is that occurring in Japan. Families of fishermen living along the coast, where they ate much more fish than other Japanese families, have a decreased incidence of coronary disease. This situation has been investigated by scientists at various laboratories in Japan. One of the most complete such investigations the findings of which are probably typical is the one carried out at the Department of Internal Medicine, Chiba University School of Medicine, Chiba, Japan, beginning in 1980. This program is well covered in a 16-page review article by Hirai et al. (1987). Only the highlights will be discussed here.

This Japanese program had three segments: (1) to develop information about the relationship between dietary ingestion of eicosapentaenoic acid (EPA) and incidence of coronary disease; (2) to determine the effects of consumption of highly purified EPA and docosahexaenoic acid (DHA); and (3) to carry out research on the effects of EPA in patients with thrombotic diseases. In this research, results were sometimes compared between individuals living in a fishing village where EPA consumption averaged 2.6 g EPA per day with those living in a farming village where average EPA was about 0.9 g EPA per day. The average deaths from coronary disease were considerably higher in the farming village than in the fishing village.

It was shown that EPA built up (after ingestion) in the phosphatidyl choline (PC) and phosphatidyl ethanolamine (EC) fractions of platelets, but the DHA did not. It was believed, however, that a considerable portion of the DHA was converted to EPA. For example, after four weeks' ingestion of DHA, a marked increase in the DHA content in PC and PE platelets occurred. The investigators concluded that both EPA and DHA contribute to antithrombotic action, although probably a somewhat different mechanism was involved for these two fatty acids. DHA seemed somewhat less effective than EPA in this regard.

A large-scale clinical study was carried out in which highly concentrated eicosapentaenoic acid ethyl ester (EPA-E) made from sardine oil was used. The clinical study was conducted with 62 patients (average age 59 years) who were suffering from various cerebrovascular and coronary diseases. The study was carried out over a 16-week period with daily doses of EPA-E being fed at levels between 1.8 and 2.7 g, depending upon the patient's body weight. Many tests such as platelet aggregation, TXB_2 production, platelet retention, bleeding time and serum lipid levels were measured. The results of this clinical test can be summarized as follows. Intake of 1.8 g per day or more of EPA can efficiently suppress platelet functions such as platelet aggregation, bleeding time, and certain rheological properties of blood and serum lipid profile. The minimum duration for intake of EPA to achieve such results is four weeks. It should be remembered that in this particular clinical test the patients were not all ones suffering from coronary diseases but also included others such as ones with cerebro-type diseases.

General Summary.
1. The intake of fish in fishing villages in Japan is two to three times as great as those living in farming-type villages, and the mortality rate due to ischemic heart disease and cerebrovascular diseases is lower in the fishing areas than in the farming areas.
2. The intake of both EPA and DHA, when taken in purified form (as EPA-E or DHA-E), each exhibits antithrombotic action, though by somewhat different mechanisms. DHA is somewhat less active than EPA.
3. In a clinical study as little as 1.8 g per day was sufficient when taken for four weeks or more to suppress such platelet functions by platelet aggregation.

Research in the United States

The largest portion of the research carried out in the United States on the effects of $\omega3$ fatty acids on coronary disease has been carried out at the University of Oregon in Portland, Oregon, by W. E. Connor and various co-workers such as Goodnight, Harris, Illingworth, and others. Connor began work at the University of Iowa on the effects of polyunsaturated fatty acids on coronary problems long before he began work at the University of Oregon. Much of his early work, which covered a wide range of topics, is summarized in a long paper (Connor and Connor 1972). Among other aspects of his work at that time were the effects of consumption of shellfish (particularly shrimp) on cholesterol uptake (Connor et al. 1963). This work showed that cholesterol could be picked up when shrimp were consumed. In this paper it was stated that all crustaceans contain large amounts of cholesterol. At this early period analytical methods for cholesterol actually included as cholesterol other harmless sterols. Whereas shrimp does contain about three to four times as much cholesterol as most fin fish, many other crustaceans may contain high quantities of other sterols yet are not always high in cholesterol.

When in 1975 Connor began work at the University of Oregon at Portland as director of the Lipid Atherosclerosis Laboratory, he and his co-workers in this group spent much of their time looking thoroughly into the relationship between dietary $\omega3$ oils and coronary aspects. Since 1975 dozens of papers have appeared by members of this group. The large volume of this research is far too great to cover here in any detail, but a few examples will be mentioned.

In his research in the 1960s at the University of Iowa, Connor carried out work on the consumption of shrimp, which was rightly described as being relatively high in cholesterol. It also implied that other shellfish were high in cholesterol and would result in equally undesirable effects. One of the aspects of the work covered early at the University of Oregon Laboratory was tests using men who consumed several different shellfish (Connor and Lin 1982). By this time analytical techniques had been developed so that cholesterol and other sterols could be accurately measured.

In this work, it was shown that even when very large amounts of clams, oysters, or scallops (1 lb per day) were fed, no increase in plasma cholesterol levels occurred. These shellfish contain considerable quantities of sterols other than cholesterol, yet the cholesterol levels are relatively low (50–60 mg per 100 g). On the other hand, in crab, lobster, and especially shrimp, the sterols are almost all cholesterol. When large quantities (about 1 lb per day) of these are consumed, the serum cholesterol level rises but only to a relatively small extent. From these experimental results it appears that if one consumes shellfish to anything like a reasonable extent, there is no likelihood of their causing any undue effect on serum cholesterol levels.

Connor and Connor (1989) have published a long review paper on diet, atherosclerosis, and fish oil. They discuss how dietary cholesterol enters the body via the chylomicron pathway and is removed as a component of chylomicron remnants. The major portion of this report, however, deals with the effects of fat, particularly $\omega 3$ fatty acids. The paper describes work not only carried out in the author's program but also, to some extent, that of others. Much of their own work was carried out with salmon on salmon oil, and in this regard it differs from that of most other research.

A portion of very recent research coming from the program at the University of Oregon concerns not effects on heart disease but rather changes within the retina and brain resulting from the presence of $\omega 3$ fatty acids. This work will be discussed in a later section.

A considerable number of other investigators in the United States are carrying out research concerning the effects of fish oil and its content of $\omega 3$ fatty acids on human or animal health. Some of these will be discussed in later sections of this chapter.

Activities of the National Marine Fisheries Service. The National Marine Fisheries Service (NMFS) of the U.S. Department of Commerce has a memorandum of understanding with two other U.S. governmental agencies, the National Institutes of Health (NIH) and the Alcohol, Drug, and Mental Health Agency (ADAMHA). Under this agreement the NMFS Laboratory at Charleston, South Carolina, will provide a long-term, consistent supply of test materials in order to facilitate the evaluation of the role of $\omega3$ fatty acids in health and disease. A subcommittee, Nutrition Coordinating Committee, of NIH, the Fish Oil Test Materials Advisory Committee, provides the review and approval mechanism for the distribution of quality-assured/quality-controlled test materials (Van Dolah and Galloway 1988) to researchers. The applicants are researchers who are funded by NIH, ADAMHA, and other research organizations.

The methods used for preparing the test materials—which may consist, for example, of fish oil fatty acid concentrate mixtures or purified individual $\omega3$ fatty acids—were developed in part by procedures developed at the Charleston Laboratory and at two other NMFS Laboratories, one at Gloucester, Massachusetts, and one at Seattle (Stout and Spinelli 1987; Spinelli et al. 1987). At the Charleston Laboratory a new wing of the building was constructed containing very large-scale equipment for manufacturing large quantities of the test materials. This new unit was dedicated on September 16, 1988.

Research In Other Countries

In England a relatively large number of $\omega3$ investigations were stimulated by the offer of the Seven Seas Health Care Ltd., manufacturer of $\omega3$ capsules (MAXEPA) to furnish to research groups free samples of their product. Other than the fact that MAXEPA contains about 18% EPA and 12% DHA any further analysis has been unavailable. In some instances investigators have made their own fatty acid profile, but there was indication that the fatty acid composition of MAXEPA may have varied over a period of years. Most of the investigations from this work involving the use of MAXEPA capsules involved supplying patients in a hospital with varying numbers of MAXEPA capsules and then measuring certain effects to determine how much these effects varied from patients not taking the MAXEPA. When if, as in most cases, the effect on coronary disease was at issue, changes were noted in such factors as the patients' bleeding time, degree of platelet aggregation, and serum lipid levels. Results of many of these British MAXEPA studies have been reported at a MAXEPA research conference (Durie 1984).

The results of these many tests have in general supported other previous studies, showing that when $\omega3$ MAXEPA tablets are consumed, bleeding time is increased and other indications show that platelet aggregation is diminished. In addition to the various tests in Great Britain based on use of MAXEPA capsules, of course, many other investigations have been and are being carried out (e.g., Sanders 1985).

In Canada a great deal of research on fish oils in general has been carried out by R. G. Ackman and associates at the Technical University of Nova Scotia in Halifax. Earlier, Ackman had been in charge of all fish oil work at the Canadian government's laboratory in Halifax (now discontinued). The largest portion of Ackman's research has been related to the analysis of fatty acids and the development of methods for their extraction or concentration from fish. He has undoubtedly done more research in this field than anyone else anywhere. In the Selected Bibliography on Fish Oils (Bauersfeld and Winemiller 1985), covering all research on fish oils from 1878 to September 1985, Ackman is listed as senior author of 197 research papers. This does not include many others of which he was a junior author.

Much of what is known today about the fatty acids in fish has resulted from research by Ackman. An example of his expertise in this area is the 63-page chapter published in a book (Ackman 1982).

Other research goes on elsewhere in Canada. For example, several papers have been published from the Department of Nutritional Sciences, University of Guelph in Ontario; for example, Mahadevappa and Holub (1987).

In Germany considerable research has been carried out by P.C. Weber and co-workers at the University of Munich. In their work, they frequently used mackerel as a source of $\omega 3$ fatty acids. Cod-liver oil has also been used. These investigators devised new theories regarding the chemical mechanism involved during the formation of eicosanoids in humans from $\omega 3$ fatty acids, based on a phospholipid fraction (von Shacky et al. 1985). This theory is enlarged upon by Weber et al. (1986).

Of course in the many other countries not mentioned above, quite a few investigations on $\omega 3$ and heart disease have been carried out. Examples of these are Nestel et al. (1987), in Australia; Hornstra (many references, e.g., Hornstra 1984) in the Netherlands; Budowski (1988) in Israel; Gibney and Connolly (1988) in the Irish Republic; Tilvis et al. (1987) in Finland; and Sametz and Juan (1985) in Austria. It is thus evident that research is being conducted worldwide on various aspects of the effects of $\omega 3$ fatty acids and fish oils on coronary disease.

EFFECTS OF $\omega 3$ FATTY ACIDS ON DISEASES OTHER THAN THOSE OF THE HEART

By far the greatest amount of research on $\omega 3$ fatty acids and disease has been carried out on the effects on heart disease. Nevertheless there have been and continue to be considerable efforts made to investigate effects of fish oil and its content of long-chain ω3 fatty acids upon many other diseases. In fact research has proceeded on so many different such types of diseases that, although on the whole a great many papers have been published, the amount of work on any one such disease is still far from being nearly as adequate as is the case for coronary heart diseases. Furthermore, research on mechanism of the action of ω3 fatty acids in these other diseases is at present at such an early stage that it will doubtlessly be a very long time before we have as good an idea of what is going on as is now known about the mechanism of the reactions for coronary-type diseases.

Inflammation Diseases

A good introductory article to the action, in general, that results in diminishing the undesirable effects of inflammatory diseases has been published by Higgs (1986). Higgs is connected with Welcome Laboratories, which carries out research for the British drug industry, so his approach is a very general one and does not include discussion of ω3 fatty acids. His paper considers the role of both prostaglandins and leukotrienes. With respect to leukotrienes he points out that Hammarstrom et al. (1975) were the first to show that lipoxygenase activity occurs in inflammation. He discusses in some detail the role of the mechanism causing inflammatory diseases, but it is obvious that present knowledge is insufficient to give a complete picture of what is going on.

Rheumatoid Arthritis.   As mentioned in Chapter 10, as early as the 1780s a 10-year study had shown that arthritis could be very beneficially affected by consumption of cod-liver oil. In that study, nothing was known about the mechanism of this effect, yet the study clearly demonstrated that the consumption of a fish liver oil could greatly diminish the progress of arthritis.

A number of investigations, starting in the late 1970s, have seemed to indicate that these 200-year-old findings had a definite reason for occurring; probably the most recent study of Kremer and Jubiz (1987) gives the best proof based on modern research methods that rheumatoid arthritis can be benefited by the consumption of fish oil. Thirty-three patients, all of whom had had rheumatoid arthritis for an average of 13 years, were fed for 14 weeks either MAXEPA or placebo capsules. The MAXEPA capsules provided 2.7 g of eicosapentaenoic acid and 1.8 g of docosahexaenoic acid per day. After 14 weeks all patients were fed placebo tablets. Then for the final 14 weeks, those who initially had been taking the MAXEPA were fed placebo tablets and those who initially had been taking the placebo tablets were fed MAXEPA tablets. In all cases, at the end of 14 weeks all of the patients who had been taking the MAXEPA showed a decrease in the number of tender joints. Also the time after awakening in the morning before the first symptoms of joint stiffness occurred was increased for those who had been taking the MAXEPA tablets.

Nephritis. Studies have been made recently involving inflammation of the kidney. Two studies using animals were made, one by Thais and Stahl (1987), the other by Robinson et al. (1987) using rats and mice, respectively. In the first of these two studies the source of the ω3 fatty acids was cod-liver oil, that of the second one being menhaden oil. In each case there was a significant reduction in the severity of glomerular nephritis when fish oil was included in the diet.

Lupus Erythematosis. This disease has symptoms ranging from a minor skin disorder to severe kidney damage. Several investigations, including those by Kelley et al. (1985) and by Accinni and Dixon (1979), have indicated that ω3 fatty acids or fish oil can favorably affect this disease.

Multiple Sclerosis. As mentioned in Chapter 10, there is considerable evidence, based largely on statistics, concerning the incidence of multiple sclerosis in different countries where the diet differs which seems to show that the presence of much ω3 in the diet may possibly result in a lower incidence of this disease.

Very recently a paper (Bates et al. 1989) was published involving a long-term study of 292 individuals, all of whom had multiple sclerosis; about half consumed ω3 concentrates and the other half did not. The results indicated that although the difference was not significant at the usual 95% confidence level, nevertheless there was a trend in favor of the group taking fish oil. For example, after two years, 79 patients were the same or better compared to 65 in the control group. Also 82 control patients were worse compared to 66 in the group consuming fish oil.

Strokes

Among Greenland Eskimos, strokes were one of the leading causes of death. When comparing the incidence of chronic diseases in Greenland as compared to those among Danes, Kromann and Green (1980) observed 25 cases in Greenland, whereas among Danes the rate would have been anticipated as only 15. This would seem to indicate that the high consumption of ω3 long-chain fatty acids, which have been assumed to be a primary cause for reduction in deaths in Greenland from heart disease, did not have an analogous effect on strokes.

On the other hand, studies conducted in Japan by Hirai et al. (1987) indicated that among Japanese, consumption of $\omega 3$ fatty acids was of value both for volunteer participants suffering from either heart disease or incidence of strokes. In this experiment the participants, some who had problems with strokes and some with heart disease, were selected from two areas. One group was from fishing villages, where consumption of fish was very high. The other group was from a farming area, where relatively little fish was consumed. It is stated that "the mortality rate due to ischemic heart disease and cerebrovascular disease was lower in the fishing area than in the farming area." Of course it is entirely possible that in Japan there are factors other than diet that might bear upon the difference between mortality rates in the fishing versus farming areas and that did not apply to conditions in Greenland.

Another possible beneficial effect of $\omega 3$ fatty acids on strokes is the possibility that consumption of $\omega 3$ fatty acids, quite regardless of whether it might reduce mortality rates due to strokes, might have a beneficial effect in reducing the damage done to cerebral tissue. Based on experiments conducted on animals (strokes in cats), Lands (1982) showed that such reduced tissue damage did occur. This might also apply to humans with strokes. Thus consumption of fish oil $\omega 3$ fatty acids may reduce tissue damage following a stroke whether or not it would affect mortality rates.

Budowski (1988) suggests that $\omega 3$ fatty acids may act by modification of leukocyte function via inhibition of the lipoxygenase pathway.

Cancer

The fact that prostaglandins may be involved in cancer has been known for some time. Williams et al. (1968) were probably the first to mention this as a possibility. Since then a fair amount of research has been carried out, much of it dealing with breast cancer. Karmeli (1987), who has herself conducted considerable research along this line, has reviewed results on cancer research to date. As she points out, epidemiological investigations have shown a relationship between the amount and type of dietary fat and mortality from breast cancer.

A number of projects have looked into the mechanism leading to the effect of fish oils (e.g., menhaden oil or fish oil concentrates such MAX-EPA) toward reducing incidents of fatal breast cancer. In most instances, as with coronary disease, apparently eicosapentaenoic acid alters the oxidative mechanism so as to increase the formation of prostaglandins favorable toward reducing the incidence of breast cancer. The results so far accumulated are not, however, so well understood as is the case with coronary events. Considerably more work is needed.

In addition to research studies on breast cancer carried out by Karmeli both at the Memorial Sloan-Kettering Cancer Center and more recently at the Department of Nutrition, Rutgers University, other projects along similar lines are under way elsewhere. For example, Carter et al. (1987), at Roswell Park Memorial Institute, have a study along these lines, as do Cohen (1987) at the Naylor Dana Institute for Disease Prevention, Stampfer et al. (1987) at Harvard, and Cave and Jurkowski (1987) at the University of Rochester School of Medicine. Some of these projects carry out research with animals, others with humans. When further progress has been made at these and other investigational institutes, we should know a great deal more about this subject.

Breast cancer is not the only type of cancer on which ω3 fatty acids or fish oil may have favorable effects. Another field where work is well under way is the investigation of effects on colon cancer. A brief review of this field has been made by Reddy (1987). As he indicates, the first suggestion that the type of dietary fat might be of significance came from a paper by Wynder and Shigematsu (1967). This was followed by work carried out by Hill et al. (1971), which showed definitely that the type of dietary fat could beneficially affect the incidence of colon cancer. Since 1980 Reddy and co-workers have published a series of papers. These papers show that menhaden oil in the diet results in less colon cancer than when it is absent and the main dietary fat is corn or sunflower oil or lard or beef tallow. It is believed that the fish oil may possibly promote the formation of certain prostaglandins that could inhibit the development of colon cancer. Similar research by several other laboratory groups are also under way; see for example, Broitman et al. (1987).

Skin Diseases

A small amount of research has been carried out indicating that probably dietary fish oils or ω3 fatty acids may be of value in alleviating certain skin diseases. Two papers, Bradlow et al. (1985) and Ziboh et al. (1985), indicate that psoriasis can be relieved by dietary intake of sources of ω3 fatty acids. In neither of these studies was the extent of relief great, but it was of statistical significance.

Rhodes (1984) describes some experiments in which individuals suffering from eczema were treated either by feeding them MAXEPA tablets or by applying externally a salve containing MAXEPA. In both cases some improvement was obtained over controls who did not have any MAXEPA treatment.

It also might be noted that when the degree of psoriasis suffered by Danish individuals is compared to that of Greenland Eskimos, there is 20 times as great an incidence in the population of the Danes as for the Eskimos (Kromann and Green 1980).

Hypertension

There is considerable evidence indicating that individuals consuming fish oil or $\omega3$ fatty acids ordinarily may have lower blood pressure than those who do not. This subject is well treated in Chapter 9 of Lands (1986).

$\omega3$ Fatty Acid and the Brain and Retina

Although it has long been known that the $\omega3$ fatty acid docosahexaenoic acid was involved with the retina, until recently few comprehensive investigations have been made linking $\omega3$ fatty acids to the retina or to certain needs of the brain. Recently such a paper has been published (Neuringer et al. 1988). This paper suggests that $\omega3$ fatty acids carry out certain functions in the brain and retina that cannot be accomplished by $\omega6$ fatty acids, and that, thus, $\omega3$ fatty acids should be classified as essential fatty acids. Connor (1989) has suggested that this field of research, involving $\omega3$ fatty acids and certain applications to functioning in the brain and retina, may possibly be of greater significance than their application to their effects in various diseases. He believes that in the future much more research will be carried out on the action of $\omega3$ fatty acids in the brain.

MEETINGS FOR DISCUSSIONS AND PRESENTATIONS ON EFFECTS OF $\omega3$ FATTY ACIDS

There have been a number of meetings at which papers were presented on effects of $\omega3$ fatty acids on health and disease. Usually after each such meeting a book containing the papers given at the meeting is printed. In this section, information is given on five such major meetings.

The first such meeting was held in London in October 1981 and was entitled Nutritional Evaluation of Long-Chain Fatty Acids in Fish Oil. This meeting was held to discuss the possible harmful effects of consuming fish oils that contain the monoene fatty acid with 22 carbons and one double bond. The fatty acid of this type that occurs in fish oil by far to the largest extent is cetoleic acid. In vegetable oils, particularly in rapeseed oil, there was at one time a different C22 : 1 fatty acid, erucic acid. It is an isomer of the cetoleic acid which occurs in fish oils. At that time, it was known that erucic acid could be quite harmful. The question arose as to whether the cetoleic acid which occurred naturally in fish oils and which during hydrogenation might form, would in any way simulate the harmful results that occurred with the consumption of rapeseed oil with its content of the harmful erucic acid. Nearly all of the papers given at that meeting dealt with this problem.

Since the meeting was largely devoted to the possibility of potentially harmful effects of fish oil, the sponsors of the meeting decided it would be well to include some papers on potentially valuable components of fish oil. The work in the previous decade carried out largely in Denmark on $\omega 3$ fatty acids was not at that time as generally known as it is today. Therefore, three papers were presented at the end of the meeting. One of these was by Dyerberg, who had been playing an important role in the work with Greenland Eskimos. Another paper was by Lands, who was one of the first investigators in the United States to look into the nutritional properties of $\omega 3$ fatty acids. The third paper dealt with the early work of Averly Nelson, whose 20-year study involving consumption of fish oils showed a greatly lowered mortality rate from heart disease. Nelson had published his work in a relatively obscure journal and had died almost at the same time as its publication, so his results were almost unknown. Maurice Stansby, who had been in close contact with Nelson and was quite familiar with his project, wrote a short chapter on Nelson's work.

The results of this meeting were published in 1982 (Barlow and Stansby 1982). The inclusion of the above-mentioned three chapters drew the attention of the scientific community to the need for more work on $\omega 3$ fatty acids of fish and their relation to heart disease. It was, therefore, planned to hold some future meetings to be devoted exclusively to these aspects.

The next major meeting held to discuss research on effects of $\omega 3$ fatty acids on health and disease was a conference at Hull College of Higher Education at Hull, England. It was sponsored by Seven Seas Health Care Limited (manufacturers of MAXEPA), and the meeting took place on June 20–22, 1983. It was attended by 46 individuals, 45 of whom were from Great Britain and one from West Germany. A total of 24 talks were given. These were presented under the following sessions: I. Background; II. Platelet Function and MAXEPA; III. MAXEPA and Lipid Metabolism; and IV. Wider Aspects of $\omega 3$ Nutrition. Diseases covered included coronary heart diseases, eczema, multiple sclerosis, and high blood pressure.

The papers presented at this meeting were edited by Durie and published by the *British Journal of Clinical Practice* as supplement 31 to volume 38, number 5, 1984 (Durie 1984). The third such major meeting was held at Reading, England, July 16–18, 1984. It was sponsored by General Mills Co., the United States Department of Commerce (Fish and Wildlife Service), the International Association of Fish Meal Manufacturers, Merck Co., Sharpe and Dolme Co., Seven Seas Health Care Ltd., and R. P. Scherer Corp., and it was entitled Conference on N-3 Fatty Acids. There were 91 attendees from as far away as Australia and Japan, and 37 papers were presented on a wide range of topics. These papers were never published, but all attendees received a copy of an elaborate program of 142 pages containing copies of each of the papers presented at the meeting.

The fourth major presentation was held in Washington, D.C., June 24–26, 1985. It was sponsored by the National Institute of Health's Nutrition Coordination Committee, by the National Marine Fisheries Service (NOAA, U.S. Department of Commerce), and by the National Fisheries Institute. There were 21 papers presented dealing with a wide range of topics. These papers were all published in book form by Simopoulos et al. (1986).

The fifth major presentation was held in Biloxi, Mississippi, May 14–17, 1987. It was called AOAC Short Course on Polyunsaturated Fatty Acids and Eicosanoids (1987). The designation "short course" is probably misleading because it actually consisted of 35 papers, each presented by a scientist, plus 59 poster presentations. A great many aspects of the subject were covered at this meeting. For example, effects of ω3 fatty acids on coronary diseases and on many other diseases such as arthritis, nephritis, breast cancer, eczema, psoriasis, and asthma were discussed. The papers presented at this meeting were published in a book edited by Lands (1987).

BIBLIOGRAPHICAL REFERENCES

Undoubtedly the most voluminous set of bibliographical references on fish oil is one entitled "A Selected Bibliography on Fish Oils" by Bauersfeld and Winemiller (1985). This bibliography covers all references on fish oil articles published from 1878 to 1985. A total of 5700 articles are listed. As an example, the author listed with the largest number of publications on fish oils is Dr. Robert Ackman, and he has references to 285 publications in this bibliography. This publication has two disadvantages. Many of the references of interest to nutritional properties such as of ω3 fatty acids have been published since 1985. Also the listings are arranged alphabetically by author with no reference to the subject covered other than what is in the title of the paper. Although this bibliography was published in 1985, the authors have been updating it frequently. Unfortunately, none of the updated versions has, as yet, been published.

Another bibliography, published in 1988, is available. Not only is it more current with respect to recently published articles, but also the subject of the articles is not fish oils in general but rather the effects of ω3 fatty acids on health and disease. It is a part of a review article on this subject (Budowski 1988). At the end of the article there is a list of 299 references.

Another similar bibliography covers the subject of ω3 fatty acids essential for the retina and the brain (Neuringer et al. 1988). It contains a reference section with a listing of 170 references.

A large number of references each with abstracts of the content of that reference is given in a popular-type book by Miller et al. (1984).

SUMMARY

Effects of ω3 Fatty Acids on Coronary Disease

The research on effects of ω3 fatty acids on heart disease is now so well documented that there can be very little doubt that such a relationship exists. As has been shown in this chapter, there is a wealth of detail now known about the mechanisms whereby arachidonate present in various foods is converted to a number of eicosanoids and how these, in turn, can result in a variety of prostaglandins which in different ways affect the aggregatory action on platelets. Much research has shown that when ω3 fatty acids are present in the diet, a significant reduction in platelet aggregation occurs which in turn can reduce the possibility of heart attacks. Research along these lines has confirmed that reduced levels of incidence of heart attacks among Greenland Eskimos as well as among Japanese fishermen and their families who ate very large amounts of fish were caused by the increased level of ω3 fatty acids in the diet of these people.

Effects of ω3 Fatty Acids on Diseases Other Than Coronary

The amount of research carried out on ω3 fatty acid effects on diseases other than coronary ones is far, far less than that for coronary-type diseases. There are so many different diseases that may be affected by ω3 fatty acids that the amount of research for any one of these many diseases is very small compared to that on heart diseases.

In the future we should expect to see a great deal more research on these other diseases. While there seems to be very little doubt that some of these diseases probably can be benefited by a diet containing ω3 fatty acids, we still know far too little about the mechanism by which such effects can be brought about.

REFERENCES

Accinni, L., and Dixon, F. J. 1979. Degenerative vascular disease and myocardial infarction in mice with lupus-like syndrome. *Am. J. Pathol.* 96:477–492.

Ackman, R. G. 1982. Fatty acid composition of fish oils. In *Nutritional Evaluation of Long-Chain Fatty Acids in Fish Oils*, ed. S. M. Barlow and M. E. Stansby, pp. 25–88. London: Academic Press.

Anthaud, B. 1970. Cause of death in 339 Alaskan natives as determined by autopsy. *Archs. Path.* 90:433–438.

Bang, H. O., and Dyerberg, J. 1972. Plasma lipids and lipoproteins in Greenlandic West Coast Eskimos. *Acta Med. Scand.* 192:85–94.

Bang, H. O., and Dyerberg, J. 1980. The bleeding tendency in Eskimos. *Dan. Med. Bull.* 27:202–205.

Barlow, S. M., and Stansby, M. E. 1982. *Nutritional Evaluation of Long-Chain Fatty Acids in Fish Oil.* London: Academic Press.

Bates, D., Cartlidge, N., French, J. M., Jackson, M. J., Nightingale, S., Shaw, D. A., Smith, S., Woo, E., Hawkins, S. A., Millar, J. H. D., Belin, J., Conroy, D. M., Gill, S. K., Sidey, M., Smith, A. D., Thompson, R. H. S., Zilka, K., Gale, M., and Sinclair, H. M. 1989. A double-blind controlled trial of long chain *n*-3 polyunsaturated fatty acids in the treatment of multiple sclerosis. *J. Neurol., Neurosurg., Psychi.* 52:18–22.

Bauersfeld, P. E., and Winemiller, L. F. 1985. A selected bibliography on fish oils. *NOAA Technical Memorandum,* NMFS-SEFC-166.

Berthelsen, A. 1940. Grønlandsk medicinsk statistik og Nosografi III det saedvanlige grønlandske sigdomsbillede. *Meddr. Grønland* 117:1–234.

Bradlow, B. A., Fretzin, D. F., Rubenstein, D., Newmark, J., Cotter, R., and Matlin, M. 1985. A double-blind trial of *n*-3 fatty acids from fish oil in psoriasis. *International Conference on Leukotrienes and Prostaglandins in Health and Disease,* Tel Aviv and Rehovot, p. 35.

Broitman, S. A., Cannizo, F., Rogers, A., and Gottlieb, L. S. 1987. Comparison of dietary marine oil and safflower oil on growth and pulmonary colonization of CT-26 implanted into bowel of mice. *Federation Proc.* 46:437.

Budowski, P. 1988. Omega-3 fatty acids in health and disease. *World Rev. Nutr. Diet* 57:214–274.

Carter, C. A., Ip, M. M., and Ip, C. 1987. Response of mammary carcinogenesis to dietary linoleate and fat levels and its modulation by prostaglandin synthesis inhibitors. In *Proceedings of the AOAC Short Course on Polyunsaturated Fatty Acids and Eicosanoids,* ed. W. E. M. Lands, pp. 253–260. Champaign, Ill.: American Oil Chemists' Society.

Cave, W. T. Jr., and Jurkowski, J. J. 1987. Comparative effects of omega-3 and omega-6 dietary lipids on rat mammary tumor development. In *Proceedings of the AOAC Short Course on Polyunsaturated Fatty Acids and Eicosanoids,* ed. W. E. M. Lands, pp. 261–266. Champaign, Ill.: American Oil Chemists' Society.

Cohen, L. A. 1987. Differing effects of high-fat diets rich in polyunsaturated, mono-unsaturated or medium chain saturated fatty acids on rat mammary tumor promotion. In *Pro-*

ceedings of the AOAC Short Course on Polyunsaturated Fatty Acids and Eicosanoids, ed. W. E. M. Lands, pp. 241–247. Champaign, Ill.: American Oil Chemists' Society.

Connor, W. E. 1989. Personal communication.

Connor, W. E., and Connor, S. L. 1972. The key role of nutritional factors in the prevention of coronary heart disease. Preventive Med. 1:49–83.

Connor, W. E., and Connor, S. L. 1989. Diet, atherosclerosis and fish oil. In Advances in Internal Medicine, ed. H. Stollerman and M. D. Siperstein. In press.

Connor, W. E., and Lin, D. S. 1982. The effects of shellfish in the diet upon the plasma lipid levels in humans. Metabolism 31:1046–1051.

Connor, W. E., Rohwedder, J. J., and Hook, J. C. 1963. The production of hypercholester-olemia and atherosclerosis by a diet rich in shellfish. J. Nutr. 79:443–450.

Durie, B. 1984. Proceedings of a symposium on MAXEPA research. Brit. J. Clin. Pract. 38, Supplement 31:1–130.

Dyerberg, J., Bang, H. O., and Hjørne, N. 1975. Fatty acid composition of the plasma lipids in Greenland Eskimos. Am. J. Clin. Nutr. 28:958–966.

Dyerberg, J., Bang, H. O., Stoffersen, E., Moncada, S., and Vane, J. R. 1978. Eicosapen-taenoic acid and prevention of thrombosis and atherosclerosis? Lancet ii:117–119.

Freuchen, P. 1915. Om. sundhedstil standen blandt polareskimoer. Ugskr. Laeg. 77:1089–1108.

Gibney, M. J., and Connolly, A. 1988. Uptake of exogenous eicosapentaenoic acid by cultured human mononuclear cells. Brit. J. Nutr. 60:13–20.

Gottmann, A. W. 1960. A report of 103 autopsies on Alaskan natives. Arch. Pathol. 70:117–124.

Hamberg, M., Svensson, J., and Samuelsson, B. 1975. Thromboxanes: A new group of biologically active compounds derived from prostaglandin endoperoxides. Proc. Nat. Acad. Sci. U.S.A. 72:2294–2298.

Hamberg, M., Svensson, J., and Samuelsson, B. 1974A. Prostaglandin endoperoxides. A new concept concerning the mode of action and release of prostaglandins. Proc. Nat. Acad. Sci. U.S.A. 71:3824–3828.

Hamberg, M., Svensson, J., Wakabayashi, T., and Samuelsson, B. 1974B. Isolation and structure of two prostaglandin endoperoxides that cause platelet aggregation. Proc. Nat. Acad. Sci. U.S.A. 71:345–349.

Hammarstrom, M., Hamberg, M., Samuelsson, B., Duell, E. A., Stawiski, M., and Voorhees, J. J. 1975. Increased concentrations of nonesterified arachidonic acid, 12 L hydroxy-5,8,10,14-eicosatetraenoic acid, prostaglandin E_2 and prostaglandin $F_{2\alpha}$ in epidermis of psoriasis. Proc. Nat. Acad. Sci. 72:5130–5134.

Higgs, G. A. 1986. The role of eicosanoids in inflammation. Prog. Lipid Res. 25:555–561.

Hill, M. J., Draser, B. S., Aries, V. C., Crowther, J. S., Hawksworth, G., and Williams, R. E. O. 1971. Bacteria and etiology of cancer of the large bowel. Lancet i:95–100.

Hirai, A., Terano, T., Saito, H., Tamura, Y., and Yoshida, S. 1987. Clinical and epidemiological studies of eicosapentaenoic acid in Japan. In Proceedings of the AOAC Short Course on Polyunsaturated Fatty Acids and Eicosanoids, ed. W. E. M. Lands, pp. 9–24. Champaign, Ill.: American Oil Chemists' Society.

Hornstra, G. 1984. Regulation of prostanoid production by dietary fatty acids. Med. Biol. (Helsinki) 62:261–262.

Karmeli, R. A. 1987. Omega-3 fatty acids and cancer: A review. In Proceedings of the AOAC Short Course on Polyunsaturated Fatty Acids and Eicosanoids, ed. W. E. M. Lands, pp. 222–231. Champaign, Ill.: American Oil Chemists' Society.

Kelley, V. E., Ferritti, A., Izni, S., and Strom, T. B. 1985. A fish oil diet rich in eicosapentaenoic acid reduces cyclooxygenase metabolites, and suppresses lupus in MRL-lpr mice. J. Immunol. 134:1914–1919.

Kremer, J. M., and Jubiz, W. 1987. Fish oil supplementation in active rheumatized arthritis: A double-blinded, controlled crossover study. In *Proceedings of the AOAC Short Course on Polyunsaturated Fatty Acids and Eicosanoids*, ed. W. E. M. Lands. Champaign, Ill.: American Oil Chemists' Society.

Krogh, A., and Krogh, M. 1913. A study of the diet and metabolism of Eskimos undertaken in 1908 on an expedition to Greenland. *Meddr. Grøland* 51:1–45.

Kromann, N., and Green, A. 1980. Epidemiological studies in the Upernavik district, Greenland. *Acta Med. Scand.* 208:401–406.

Lands, W. E. M. 1982. Experiments with strokes produced in cats. In *Nutritional Evaluation of Long-Chain Fatty Acids in Fish Oil*, ed. S. M. Barlow and M. E. Stansby, pp. 273–274. London: Academic Press.

Lands, W. E. M. 1986. *Fish and Human Health*. Orlando, Fla.: Academic Press.

Lands, W. E. M. 1987. *Proceedings of the Short Course on Polyunsaturated Fatty Acids and Eicosanoids*. Champaign, Ill.: American Oil Chemists' Society.

Mahadevappa, V. G., and Holub, B. J. 1987. Quantitive loss of individual eicosapentaenoyl relative to arachidonyl containing phospholipids in thrombin-stimulated human platelets. *J. Lipid Res.* 28:1275–1280.

Meldorf, G. 1904. Tuberkulosens udoredelse i Grønland. 26:211–288.

Miller, T. M., Williams, W. P., Jr., Gresham, V. R., and Wallace, W. B. 1984. *Fatty Fish and Human Nutrition Resource Notebook*. Gulf and South Atlantic Fisheries Development Foundation, Inc. Contract GASAFDI No. 22-19-18500. Available under "Marine Chemurgics" from National Technical Information Service 5285 Port Royal Road, Springfield, Virginia 22161.

Moncada, S., Gryglewski, R., Bunting, S., and Vane, J. R. 1976. An enzyme isolated from arteries transforms prostaglandin endoperoxides to an unstable substance that inhibits platelet aggregation. *Nature (London)* 263:663–665.

Moncada, S., and Vane, J. R. 1981. Prostacyclin: Its biosynthesis, actions and clinical potential. *Philos. Trans. Roy. Soc. London Ser. B*. 294:305–329.

Nestel, P., Topping, D., Marsh, J., Wong, S., Barrett, H., Roach, P., and Kamboris, B. 1987. Effects of polyenoic fatty acids n-3 on lipid and lipoprotein metabolism. In *Proceedings of the AOAC Short Course on Polyunsaturated Fatty Acids*, ed. W. E. M. Lands. Champaign, Ill.: American Oil Chemists' Society.

Neuringer, M., Anderson, G. J., and Connor, W. E. 1988. The essentiality of n-3 fatty acids for the development and function of the retina and brain. *Ann. Rev. Nutr.* 1988:517–541.

Norman-Hansen, C. M. 1911. Ophthalmologiske iagttagelser hos et artisk folk. *Hosp. Tid.* 54:202–205.

O'Connor, T. P., Roebuck, B. D., and Campbell, T. C. 1987. Effect of varying dietary omega-3: Omega-6 fatty acid ratio on L-azerserine induced preneoplastic development. In *Proceedings of the AOAC Short Course on Polyunsaturated Fatty Acids and Eicosanoids*, ed. W. E. M. Lands, pp. 238–240. Champaign, Ill.: American Oil Chemists' Society.

Reddy, B. S. 1987. Dietary fat and colon cancer: Effect of fish oil. In *Proceedings of the AOAC Short Course on Polyunsaturated Fatty Acids and Eicosanoids*, ed. W. E. M. Lands, pp. 233–237. Champaign, Ill.: American Oil Chemists' Society.

Rhodes, E. L. 1984. MAXEPA in the treatment of eczema. *Brit. J. Clin. Pract.* 38 Supplement 31:115–116.

Robinson, D. R., Tateno, S., Patel, B., and Hirai, I. 1987. The effect of dietary marine lipids on autoimmune disease. In *Proceedings of the AOAC Short Course on Polyunsaturated Fatty Acids and Eicosanoids*, ed. W. E. M. Lands, pp. 139–147. Champaign, Ill.: American Oil Chemists' Society.

Sametz, W., and Juan, H. 1985. Influence on a diet rich in eicosapentaenoic acid in the development of raw paw edema and information of prostaglandins I-2 and E-2. *Agents Action* 17:214–219.

Sanders, T. A. B. 1985A. The importance of eicosapentaenoic and docosahexaenoic acids. In *The Role of Fats in Human Nutrition,* ed. P. Padley, pp. 101–116. Chichester: Ellis Harwood.

Sanders, T. A. B. 1985B. Influence of fish-oil supplements on man. *Proc. Nutr. Soc.* 44:391–397.

Simopoulos, A., Kifer, R. R., and Martin, R. E. 1986. *Health Effects of Polyunsaturated Fatty Acids in Seafoods.* Orlando, Fla.: Academic Press.

Smith, J. B., and Willis, A. L. 1971. Aspirin selectively inhibits prostaglandin production in human platelets. *Nature (London) New Biol.* 231:235–238.

Spinelli, J., Stout, V., and Nilsson, W. B. Purification of fish oils. U.S. Patent #4,692,280. Sept. 8, 1987.

Stampfer, M. J., Willett, W. C., Colditz, G. A., Spezer, M. D. 1987. Intake of cholesterol, fish and specific types of fat in relation to breast cancer. In *Proceedings of the AOAC Short Course on Polyunsaturated Fatty Acids and Eicosanoids,* ed. W. E. M. Lands, pp. 248–252. Champaign, Ill.: American Oil Chemists' Society.

Stansby, M. E. 1969. Nutritional properties of fish oils. *World Rev. Nutr. Diet.* 11:46–105.

Stout, V., and Spinelli, J. Polyunsaturated fatty acids from fish oils. U.S. patent #4,675,132. June 23, 1987.

Thais, F., and Stahl, R. A. K. 1987. Effect of dietary fish oil on renal function in immune mediated glomerular injury. In *Proceedings of the AOAC Short Course on Polyunsaturated Fatty Acids and Eicosanoids.* ed. W. E. M. Lands, pp. 123–126. Champaign, Ill.: American Oil Chemists' Society.

Tilvis, R. B., Rasi, V., Viinikka, L., Ylikorkala, O., and Miettinen, T. A. 1987. Effects of purified fish oil on platelet lipids and function in diabetic women. *Clin. Chim. Acta* 164:315–322.

Van Dolah, F. M., and Galloway, S. B. 1988. Biomedical test materials program: Analytical methods for the quality assurance of fish oil. *NOAA Technical Memorandum NMFS-SEFC,* p. 211.

Vane, J. R. 1971. Inhibition of prostaglandin synthesis as a mechanism of action for aspirin-like drugs. *Nature (London) New Biol.* 231:235.

von Schacky, C., Siess, W., Fischer, S., and Weber, P. C. 1985. A comparative study of eicosapentaenoic acid metabolism by human platelets in vivo and in vitro. *J. Lipid Res.* 26:457–464.

Weber, P. C., Fischer, S., von Schacky, C., Lorenz, R., and Strasser, T. 1986. Dietary omega-3 polyunsaturated fatty acids and eicosanoid formation in man. In *Health Effects of Polyunsaturated Fatty Acid in Seafoods,* ed. Simopoulos, Kifer, and Martin, pp. 49–60. Orlando, Fla.: Academic Press.

Williams, E. D., Karim, S. M., and Sandler, M. 1968. Prostaglandin secretion by medullary carcinoma of the thyroid. *Lancet* i:22.

Wynder, E. L., and Shigematsu, T. 1967. Environmental factors of cancer of the colon and rectum. *Cancer* 20:1520–1561.

Ziboh, V. A., Miller, C., Kragball, K., Cohen, K., Ellis, C. N., and Voorhees, J. J. 1985. Significance of dietary intake of polyunsaturated fatty acids in the clinical management of psoriasis. *II International Congress on Essential Fatty Acids, Prostaglandins and Leukotrienes.* Pp. 135–136.

INDEX